Jonathan G. Wiik

and

Healthcare Evolution:
Helping Providers Get Paid in an Era of Uncertainty

"Jonathan Wiik's latest book digs further into the obstacles we face as healthcare providers and business leaders. His style of communicating with a mixture of humor and reality makes this an excellent read for all."

—Joseph J. Mikoni, Associate Vice President, Diagnostic Testing and Support Services, Boulder Community Health

"Jonathan is a highly gifted individual in the healthcare space, and he has a unique understanding of the healthcare business and revenue cycle management. Jonathan's prose is a pleasure to both listen and read. I highly recommend this book."

—Scott Becker, JD, CPA, Publisher, Becker's Healthcare; Partner, McGuireWoods, LLP

"Jonathan's smart, sincere and thoughtful approach models the strategies he advocates. His wisdom has guided me and continues to shape my approach to many aspects of healthcare."

—Kelly Clasen, Senior Director, Business Operations, Middle Park Medical Center

"Jonathan will be listened to by providers, policy-makers and payers, including each of us as patients, even though it will hurt. Without the vision of the healthcare system from above, each player will continue to make the same mistakes. Take a ride with Jonathan so each of us can see how we have contributed to this mess and learn what it means to be in alignment. Wiik is the masterful pilot we need at just the right time. Listen and align or keep doing the same thing and experiencing the same chaos. If you care about healthcare, this is a must-read."
—Craig Antico, Co-Founder and Chief Executive Officer, RIP Medical Debt

"*Healthcare Evolution: Helping Providers Get Paid in an Era of Uncertainty* is required reading for anyone interested in understanding our complex healthcare system. Jonathan's thoughtful research helps us understand how we got here; his data-rich insight helps us understand how we are performing; and his creative curiosity and passion helps us think through ideas for creating the better healthcare system that we seek."
—Brandon Childs, Vice President, Payer and Provider, Collaboration Optum

"Understanding the complexities of the healthcare industry can be daunting. Predicting healthcare's future is even more difficult. Jonathan does a tremendous job of simplifying both in his new book. It's a must-read for those operating in a world of constant change."
—Jim Bohnsack, Chief Revenue Officer, TransUnion Healthcare

"We are grappling with how to best maximize revenue for our share of the cost for healthcare services. Jonathan's insight on patient and payer behavior is invaluable—his thought leadership certainly will help us through these challenging issues."
—Jason Petrasich, Senior Vice President, Artificial Intelligence, Meduit; formerly National Vice President, Revenue Cycle, Prospect Medical Holdings, Inc.

"Getting paid as a healthcare provider has never been more challenging than it is today. The complexities associated with the seemingly simple process of payment are indeed mind-numbing. It takes someone with a keen intellect, years of hospital revenue cycle experience, a passion for this type of work and a good sense of self-deprecating humor to publish a book about this folly. Mr. Wiik is able to articulate the intricacies of the revenue cycle in a manner that becomes navigable—and this book is a clear illustration. I heartily recommend this read to our friends in the industry, both new and seasoned. We all continue to struggle with the daily changes in the revenue stream, and this timely thesis is a welcome explanation in a muddled mess."
—Timothy Cashman, Chief Financial Officer, Estes Park Health

"Jonathan's energy is contagious. He's passionate about healthcare and breaks down the challenges in a thought-provoking way."
—Leslie Richard, System Vice President Revenue Cycle, CommonSpirit Health

"At a time when clear and logical thinking about healthcare is sorely needed, this book is filled with powerful, useful tools that will help you face reality and deal with the very real problems facing healthcare today."

— Joshua L. Robinson, Chief Operating Officer, Partner, Crossroads Health, LLC

"There could be no better author of a book on both 'getting paid' and 'healthcare uncertainty.' Jonathan is an expert at the first and a savvy industry thinker on the second. In his earlier book, *Healthcare Revolution: The Patient Is the New Payer*, he clearly laid out the reality facing Americans who get sick or injured. He also made it clear the impact this would have on the provider. This time around, he describes a world of change and disruption and then—somehow—shows us how this uncertainty can be managed to the benefit of everyone. A five-star recommendation from me."

—Jerry Ashton, Co-Founder and Director, Education and Engagement, RIP Medical Debt

Healthcare Evolution:

Helping Providers Get Paid
in an Era of Uncertainty

Jonathan G. Wiik

www.linkedin.com/in/JonathanWiik

ISBN: 978-0-578-61530-1

*To all who want to make healthcare
more affordable…*

TABLE OF CONTENTS

FOREWORD

Bradley S. Tinnermon
Vice President, Revenue Cycle and Revenue Integrity
Banner Health, Phoenix, Arizona

When I was still in high school pondering my career options, I spent time with my uncle who was in hospital administration. He'd made a nice career over a 25-year period from the 1970s to the '90s and had seen many changes in our provider and payer systems during that time. He also spent time in the Middle East helping developing nations with their healthcare delivery models and launched early ambulatory surgery centers in suburban communities. He felt connected with the communities he served and strongly believed the work he did was making those communities stronger. He had a vision at the time that the Baby Boomer population would significantly impact the economy of healthcare. He proclaimed individuals with a master's degree in health administration and hotel and resort management would be well-positioned, as he saw the Baby Boomers living a life of leisure, residing in retirement communities with "built-in" healthcare and vacationing in locations with the same amenities. He also said the healthcare space is fairly recession-proof, but that it will face challenges due to the many government regulatory changes that occur.

Thirty years after those conversations and 25 years into my own healthcare career, it turns out he was wrong about the Baby Boomer resort concept, but certainly right that this would be a challenging industry. He could never have predicted the margin pressure from shifting payment responsibility to the patient and cost pressures from information technology and its subsequent security. Jonathan Wiik's first book, *Healthcare Revolution: The Patient Is the New Payer*™, does an excellent job going over the history of healthcare from a revenue cycle management (RCM) perspective and reminds us how we got here. That book is now required reading for my revenue cycle leadership team. It has helped our team focus on how to influence the business factors as opposed to react to those factors based on what we decipher in our data. Understanding what's causing a shift in the business and how payers and patients are responding to those environmental changes is the first step in evaluating the strategies we're using and considering.

Like many other health systems, Banner Health provides care and insurance to a large population in multiple settings across several states—academic hospitals, cancer centers, rural facilities, community physician groups, urgent care centers and everything in between. And like many other health systems, there's no one-size-fits-all strategy that works. What pleases the Chief Financial Officer (CFO) angers the physicians; what works for the academic physicians doesn't work for the rural facilities; and what drives revenue hurts the insurance actuary. What we can all agree on is managing health over managing care is where this delivery model needs to move. Much easier said than done, but it's undisputed that an ounce of prevention is worth a pound of cure.

Jonathan points out in his first book that we have made incredible investments in electronic health records (EHR), moved through ICD-10 and actually have the processing power to analyze this daunting amount of health data. Can we move on from this system of debating who should pay, and was it necessary to introduce an accountable system of population health? Can we not only increase life expectancy but also improve the quality of life? Are we on the verge of using all of this data and technical infrastructure to actually deliver on population health?

Most of us entered the field of healthcare like my uncle, wanting to feel connected to the communities we serve and believing we can make those communities stronger. Certainly challenged, many of us in RCM feel the pressure from communities we serve to find a better way to deliver health services. Jonathan's second book, *Healthcare Evolution: Helping Providers Get Paid in an Era of Uncertainty*, will give us all insights to consider and possibly use for positive influence, instead of reacting to what we see later.

INTRODUCTION

It's a challenging time to be a revenue cycle manager in the healthcare industry. I've been doing this for a very (very) long time, initially as a Chief Revenue Officer and more recently in my role as Principal of Healthcare Strategy at TransUnion Healthcare. And the U.S. healthcare system has always been a complex system with equally complex problems. But what I see now is an industry in utter chaos—it's exhausting, cyclical and unnecessary. To put it quite frankly, it's a mess. I've spoken with hundreds of healthcare leaders, and not a single one, if given the opportunity, stated they would go back and create this mess of a "sick-care" system we have today.

Almost three years have passed since I published my first book, *Healthcare Revolution: The Patient Is the New Payer*, which provided a big-picture view of the challenges facing healthcare providers. Unfortunately, since then, the dysfunction in the U.S. healthcare system has gotten worse—not better.

Payment uncertainty in the U.S. healthcare system has become an exhaustive burden for all stakeholders. Healthcare expenses continue to climb, with little to no effective efforts to develop a holistic, long-term strategy to curb them. At the same time, legislative reform and regulatory attempts to address shortfalls in quality, rates and outcome have stalled, perpetuating inefficiencies and onerous rules that add costs instead of removing them. As expenditures keep rising, all stakeholders—patient, provider, payer and employer—are trying to find new ways to provide access to affordable, effective healthcare in our country.

Where does this leave providers? Stuck in the middle. A healthcare provider's number one priority is to provide high-quality patient care. They're tasked with achieving the patient-centered Triple Aim outcomes defined by the Institute for Healthcare Improvement (IHI):[1]

- Improving the patient experience of care (including quality and satisfaction)
- Improving the health of populations
- Reducing the per capita cost of healthcare

Sounds simple and easy, right? But providers finding success in achieving these goals will quickly tell you it's a difficult task. Especially when the system is so out of alignment.

In addition to achieving the Triple Aim, hospitals and healthcare systems need to make sure revenue outpaces expenses and operating margins support long-term sustainability. For some hospitals, like nonprofits and safety net hospitals, controlling costs isn't a matter of protecting margin—it's a matter of survival.

As we say in the industry, "No margin, no mission." While this mantra has almost become cliché, it's taking a front seat again in strategic planning, for better or worse. When I define "margin" I'm assuming a reasonable margin (i.e., that prices and contractual or patient revenue is appropriate and fair, and at the same time, expenses are appropriate).

When you take a close look at our industry, however, red flags quickly appear in terms of fundamental differences in each stakeholder's perspective on how healthcare should be delivered and funded. What's a "reasonable margin?" What are "appropriate expenses?" Each stakeholder has a different opinion and conflicts emerge as a result of those different perspectives, resulting in an underperforming sick-care system.

The margins that stakeholders are fighting about—at least the operating margins of healthcare providers—aren't that significant to begin with. In part, that's due to the fact that the majority (56 percent) of the 5,262 community hospitals in the United States are not-for-profit.[2] Nonprofit and public hospitals, in particular, are being squeezed by increasing expenses and declining revenues.[3] However, it's not just nonprofits that are struggling. One study found that two-thirds of health systems have seen their operating incomes decline over the past three years.[4] Data from the American Hospital Association (AHA) showed by 2016, nearly one-third (30.6 percent) of hospitals had negative operating margins.[5] That's the highest percentage of hospitals with negative operating margins since 2008, in the middle of the Great Recession.

You may be asking yourself, "Really? Is it that bad?" Pay attention people—it's no wonder a 2018 survey of healthcare CEOs found financial challenges are their number one concern, ranking above all other challenges, including government mandates, patient safety and quality, personnel shortages and behavioral health addiction issues.[6]

What's behind the financial challenges facing the healthcare industry? We all have an opinion when asked. I would offer a lot of it is due to factors beyond a provider's control. For example, government healthcare reform is being legislated and then reversed so quickly it could give you a case of whiplash. The Patient Protection and Affordable Care Act (PPACA, commonly referred to as the ACA) was enacted in 2010. Six years later a new sheriff came to town who didn't care for his predecessor's healthcare reform. The new administration promptly started stripping away the foundations of the ACA—before providers even had a chance to fully adjust to all of the changes (changes in payer mix, changes in reimbursement requirements, etc.) brought about by the ACA in the first place.

But it's not just legislative reform giving revenue cycle managers headaches. Changes in technology are driving costs, too. The American Recovery and Reinvestment Act of 2009 (ARRA) authorized the Centers for Medicare & Medicaid Services (CMS) to create an incentive program (a.k.a. meaningful use) to encourage providers to adopt and use electronic health records (EHRs). Ten years later, EHR systems are no longer optional. Implementing, maintaining, integrating and upgrading these complex solutions has increased the cost of doing business for healthcare organizations. I'm not in a position to judge whether or not the clinical outcomes have been worth it—my expertise is in revenue cycle management (RCM), not clinical practice. But with respect to the financial impact of EHRs, one study found administrative costs associated with EHR-based billing and insurance-related activities ranged from $20.49 for a single primary care visit to $215.10 for an inpatient surgical procedure.[7] That's six- to seven-figure costs annually—for hardware and software—and they directly impact the bottom line. (Ask any CFO for the ROI on their HER ... let me know what they say.)

The meaningful use program was implemented with the best of intentions, but we're now at a point in time that some people in the industry refer to as the "meaningful use hangover." (Some physicians have taken that a step further and now refer to it as "meaningless use.") The meaningful use program was successful in terms of encouraging providers to adopt EHRs—the most recent data show 96 percent of all nonfederal acute care hospitals have adopted certified health information technology systems.[8] On the other hand, interoperability across the industry is still a long way from becoming reality. And more important for RCM professionals is the fact the meaningful use reform failed to address any aspect of healthcare finance. After all, clinical interactions happen in the context of payment systems: One must get paid to sustain the system. Yet when the simplest of RCM workflows and tasks are attempted within the EHR structure, staff members consistently struggle to make it work.

When writing 2017's *Healthcare Revolution,* I evaluated significant societal trends impacting U.S. healthcare costs, including the aging population (the "silver tsunami"), an increase in the prevalence of chronic disease, the rising cost of pharmaceuticals, and costs associated with keeping up with advances in clinical technologies. While these trends provide context for the increasing challenges of RCM in the healthcare industry, the fact is these challenges are beyond the control of a revenue cycle manager (RCM superpowers notwithstanding).

Given the impact and scope of these legislative, technological and population health trends, it may seem the only option revenue cycle managers have is to throw their hands up in surrender.

But fear not, my revenue cycle brothers and sisters—I'm here to tell you there *are* strategies a revenue cycle manager can employ to protect revenue and minimize revenue leakage, even in the midst of the chaos that defines the U.S. healthcare system today. Revenue cycle managers *can* have a significant impact on a healthcare organization's revenue picture, if they have a clear understanding of what the new challenges are—and if they're equipped with the resources and tools available to help them deal with these challenges.

The first step in facing these RCM challenges is to admit the old assumptions underpinning the traditional approach to RCM no longer apply. Break all the rules. Some of the no-longer-applicable assumptions plaguing our industry are the following:

Assumption 1: The patient has health insurance coverage that will fully cover their care.

Fact: The uninsured rate has dropped to around 10 percent and hovers in the mid-teens (depending upon which measure you use) since the passage of the ACA.[9] So while it might be true that you can expect 9 out of 10 patients who enter your door will have some form of insurance coverage, it's also true few of today's patients have coverage that will *fully* cover their care. In fact, according to survey data from the Commonwealth Fund, 29 percent of adults who were insured all year in 2018 were underinsured. That means because of high deductibles and/or high out-of-pocket costs, they're "more likely to struggle paying medical bills or to skip care."[10] And if the patient is covered by Medicaid or Medicare, you also may be looking at underpayments that don't align with the actual cost of care (more on that later). If they're covered by commercial insurance—well, as commercial insurers have attempted to hold the line on costs, they've added more requirements to evaluate whether or not the care should be covered (e.g., medical necessity, pre-authorizations), which can impact the amount of payment you actually receive. And the balance left to the patient? We'll get to that in assumption 3.

Assumption 2: Insurance will pay the claim.

Fact: Have you noticed your denials rate going up? It seems to be
a large trend in the industry, and it's not just your
organization that's seeing a wave of denials. An analysis by
the Advisory Board revealed the median 350-bed hospital
experienced an increase in denial write-offs from $3.9
million in 2011 to $7 million in 2017.[11]

Assumption 3: The patient will pay the balance after insurance
(BAI).

Fact: As I pointed out in *Healthcare Revolution*, patients are the
new payers. Insurers and employers have shifted costs to
patients via higher deductibles, larger copays and higher
coinsurance responsibilities, so revenue collected directly
from patients is making up a bigger piece of the overall
revenue picture.[12] In fact, over the past decade the amount
of provider revenue from patients has increased from less
than 10 percent to more than 30 percent.[13] The intent of this
effort was to ensure patients have some skin in the game, so
they would make better financial choices regarding their
care. Great idea, but the implementation led to unintended
outcomes—patients are horrible payers. They take longer to
pay when they do pay—if they pay at all—and they
subordinate medical bills to other bills. Studies show
patients rank paying medical bills below paying their
mortgage or rent, utilities, car payments, and even their
cable, cellphone and internet bills.[14] Patients also put off
going to the physician if costs are too high. This creates a
"train wreck" scenario—now the patient is *really* sick by
the time they enter the system and it's *really* expensive to

treat them. That's why I say "Death to the deductible!" It's not working as *intended*.

So how does a revenue cycle manager fight back when all the traditional assumptions have been upended? The first step in any recovery process is admitting there's a problem (i.e., acknowledging the healthcare ecosystem has changed so significantly that old assumptions no longer apply).

The next step is to resolve to do things differently and move forward. A mantra I've always loved is "If you always do what you've always done, you always get what you've always gotten." As I've visited with providers around the country, I've sometimes been surprised by how many healthcare providers hold onto the "We've always done it this way" mantra. These simple words, when spoken and followed religiously, can represent the last words before a ship sinks. With providers, this sentiment sometimes takes the form of "This is how we've always delivered care, and this is how we're going to continue to deliver care, regardless of the cost." We could be talking about any number of business strategies, from providing patient estimates at the time of service to developing and deploying a digital engagement portal for patient payments. Too often, providers respond to these types of ideas with the same old objections that ultimately boil down to "But this is the way we've always done it."

In my RCM experience, I've observed providers are sometimes reluctant to examine the business decisions and strategies that can contribute to their financial struggles. Yes, declining margins can be the result of factors beyond a provider's control—like changes in regulations, technology and population health. But providers have the ability to make business choices in response to those external changes, which can help them navigate these challenging times.

In my life outside of RCM, I enjoy many outdoor activities. One of those activities is white water rafting. I am, in fact, a certified white water rafting guide instructor. The turbulence a person encounters in white water rafting is in some ways very similar to the turbulence healthcare providers are experiencing in the industry right now. When I'm training people to become raft guides, I point out that you have to *choose* where you go on the river. *Not* choosing your route is also a choice. And if you choose to not act, you're eventually going to hit something with your boat and very bad things are going to happen quickly.

The same is true in healthcare. We have to be willing to move forward as an industry—we cannot stay where we are and be silent. It's mission critical for us to adapt to the changing healthcare environment by doing some things—maybe a lot of things—differently than we've done in the past.

Unexamined business practices—and unsubstantiated assumptions—have always been the enemies of effective business strategies. The best way to change ineffective business practices is to learn about alternative ways of doing things. That's part of what this book is about.

In my current role at TransUnion Healthcare, I've had the privilege of visiting hundreds of hospitals and talking to hundreds of hospital executives. I've learned a few things about different ways of approaching RCM. I've learned about new strategies for addressing this turbulent healthcare environment in ways that help providers create "frictionless" payment systems. I talk about these solutions—both those available now and solutions on the horizon—throughout this book.

The best way to fight assumptions is with information: facts, figures and, most of all, actionable data. As one of my favorite process improvement gurus, W. Edwards Deming once said, "In God we trust, all others must bring data."[15] That's also what this book is about: Giving you the context you need to make the case for data-based revenue cycle process improvements at your organization.

Revenue cycle managers have their own version of the IHI's Triple Aim. The RCM version is to get paid the highest possible amount, in the shortest amount of time, for the lowest cost. But right now, the healthcare delivery system is not aligned with those outcomes. And it doesn't look like the turbulence in the U.S. healthcare system is going to resolve any time in the near future. Until the time all stakeholders in the system are working together to tackle healthcare costs, providers are going to find themselves stuck in the middle of a sick-care system. Providers are going to have to implement proactive RCM strategies in self-defense until the U.S. healthcare system is righted and reimbursement practices align with the best interests of all stakeholders—including patients, providers and payers.

My goal in writing *Healthcare Evolution: Helping Providers Get Paid in an Era of Uncertainty* is to share what I've learned with you, provide some context as to why traditional approaches no longer apply, and suggest some effective strategies for addressing the new realities of healthcare RCM. The message I hope you take away from this book is this: Despite the disorder in the system, there are meaningful actions you can take and effective strategies you can deploy to establish a frictionless payment system that will both protect your organization's revenue and empower your patients.

SECTION ONE

WHAT IS GOING ON?

CHAPTER 1

THIS IS NOT WORKING

The current state of the U.S. healthcare system is … broken. "Oh, it's great. Don't you love it?"—said no one, ever. You get an eye roll, a sigh or a political discussion that can separate the closest of friends. Our healthcare system is dysfunctional, folks, no matter what perspective you view it from. Whether you are a patient, provider, payer or employer—it is clear the current system is most certainly not working.

Let's get real and talk turkey about the numbers. Regardless of what measures you use, the statistics don't look good. Costs are out of control. Outcomes are poor—for many reasons. Payment is *not* clear. Hospital and health systems' traditional approaches to increasing revenue are no longer effective (it's a lot like building another wing on a plane). I know that you've heard and know this stuff. If you're a provider, you live it every day. And maybe you're sick of hearing about the situation— all problems, no solutions, and it can't be fixed. But in case you need a reminder about just how bad things are, this chapter will refresh your memory.

Costs Are Out of Control

Spending related to healthcare currently makes up 17.9 percent of the gross domestic product (GDP) in the U.S.[16] This means out of every dollar of economic activity that occurs in the U.S., 18 cents—nearly one-fifth of the total—is spent on healthcare.

Between 1970 and 2018, U.S. health spending rose from $355 per capita to $11,172—an increase of over 3,000 percent.[17] To put that in perspective, the average price of a sedan in 1970 was $3,543.[18] Multiply that number by 3,000 percent and if you were to buy that same car today, it would set you back $106 thousand. As I pointed out in *Healthcare Revolution: The Patient Is the New Payer*, if the price of eggs had increased at the same rate as the U.S. per capita cost of healthcare, a dozen eggs would now cost more than $55.[19] Thank goodness neither vehicles, nor eggs, have followed the same cost curve as healthcare!

Whether you look at the per capita increase in U.S. health expenditures in terms of current or constant (adjusted) dollars, the trajectory is alarming (figure 1.1).

Figure 1.1 Total National Health Expenditures, U.S. $ per Capita, 1970–2018

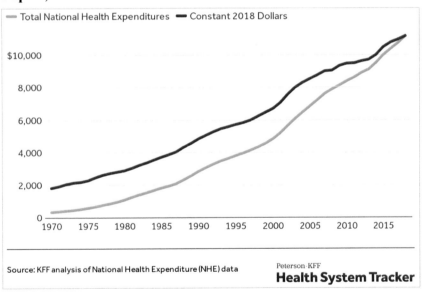

Source: "How does health spending in the U.S. compare to other countries?" Peterson Center on Healthcare and Kaiser Family Foundation. Peterson-KFF Health System Tracker. December 7, 2018. https://www.healthsystemtracker.org/indicator/spending/per-capita-spending/

The curve looks like the flight path of a space shuttle after launching from Cape Canaveral. We've experienced huge, skyrocketing costs and the United States is the best at spending the most. To put that in context, note U.S. spending per capita is significantly higher than comparable wealthy countries (figure 1.2). For example, in 2017, health spending per person in the U.S. was 28 percent higher than the next highest per capita spender, Switzerland.[20]

Figure 1.2 Health Consumption Expenditures per Capita, U.S. Dollars, PPP Adjusted, 2017

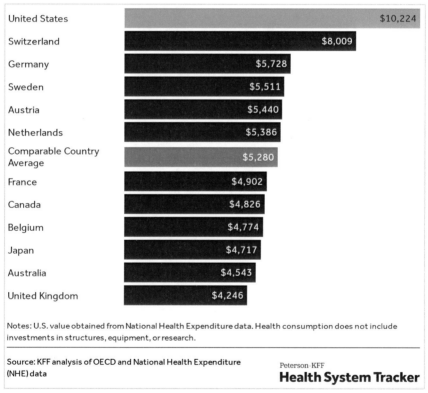

United States	$10,224
Switzerland	$8,009
Germany	$5,728
Sweden	$5,511
Austria	$5,440
Netherlands	$5,386
Comparable Country Average	$5,280
France	$4,902
Canada	$4,826
Belgium	$4,774
Japan	$4,717
Australia	$4,543
United Kingdom	$4,246

Notes: U.S. value obtained from National Health Expenditure data. Health consumption does not include investments in structures, equipment, or research.

Source: KFF analysis of OECD and National Health Expenditure (NHE) data

Peterson-KFF
Health System Tracker

Source: Bradley Sawyer and Cynthia Cox. "How does health spending in the U.S. compare to other countries?" Peterson Center on Healthcare and Kaiser Family Foundation. Peterson-KFF Health System Tracker. Dec. 7, 2018. https://www.healthsystemtracker.org/chart-collection/health-spending-u-s-compare-countries/

If line charts and bar graphs don't alarm you, perhaps big numbers will. U.S. National Health Expenditures (NHE) grew to $3.5 trillion in 2017.[21] The Centers for Medicare & Medicaid Services (CMS) estimate at the current rate—and under current law—national health spending will reach nearly $6.0 trillion by 2027.[22] Is American healthcare that *different*? Why are *we* so expensive? Read on.

Delivery Is Inefficient

The U.S. healthcare delivery system is extremely inefficient. This is partly due to our fragmented approach to healthcare. For better or worse, the U.S. doesn't use a centralized model for healthcare delivery. We don't have a centralized payment model (i.e., single-payer), either. And we don't maintain a centralized repository for healthcare data (although part of the impetus for meaningful use was to nudge healthcare providers in this direction). We don't have *a* healthcare system, we have healthcare "systems" that don't play nice in the sandbox together. More on that later.

The upside of this is the fact U.S. consumers have a variety of choices when it comes to healthcare. The downside is the delivery of healthcare services—and the very mechanisms by which providers get paid for those services—are plagued by inefficiencies that inflate costs. Let's identify just a few of these inefficiencies here:

Consumers Aren't Educated About Where to Obtain Care

Think of how many different places healthcare consumers can go to get healthcare services in the U.S. They can go to a public health clinic. They can go to a retail clinic that's set up in a local grocery store or pharmacy chain. They can go visit their primary care physician (during regular office hours) in a big medical building downtown. They can go to a nearby urgent care clinic. They can go to the emergency department (ED), which may or may not be associated with the local community hospital. (It might even be one of the new, freestanding EDs that have become so ubiquitous lately.) They can also, of course, go directly to the local community hospital—which may be either a public, not-for-profit or for-profit facility. And now that technology has entered the picture, it's sometimes also possible for patients to email their physician and/or nurse, or even set up a phone or video consultation.

No wonder the consumer is confused about where to go. The problem is that the consumer's decision about *where* to go for healthcare services is not communicated. We, as consumers, often go to what is in front of us. We use our phone, call a friend or remember a place we drove by last week, and decide, "they're open, let's go there."

All of this can have tremendous cost consequences down the road—cost consequences which the patient, provider and/or the payer end up paying for. But the patient isn't necessarily aware of those cost consequences, due to the complexity and lack of transparency within the system. And even when the patient is aware of cost differences, sometimes immediate access preferences or needs (e.g., "I know I can go to the ED and get seen today or … I have to wait two weeks for an appointment with a primary care physician") override cost concerns.

The reality today is: Treatment for the same condition (a sore throat, for example) can cost more than five times as much in an ED versus an urgent care center (figure 1.3).

Figure 1.3 Emergency Room Cost Versus Urgent Care Cost

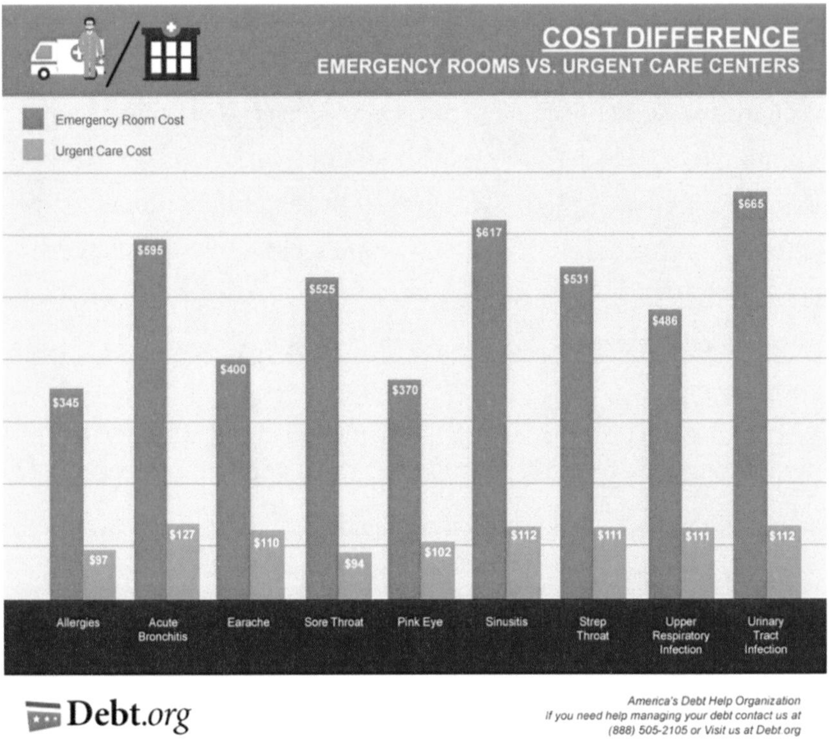

COST DIFFERENCE
EMERGENCY ROOMS VS. URGENT CARE CENTERS

Emergency Room Cost
Urgent Care Cost

	Allergies	Acute Bronchitis	Earache	Sore Throat	Pink Eye	Sinusitis	Strep Throat	Upper Respiratory Infection	Urinary Tract Infection
Emergency Room Cost	$345	$595	$400	$525	$370	$617	$531	$486	$665
Urgent Care Cost	$97	$127	$110	$94	$102	$112	$111	$111	$112

Debt.org

America's Debt Help Organization
If you need help managing your debt contact us at
(888) 505-2105 or Visit us at Debt org

Source: Bill Fay. "Emergency Rooms vs. Urgent Care Centers." Debt.org. (n.d.)
https://www.debt.org/medical/emergency-room-urgent-care-costs/

Was the care five times better? This is an extreme cost variability, simply based on where care is received and who provided it. Data from the Centers for Disease Control and Prevention (CDC) show the U.S. records 145.6 million emergency department visits a year.[23] Of those, 42.2 million (29 percent) are injury related.[24] Out of the total number of visits, less than 9 percent (12.6 million) result in hospital admission and less than 2 percent (2.2 million) result in admission to a critical care unit.[25] This tells me the ED attached to the hospital or the ED in general was "too much" care. Too much in terms of supplies; too much time spent; too much in dollars billed. This overuse of resources comes at the expense of the patient, provider and payer.

ED overutilization can drive tremendous costs in a hospital or health system. One study estimated between 13 and 27 percent of ED visits in the U.S. could be managed in physician offices, clinics and urgent care centers at a savings of $4.4 billion annually.[26] Another study found six common chronic conditions (asthma, chronic obstructive pulmonary disease, diabetes, heart failure, hypertension and behavioral health conditions) represented almost two-thirds of ED visits in 2017.[27] And, out of those, 4.3 million visits (1 in 3) were preventable and could have been treated in a less expensive outpatient setting.[28]

I'm a big fan of urgent care centers—they provide much of what a patient needs for self-directed care (that is, the patient seeking care somewhere on their own). I don't think we will see physician's clinics holding 24/7 hours like a Walmart anytime soon, so let's turn to urgent care centers. They're much more efficient and they cost *a lot* less. UnitedHealthcare measured the difference and found the average cost for an urgent care visit (nationally) is $205 versus $2,582 for an emergency visit.[29] Ten times the cost, people! Yes, I'm applying generalizations, and yes, EDs are necessary and important.

What I'm saying is when you look at the big picture, *a lot* of what happens in an ED could happen in an urgent care setting. But patients go to the ED because it's all they know, or what they want, not because of what it costs. We don't purchase any other goods that way, but with healthcare, we go to the ED too often, for the wrong reasons, and ultimately pay too much for it.

Regulations Complicate Matters

Regulations—such as the Emergency Medical Treatment and Active Labor Act of 1986 (EMTALA)—can also complicate the issue of making sure patients are treated at the appropriate level of care. EMTALA is a federal law that ensures public access to emergency services regardless of an individual's ability to pay. EMTALA applies to all Medicare-participating hospitals that offer emergency services.[30]

The implication of EMTALA for providers is hospitals have an obligation to screen and stabilize anyone who presents to the hospital campus and requests emergency services, regardless of their ability to pay.[31,32] An unintended consequence is too many patients receive treatment at one of the most expensive sites of care in the healthcare system—the ED—even when their healthcare situations don't require it. As payers crack down on medical necessity criteria and contractual requirements, providers are once again caught in the debate between volume and value of care. Overutilization of the ED may generate additional revenue for ED physicians, however EDs also generate a disproportionate amount of bad debt and uncompensated care. According to a report by the Heritage Foundation, 42 percent of self-employed physicians reported "a major portion of their bad debt is attributable to delivery of medical services required by federal law, amounting to $4.2 billion annually."[33]

The Level of Care Happens for Too Long at the Wrong Place

EDs aren't the only place where misaligned levels of care occur. For example, patients are often held in hospitals longer than they need to be. When a patient no longer requires acute care, that patient should be transitioned home, or if unable to care for themselves, moved to a post-acute facility. Skilled nursing facilities (SNFs) and long-term acute care facilities (LTACs) have nurses who are trained specifically to treat ongoing nonacute conditions such as wound care, infections, respiratory therapy, ambulation, nutrition and related conditions. The cost package in SNFs and LTACs is a lot lower than the cost of care in an acute care facility.

Once that "wrong" level of care has been provided, there is no way to walk it back. The cost has been incurred, and somebody has to pay it. Whether that's a sore throat that ended up in the ED, or a long-term care patient who stayed too many days in an acute-care hospital—a higher-than-necessary cost has been incurred. Costs related to the "wrong" level of care are significant cost drivers in the U.S. healthcare system. As a recent Healthcare Financial Management Association (HFMA) article noted, "… organizations can achieve material savings from having the ability to place such high-cost patients in more appropriate settings such as a long-term acute care hospital or SNF, in a timely manner."[34]

Fragmented and Episodic Patient Care Leads to a Fragmented and Episodic Payment System

The fragmentation and inefficiencies in the healthcare delivery system also impact the way payments work. No matter who the payer is—the government, employer, a commercial payer or the patient—they're paying for that inefficiency.

An analogy I use is every episode of care is like a single opaque jar for each patient. You can take one jar off the shelf, unscrew the lid, dump out the contents and examine them all individually. But this just represents one episode of care.

Now imagine a whole wall of opaque jars. And some of these other jars are related to the same patient, but you can't see into them. You can't see which of the other jars might contain something that's related to this particular episode of care. You can't see the patient's context, in terms of coverage, outcome and payment. What barriers exist for good payment on that claim? Is this particular patient a high utilizer of services? Is this likely to be a high-cost patient?

Providers don't know because they don't have that context. Providers are looking through a porthole at what is happening right now with the patient, rather than getting a holistic view. If they *did* have that context, patients, providers and payers could work together to find the best outcome for the most affordable cost. But our system isn't set up for efficiency. The way it's set up now means providers are having a "one-off" with each encounter.

There Are a Lot of Different Payers Out There (With a Lot of Different Rules)

In addition to the disjointed, episodic nature of the healthcare delivery system, the sheer number of payers in the U.S. system also factors into the complexity. Just take a moment to think about how many different healthcare payers there are—if you are a revenue cycle management (RCM) professional, this is something you're probably intimately familiar with. There are the big five: UnitedHealth Group, Anthem, Aetna, Cigna and Humana. There are lesser-known payers like Centene Corporation, Health Net, WellCare Health Plans, Molina Healthcare and Magellan Health. And there are many you may not have encountered—yet. In fact, according to the Insurance Information Institute (III), there were 907 health insurance companies in the U.S. in 2017.[35] Of course, each insurer may have dozens of plans, representing thousands of health plans across our country.

And health insurance companies aren't the only payers out there. There are the government payers, like Medicare and Medicaid. There are other public plans for special groups, such as the Veteran's Administration. There are employer-based plans. There are self-funded plans. There are ancillary payers that come into play, like auto insurance claims and dental insurance claims. There are primary payers and secondary payers. And then, of course, there's the patient payer.

Not only are there hundreds of payers to deal with—there are the different payers' rules and policies to navigate as well. Do you think these 900-plus payers, with their hundreds of different plans, have similar rules? As an RCM professional, you're well aware the opposite is true. Most payers—and payer plans—have very different rules in place, making it extremely difficult for providers to manage consistently. This drives up administrative costs and also forces inconsistent payment. Thousands of plans translate into literally tens of thousands of pages of policy minutiae providers have to deal with, covering everything from pre-authorizations to medical necessity to length of stay. (I'll have more to say about this when I address denials, in chapter 3).

Providers Aren't Incentivized to Provide Efficient Care ... Yet

Although there's a lot of talk about value-based care in the healthcare industry, the industry still largely operates in a fee-for-service (FFS) market. In the FFS reimbursement model, providers are paid for each service performed. This incentivizes providers to maximize the number of services offered because they are paid for each individual diagnostic test, procedure and treatment they provide. Incentivizing providers to maximize the number of services they provide isn't cost efficient. It isn't tied to better outcomes, either. But it's the way the system currently operates.

The movement toward value-based care—where reimbursement is tied to patient outcomes, rather than the volume of services provided—was supposed to change all that. CMS, as it often does, has tried to lead the way on value-based care by implementing a number of programs designed to nudge providers in that direction.[36] CMS programs like the Hospital Value-Based

Purchasing (VBP) Program, the Hospital Readmission Reduction Program (HRRP) and the Hospital Acquired Condition (HAC) Reduction Program are designed to start linking payment to patient outcomes, instead of services performed. But as we will see in chapter 2, the value-based care reimbursement model hasn't gained much traction in the industry.

Outcomes Are Poor

Despite how much money the U.S. is spending on healthcare and despite the abundance of healthcare facilities available in the U.S., our healthcare outcomes aren't anything to write home about. One way to measure healthcare outcomes is to use the Healthcare Access and Quality (HAQ) Index developed by the Institute for Health Metrics and Evaluation (IHME).[37] The HAQ index takes into account "causes from which death should not occur in the presence of effective care to approximate personal healthcare access and quality by location and over time."[38] Another way to describe the HAQ index is "amenable mortality," which means mortality rates that can be impacted by access to quality healthcare.

HAQ ratings are calculated on a scale from 0 to 100, with higher scores meaning high quality and access (lower mortality rates for causes amenable to healthcare) and lower scores meaning lower quality and access. The most recent data pegs the U.S. at 88.7.[39] Not a bad score, right? That's a B+ on a standard grading scale. Do you want B+ healthcare?

The problem is the U.S. is drawing a B+ when its peers are getting As. The average HAQ score for comparable countries is 93.7—a solid A on the grading scale. HAQ ratings for comparable countries range from 96.1 for the Netherlands to 90.5 for the United Kingdom (figure 1.4). We spend more money on healthcare than any other industrialized country and have a B+ to show for it. We've got some catching up to do.

Figure 1.4 Healthcare Access and Quality Index Rating, 2016

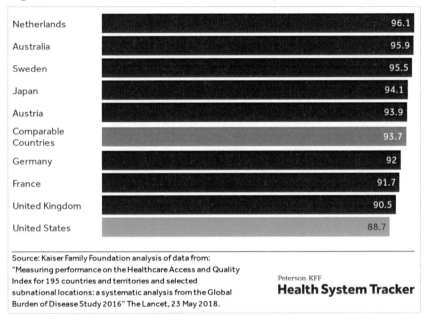

Source: Kaiser Family Foundation analysis of data from:
"Measuring performance on the Healthcare Access and Quality
Index for 195 countries and territories and selected
subnational locations: a systematic analysis from the Global
Burden of Disease Study 2016" The Lancet, 23 May 2018.

Peterson-KFF
Health System Tracker

Source: Bradley Sawyer and Daniel McDermott. "How does the quality of the U.S. healthcare system compare to other countries?" Peterson Center on Healthcare and Kaiser Family Foundation. Peterson-KFF Health System Tracker. March 28, 2019. https://www.healthsystemtracker.org/chart-collection/quality-u-s-healthcare-system-compare-countries/

The Usual Strategies Don't Work

As a result of this topsy-turvy system, the usual strategies no longer work. In fact, many of the traditional strategies for getting ahead of costs are now actually inflating costs, rather than bending the cost curve. We've made things worse, not better: a healthcare-cost backfire.

Higher Deductibles Don't Lead to Better Patient Choices

The high-deductible health plan (HDHP) experiment is over. Higher deductibles don't help patients make better choices about healthcare. One study found only 4 percent of enrollees with HDHPs compared costs across healthcare professionals during their last use of medical care, in comparison to 3 percent of enrollees without HDHPs who compared costs.[40] That's a difference of only 1 percent in healthcare shopping behavior!

So enrollees with HDHPs don't shop smarter for healthcare, but many of them actually *postpone* seeking healthcare instead, which doesn't help at all. High deductibles incentivize patients to postpone getting care until they're really sick and therefore more expensive to treat. A 2017 study of patients with diabetes found those with HDHPs postponed needed care due to cost concerns, and then ended up with increased emergency department visits due to preventable acute diabetes complications.[41] In fact, annual emergency department acute complication visits for low-income HDHP members increased by 21.7 percent in the year after transitioning to HDHPs, compared to the control group, who remained in low-deductible plans.[42]

And if the patient eventually does come in for care, but the deductible is unaffordable, that just leaves the provider with bad debt. There is no scenario in which HDHPs result in positive outcomes—for patients or for providers. That's why I say "Death to the deductible." It doesn't work for anybody.

Heads in Beds Doesn't Work Anymore

Some providers are still trying to capture market share by increasing the number of healthcare facilities available, and in some cases increasing the number of available beds in those facilities. But does an increase in the number of healthcare facilities or number of beds translate to better care and lower costs? The evidence would seem to indicate it doesn't.

In case you're wondering, according to the American Hospital Association (AHA) there are a total of 931,203 staffed beds across all U.S. hospitals.[43] Of those, 798,921 beds (about 86 percent) are in community hospitals (nonfederal, short-term general and other special hospitals).[44] The total number of beds has actually dropped slightly over time, from 3 beds per 1,000 population in 1999, to 2.5 in 2017.[45]

Is this enough? Too many? Too little? Interestingly, the U.S. ranks lower than average in terms of hospital beds per 1,000 population in comparison to other countries (figure 1.5).

Figure 1.5 Total Hospital Beds per 1,000 Population, 2016

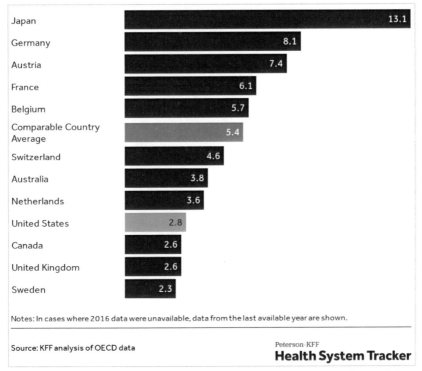

Notes: In cases where 2016 data were unavailable, data from the last available year are shown.

Source: KFF analysis of OECD data

Peterson-KFF
Health System Tracker

Source: "Hospital beds per capita." Peterson Center on Healthcare and Kaiser Family Foundation. Peterson-KFF Health System Tracker. (n.d.)
https://www.healthsystemtracker.org/indicator/quality/hospital-beds-per-capita/

While it's true that low availability of hospitals or hospital beds can potentially contribute to higher prices, this doesn't seem to be the case for the U.S. at the national level (although hospital closures in rural areas are becoming a bigger problem). Alongside the decline in the number of beds per capita, the hospital occupancy rate has declined as well. In 1980, the U.S. hospital occupancy rate was 77.7 percent; by 2017, it had dropped to 65.9 percent.[46]

How does unused capacity impact healthcare costs? At the provider level, unused hospital beds are a waste of resources due to flexible staffing plans where the caregivers "flex" as the hospital census changes. Nurse-to-bed ratios, which are often driven by contracts or policy, are inflexible and can drive costs in fixed-staffing environments when the hospital is only half full.

At the regional level, things get even more interesting. A Dartmouth Atlas Project study of the relationship between healthcare spending and quality of care identified a phenomenon called "supply-sensitive care" in high-spending regions of the country.[47] Supply-sensitive care is defined as "discretionary care that's provided more frequently when a population has a greater per capita supply of medical resources."[48] The effect is as follows:

> In regions where there are more hospital beds per capita, patients will be more likely to be admitted to the hospital—and Medicare will spend more on hospital care. Where there are more intensive care unit beds, more patients will be cared for in the ICU—and Medicare will spend more on ICU care. The more CT scanners are available, the more CT scans patients will receive—and so on.[49]

The researchers further note "studies that have looked at the additional services provided in high-spending regions have shown the higher volume of care doesn't produce better outcomes for patients."[50] Unused capacity can actually accelerate utilization in ways that aren't correlated with better patient outcomes.

More Facilities Doesn't Equate to Better Outcomes—Or Lower Costs

So perhaps we should be alarmed, not reassured, at other types of "capacity building" occurring in the U.S. healthcare system. We're seeing a lot of ways providers are reaching out to meet the patient by making it easier for them to access care, but some of these strategies are driving costs up. For example, the number of Medicare-certified ambulatory surgery centers (ASCs) increased from 5,105 in 2010 to 5,532 in 2016, an increase of 8 percent in 6 years.[51] Now, a lot of this growth is attributable to a larger trend of moving many surgeries from the inpatient setting to the outpatient setting, but it still represents an increase in capacity.

The number of urgent care clinics is growing rapidly as well, increasing from 6,946 in 2015 to 8,285 in 2018, representing a 19 percent increase in just 3 years.[52] Even more alarming—at least, alarming to the Medicare Payment Advisory Commission (MedPAC)—has been the rapid growth of stand-alone EDs.

> "There has been a growth in free-standing emergency departments in urban areas that does not seem to be addressing any particular access need for emergency care," said James Mathews, executive director of MedPAC. The convenience of a neighborhood emergency department may even induce demand, he said, calling it an "if you build it, they will come" effect.[53]

In 2018, MedPAC even recommended changing Medicare's payment policies so freestanding EDs (FSEDs) wouldn't be allowed to collect the same "facility fees" which hospital EDs are entitled to.[54] The number of FSEDs is currently estimated to be more than 500.[55] That may seem like a small number, but FSEDs can have a disproportionate impact on healthcare costs.

A Colorado-based study found patients were using FSEDs, rather than urgent care centers, for non-life-threatening conditions, and paying significantly more as a result.[56] FSEDs treat many of the same conditions that could be treated in an urgent care center, but in some cases, charge up to 35 times as much for the same condition (figure 1.6).

Figure 1.6 Costs at Stand-Alone Emergency Departments Versus Costs at Urgent Care Centers in Colorado, 2014

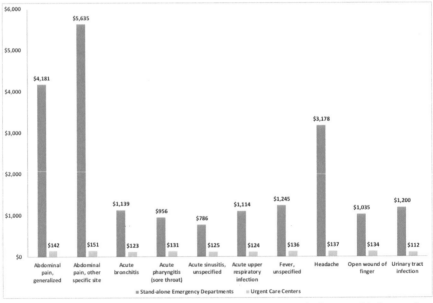

Source: Medicare Program Advisory Commission (MedPAC). Report to the Congress: Medicare and the Health Care Delivery System. Chapter 8: Stand-alone emergency departments, Figure 8-3 (Data from Colorado Center for Improving Value in Health Care, 2016). June 2017. Accessed June 25, 2019. http://www.medpac.gov/docs/default-source/reports/jun17_ch8.pdf

The authors of a 2017 article about FSEDs, which was published in the *Annals of Emergency Medicine*, came to the following conclusion:

… freestanding EDs will continue to proliferate in areas in which there are few restrictions, potentially creating more supply than demand. Health services research demonstrates that geographic proximity to an ED can induce demand and suggests that freestanding EDs may not be pure substitutes for emergency care at a hospital-based ED because patients may be more likely to seek care at a conveniently located freestanding ED. To the extent that freestanding EDs increase utilization without improving outcomes, their presence can drive up costs for insurers and, ultimately, patients who pay those premiums.[57]

Lots of building is going on—lots of expensive access points, like FSEDs, are being built as providers try to meet the patient where they are, while preserving or gaining market share. But outcomes aren't improving, and costs are going up. So, what are we really accomplishing?

Nobody Wins

In the current U.S. healthcare scenario, nobody wins. Patients don't experience the best possible outcomes; payers keep trying to offload costs; and providers are stuck with the task of trying to provide quality care in the context of a payment system that hasn't figured out how to incentivize efficient, coordinated care.

Our layered approach to healthcare delivery has contributed to the development of a "sick-care" system, rather than a healthcare system. What do I mean by a sick-care system? I'll explain more about that in chapter 2.

CHAPTER 2

SICK CARE, NOT HEALTHCARE

Our current healthcare model is simply not set up to manage costs from an "outcome" standpoint. It's not healthcare; it's *sick* care. If we all kept up on our annual primary care visits and started there for all of our other care, we'd be in a much better place. In a true *healthcare* system, patients would proactively take care of their health, with the support of healthcare resources. But the reality is, most patients are disengaged from the healthcare system and interact with it only sporadically.

Hospitals are then placed in the awkward position of taking a "Let's fix what happened and we hope we don't see you again" approach. What I mean by that is: Hospitals want good long-term outcomes for patients. They want to address patients' healthcare problems with care plans that are effective for the long term, whether that means successfully delivering a baby or rehabilitation after a heart attack.

One of the issues, however, is the majority of healthcare delivery models are set up to react versus proactively planning for care. An uneventful delivery of a healthy infant means a one-time visit and some routine postnatal care; a heart repair may mean surgery followed by cardiac rehab.

But chronic disease management—like chronic diabetes management—is not a "one-and-done" issue. Hospitals, with their episodic care models, are not typically set up to deal effectively with chronic disease.

Healthcare payments are also—for the most part—based on this episodic principle (i.e., a fee-for-service or "pay-as-you-play" model). In our current sick-care structure patients enter the system when they're already ill and have "blind" encounter-based episodes (remember the jars?), so treatment is often repetitive and over-used, driving high costs. Patients also need a simple solution, and often we go overboard to meet their needs. Think of it in terms of engines—the patient needs to find a motor for a lawnmower, and the hospital ends up delivering a finely tuned racing engine for a Ferrari. Why are we stuck in the sick-care model of doing things? Let me count the ways.

Current Payment Models Reward the Wrong Things

We still live in a fee-for-service (FFS) world. For the most part, hospitals are still paid by the episode of care—essentially, they're paid by the hour and not by the job. More patients drive more revenue. More procedures drive more revenue. More MRI and CT scans drive more revenue. More admissions drive more revenue. And on and on. And as we saw in the last chapter, reimbursement is also tied to site-of-service (i.e., go to an urgent care center with a headache and you might end up paying $137). Go to the ED with that headache and you might end up paying $3,178, or 23 times as much to treat the exact same condition.[58] Neither of these approaches—more services, nor services provided in a facility that offers an excessive level of care—are correlated with better patient outcomes.

There certainly has been a trend to transition from fee-for-service to fee-for-value (i.e., value-based care), yet providers are still holding tightly onto fee-for-service models. They don't want to lose it, partly because they know *how* it works and has for decades—just ensure the insurance carriers play ball, and it's the same game. It's predictable and carries relatively low risk. Do a test or admit a patient and get paid. Build a freestanding ED (FSED) and get paid (whether it was needed or not).

This traditional view of trying to grow revenue from a patient volume standpoint amazes me. Build it and they will come. That said, some providers—when petitioned—agree the "build it and they will come" strategy is old news. They know they must control costs and be both efficient and attractive to consumers with a complete offering. But I still see so many hospitals and freestanding care centers across the street from one another. Healthcare is not Starbucks, gang. There's a cost to all that building and it's even more significant in healthcare. Building new facilities or FSEDs and even investing in mergers and acquisitions adds plant costs, which are then passed on to healthcare purchasers—including patients and employers. We may have added volume and access with all this building, but we may or may *not* have had an incremental increase in quality. All of these strategies are predicated on increasing revenue by increasing market share and patient volume, but they dramatically increase healthcare delivery costs as well.

Outcomes Models—We Are Not There Yet

As I mentioned in chapter 1, value-based care was supposed to address the inefficiencies in the system. One of the reasons our healthcare system is so out of whack is the incentives are not aligned. Aligning payment with outcomes (value) instead of merely the number of services provided (volume) is supposed to balance the system. The theory is that by rewarding or otherwise incentivizing providers using a pay-for-performance model, there would be a greater ability to control costs. But the truth is value-based care is still in its infancy, and most providers haven't adopted it to the level that would make a significant impact on cost. As an industry, we are talking a lot about it but not many providers are actually willing to do it effectively.

Imagine if the airlines charged this way: "Well, the plane got you halfway to your destination, but here is the bill for the fuel, the pilot, flight attendants and baggage handlers. We can get you home soon but even though you paid your base fare (a.k.a. "insurance premium"), you need to pay more now for all this other support." I'm astounded that our industry has allowed this for so many years. Airlines are starting to nickel and dime consumers too, for cost-control purposes. Consumers have accepted this in the airline industry because it has resulted in lower fares and because consumers knowingly agree to these individual charges in advance, when they purchase their tickets.

In healthcare, it's the opposite. You get an itemized bill *after the fact* that may include providers, services and/or supplies that you had no input in choosing at the front end of care. The healthcare industry needs to look at getting paid for what we do holistically, being fair to payers and to healthcare buyers, with patient outcomes as the keystone of the effort. (See chapter 6 for more details on the various types of value-based care models currently in place.)

Adoption of Value-Based Care Models Is Growing—But Still Low

A study by the Health Care Payment Learning & Action Network (LAN) found as of 2017, a little more than one-third of total U.S. healthcare payments were tied to alternative payment models (APM).[59]

The study revealed:

- Forty-one percent of healthcare dollars were solidly in traditional fee-for-service or other legacy payment models, not linked to quality and value

- Twenty-five percent of healthcare dollars were in fee-for-service plans linked to quality and value (for example, pay-for-performance or care coordination fees)
- Thirty-four percent of healthcare dollars were in shared savings, shared risk, bundled payment or population-based payments (a.k.a. value-based care plans)[60]

The LAN's goal was to see 50 percent of U.S. healthcare payments tied to APMs by the end of 2018.[61] Although the industry is moving in this direction, it's moving slowly—too slowly. Of all industries, healthcare feels the most pain in cost and outcomes, yet our industry is reticent to move to correct them. We must change the care delivery and payment models to drive down cost and pay on outcomes and necessity versus reimbursing for each procedure performed no matter how many times or how ineffective.

The "Healthcare Quality Stick" Is Not Meaningful to Most Consumers

Ever need to measure something? What do you do? You go get a tape measure, a thermometer or the appropriate tool and get moving. In more complex scenarios, you may talk about needed metrics or key performance indicators (KPI). The point is, you measure it. Why is healthcare so hard to measure? For value-based care to work, we need to have a "quality stick" we all agree on. How do we legitimately measure and quantify *quality*, and then, how do we define *quality* healthcare in a way that's meaningful to the patient? This debate has been going on for decades. A number of different measures have been put forth, including:

- Measures advanced by the Agency for Healthcare Research and Quality (AHRQ), an agency of the U.S. Department of Health and Human Services

- Centers for Medicare & Medicaid Services (CMS) Star ratings, which comprise performance measures from the Healthcare Effectiveness Data and Information Set (HEDIS), the Consumer Assessment of Healthcare Providers and Systems (CAHPS) patient surveys, the Medicare Health Outcomes Survey (HOS), Prescription Drug Program and CMS administrative data[62]
- The Leapfrog Group's hospital performance data and hospital comparison tool[63]
- Healthgrades.com

Are these measures actually helpful or meaningful? Each measure uses different metrics, which leads to apples to oranges comparisons. Many of the measures rely on "technical aspects of healthcare quality (for example, hospital-wide mortality, complication and infection rates)," which may not be meaningful to individual consumers.[64] In addition, all of the comparisons are internal to the U.S. health system. Is that appropriate? Do we consider the U.S. system to represent the model health system?

Does it even matter? Consumers, for the most part, seem to be ignoring these quality measures and data resources. Studies consistently show "referrals from friends, family, and providers are the most important sources of information when choosing a new doctor."[65] Did you look it up or did you just go?

Many providers also protest that some of the metrics don't take into account important variables (how sick a population the provider treats, comorbidities, specializations) which can impact the "grade" a provider receives on these measures.[66] And some providers have discovered ways to manipulate quality reporting data.[67] If I hear "But my patients are sicker" one more time, I'm going to lose it. All providers have "sicker" patients, and we all must deliver high-quality care at a lower cost.

Providers Can't Fix Everything

Physicians aren't wizards with magic wands. They have their own sphere of influence, typically in a narrow field of practice, and they take the opaque "care" jars off the shelf, one jar at a time. There are many aspects of care physicians have no leverage over which absolutely do contribute to the cost of care. If you talk to physicians, they'll tell you they're handling this piece and are doing the best they can with what they have. More innovative physicians may have expanded their sphere to look upstream to include preventative care. But most just do their part, within the existing siloed structure of healthcare. Aspects of care that physicians and providers don't have any control over include the following:

The Prevalence of Chronic Disease

As I pointed out in my first book, according to the Centers for Disease Control and Prevention (CDC), 6 out of every 10 adults in the U.S. has a chronic disease.[68] Four out of every 10 adults have 2 or more chronic diseases.[69] The CDC further notes that chronic diseases—heart disease, cancer, chronic lung disease, stroke, Alzheimer's disease, diabetes and chronic kidney disease—are the leading causes of death and disability in the U.S. and a major driver of healthcare costs.

In fact, Americans with one or more chronic conditions account for 90 percent of all healthcare spending.[70] A little more than 1 in 10 Americans (12 percent) has multiple chronic conditions (5 or more).[71] This 12 percent of the population accounts for 41 percent of total healthcare spending.[72] Captain Obvious says we need to fix this before we fix anything else.

Many chronic diseases are linked to lifestyle choices. Using tobacco, poor nutrition choices, lack of exercise and excessive use of alcohol all contribute to chronic disease. This means that providers are on the receiving end of an increasingly sicker population, which increases the need for services and the complexity of care. In this sick-care system, providers have few means and little incentive to reach out to populations with preventative care measures.

This is a problem at the patient and system level. At the patient level, patients are disengaged in their healthcare from a lifestyle and financial engagement piece. It's an afterthought for most and dismissed by some: "I'll use it when I need it, and I'll find out how much it costs when I get billed." "I have insurance, I'll be fine." "I'm healthy and don't need it." Patients have a choice in where they go for care, where they research the costs, what insurance they purchase and many other factors. From a personal standpoint, they also have a choice in lifestyle—and if it is unhealthy, then healthcare costs will be much higher.

It's a problem at the system level because chronic disease requires a very different treatment approach than traditional acute care. A diabetic patient who presents with severe hypoglycemia or "insulin shock" may come to the emergency department (ED) and need treatment to stabilize their blood glucose level. Hospitals are well-equipped to deal with acute care emergencies such as these.

But the bigger picture reveals that unless the patient is also given tools and resources to manage their lifestyle, diet and diabetes appropriately, they'll end up back in the ED again. As I've already pointed out, the ED is the most expensive place to get care. Add the cost of ED care to the ongoing nature of chronic disease and you have an impending disaster of unnecessary healthcare costs.

Patients need to take an active role in their own care, because providers can't fix everything for everyone. Acute care hospitals are designed to treat acute care episodes, not manage chronic care patients.

The Role of Social Determinants of Health

Social determinants of health (SDOH) is a big buzzword in the industry right now. SDOH refers to the reality there are many social, environmental and economic variables that impact an individual's health, arguably more than our healthcare system can ever fix. In fact, one study concluded healthcare accounts for only 10 percent of premature deaths, but patient behavior, social circumstances and environmental exposure combined account for 60 percent of premature deaths (figure 2.1). Notably, genetic predisposition accounts for 30 percent of premature deaths.

Figure 2.1 Proportional Contribution to Premature Death

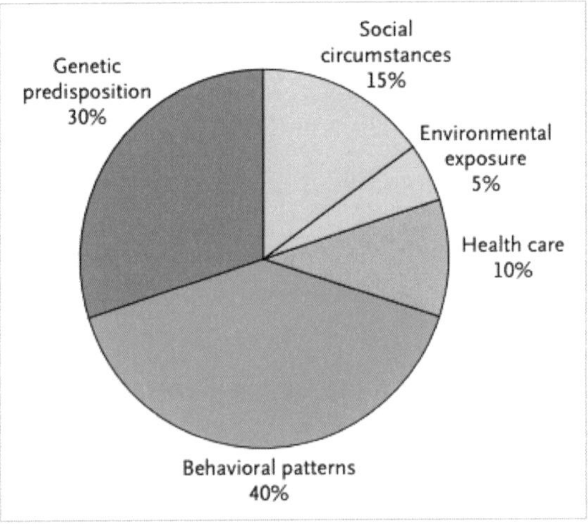

Source: Steven A. Schroeder, M.D. "We Can Do Better—Improving the Health of the American People." The New England Journal of Medicine, September 20, 2007. *N Engl J Med* 2007; 357:1221-1228 DOI: 10.1056/NEJMsa073350. Accessed June 25, 2019. https://www.nejm.org/doi/full/10.1056/nejmsa073350

Social determinants of health include variables such as economic stability, a patient's neighborhood and physical environment, education, access to food, community and social supports, and healthcare (figure 2.2).

Figure 2.2 Social Determinants of Health

Economic Stability	Neighborhood and Physical Environment	Education	Food	Community and Social Context	Health Care System
Employment	Housing	Literacy	Hunger	Social integration	Health coverage
Income	Transportation	Language	Access to healthy options	Support systems	Provider availability
Expenses	Safety	Early childhood education		Community engagement	Provider linguistic and cultural competency
Debt	Parks	Vocational training		Discrimination	
Medical bills	Playgrounds			Stress	Quality of care
Support	Walkability	Higher education			
	Zip code / geography				

Health Outcomes
Mortality, Morbidity, Life Expectancy, Health Care Expenditures, Health Status, Functional Limitations

Source: Samantha Artiga and Elizabeth Hinton. "Beyond Health Care: The Role of Social Determinants in Promoting Health and Health Equity." Kaiser Family Foundation. May 10, 2018. Accessed June 25, 2019. https://www.kff.org/disparities-policy/issue-brief/beyond-health-care-the-role-of-social-determinants-in-promoting-health-and-health-equity/

These factors impact everything from premature patient mortality to how many times a patient is likely to visit the ED each year. As John Auerbach, associate director for policy at the CDC once said:

> The definitive factors in determining whether someone is in good health extend significantly beyond access to care and include the conditions in their life and the conditions of their neighborhoods and communities.[73]

For example, let's say "Joe" falls and breaks his hip. He goes to the ED, is admitted to the hospital and gets better, but he needs rehab to learn how to walk again. But he lives in a high-crime neighborhood, doesn't own a car, and lives four miles away from the nearest bus station. How will he access the care he needs?

Providers are beginning to realize that if they can identify and address these needs—in this case, Joe's need for transportation—they can improve patient outcomes. If Joe doesn't go to rehab, he might break his hip again or end up getting a post-hospitalization infection. Medicare doesn't think too highly of those outcomes and docks a hospital's payments if those things happen. So, it's actually in the healthcare system's best interest to find a way for the patient to participate in rehab—maybe even hiring Uber or Lyft to get him there—rather than risking a negative patient outcome. How many more times do you want to see Joe in your ED because you did not address SDOH?

Another example is housing. If a homeless patient can be discharged from the hospital or from the emergency department and put back on the street—that's dangerous. Providers want the patient to leave better than they came and hopefully come back in a less acute way, if at all, so that healthcare can be managed holistically. If the patient doesn't have a stable place to get better, they're more likely to experience negative outcomes, such as getting an infection—then they boomerang back to the ED.

Many providers are beginning to pick up on this, and so they are doing things like buying apartment complexes or partnering with shelters to set up respite programs. Sometimes it's worth spending $500 to give a patient a few days in a hotel room to recover safely so they don't end up back in the ED—costing the provider $6,000—in the next week. That's a no-brainer.

There are a wide range of use cases like this, where it's not only in the patient's best interest but also in the provider's best interest to identify and address those other variables that impact patient outcomes.

Failing to address an SDOH factor can contribute to overutilization (accessing more healthcare services more often than necessary) and "wrong" levels of care (accessing healthcare services that treat at a higher level of acuity than is called for), which are two major contributors to healthcare costs. Getting upstream of these issues—and focusing on healthcare, not sick care—is the key to changing the healthcare paradigm.

Twenty-five years ago, the role of SDOH wasn't as significant to providers, because in a fee-for-service world, the more services you provided, the more you got paid. But now, payers like Medicare have started moving toward payment on *outcomes* instead of *volume*. They have implemented rules that penalize providers for hospital readmissions within 30 days or for hospital-acquired infections. Today, SDOH can be extremely significant to revenue cycle leaders: in today's environment, ignoring SDOH can directly impact the bottom line.

Another aspect of SDOH that merits attention is the nation's investment in programs and services that mitigate SDOH factors. If you compare the holistic healthcare spending in the U.S. to other countries, like Sweden, Germany or the U.K., you find the U.S. spends much less on social services and much more on healthcare (figure 2.3).

Nations that are members of the Organization for Economic Cooperation and Development (OECD) spend an average of $1.70 on social services for every $1 spent on health services, while the U.S. spends only 56 cents on social services for every $1 spent on health services.

Figure 2.3 Health and Social Care Spending as a Percentage of GDP

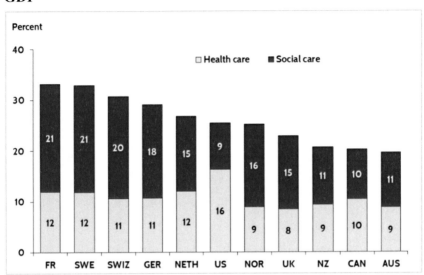

Source: Stuart M. Butler, Dayna Bowen Matthew and Marcela Cabello. "Re-balancing medical and social spending to promote health." USC-Brookings Schaeffer on Health Policy. February 15, 2017. Accessed July 2, 2017. http://brook.gs/2lLn7BB

Other countries have this figured out. They understand that addressing things like housing, transportation, nutrition and other elements of SDOH is actually going to decrease the amount providers spend on healthcare services over the long term. They understand the patient must be treated holistically—not just the disease—and they're investing in that approach.

The Patient Is Disengaged

Patients can be disengaged from their own care in a number of ways: they may be disengaged from their own role in keeping themselves healthy and making healthy lifestyle choices that offer protection from chronic disease; they may be disengaged from the true cost of their care; and they might be intimidated by the complexity of costs and coverage. I believe one of the reasons healthcare in the U.S. is chaotic is we are complacent.

As patients, we care only indirectly about cost and quality—as long as someone else is paying and our neighbor vouched for the provider's competency. We accept whatever is given—freely. We also, for the most part, don't engage with the system unless something goes wrong.

The Healthcare System as a Safety Net Instead of Health Partner

Many patients view the healthcare system as a safety net system—a place to go only when things go wrong, rather than a place to go for maintaining or improving their health even when they don't have any emerging problems. They show up at the ED for emergent problems that could have been headed off earlier, in a less urgent stage of care.

In the United States however, patients actually visit the doctor less frequently than in comparable countries, as illustrated in the chart below (figure 2.4).

Figure 2.4 Doctors Consultations, per Capita, in All Settings, by Country, 2015

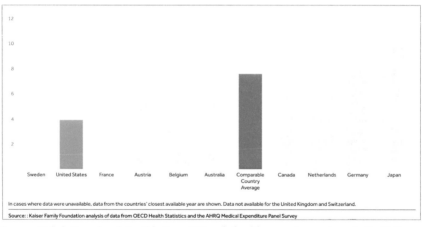

In cases where data were unavailable, data from the countries' closest available year are shown. Data not available for the United Kingdom and Switzerland.

Source: : Kaiser Family Foundation analysis of data from OECD Health Statistics and the AHRQ Medical Expenditure Panel Survey

Source: Rabah Kamal and Cynthia Cox. "How do healthcare prices and use in the U.S. compare to other countries?" Peterson Center on Healthcare and Kaiser Family Foundation. Peterson-KFF Health System Tracker. May 8, 2018. https://www.healthsystemtracker.org/chart-collection/how-do-healthcare-prices-and-use-in-the-u-s-compare-to-other-countries/

So not only is healthcare delivered in an episodic manner; patient behaviors around accessing care are episodic as well. For example, the patient hurts his ankle, goes to the closest FSED, gets that ankle fixed and then walks out. The patient will likely never see that particular provider again. The system *delivers* care episodically and the patient *consumes* care episodically. Neither one is invested in the holistic picture, and that impacts costs.

Patients Are Disengaged from the Cost of Their Care

Patients are very often also disengaged from the cost of their care. In some ways, the industry has historically encouraged patients not to worry about the cost of their care beyond knowing whether they have insurance coverage or not. The third-party payment system has hidden costs and inflation in pricing. In the not-so-distant past, the only thing patients needed to know was whether or not they had health insurance coverage and their small copay, and that was the end of it. When I speak publicly, I often ask a rhetorical question: "Why is our healthcare so expensive?" The audience often blames the usual suspects—Big Pharma, the aging population, technology, hospital and insurance profits, the uninsured, etc. I then say, "Yes, that's part of it, but most of it is your fault" (pointing at the crowd ... which is followed by gasps). I continue with, "For years you saw a number at the top of your statement getting larger and larger, but you didn't care, because your portion—down on the bottom—didn't get bigger. Now it has and now you care, but it may be too late. You now pay $55 for a dozen healthcare eggs and are not happy."

The employer-based health insurance system that evolved in the U.S. put the responsibility for providing healthcare coverage on employers, not on individual patients. Benefits and coverage were negotiated between the employer and the third-party payer. All patients had to do was check a box during the annual enrollment period. Patients weren't clamoring for cost transparency, because the costs were largely invisible to them— their employers paid the bulk of the insurance premium, and when patients did receive care, out-of-pocket (OOP) costs were minimal.

But healthcare doesn't work like that anymore.

That model—of minimal patient engagement in their own healthcare costs—set us up for the growing pains the patient is experiencing today. It created unrealistic expectations. In what other industry can you get served first, and not worry about costs until much, much later, if at all? Imagine going out to eat, maybe at one of those fancy places with no prices on the menu. You have a food expert (think "physician" here) order everything for you from the menu—the finest wines, steak and lobster—and all that food just keeps coming. After you've had your fill, you say, "Oh, don't give the bill to me—I have dining insurance. They'll cover it." The bill comes with an astronomical tab, but all you owe is the tip (a.k.a. the copay). What would the restaurant industry look like today if consumers relied on third-party payers to cover their costs? I'll tell you one thing: a system like that would encourage overutilization. People could order too much and overeat without fiscal consequences—and as a consequence, there would be a lot of food wasted, and our national obesity problem would probably be a lot worse, because consumers would be separated from the financial consequences of their behavior.

That's how healthcare has worked (ahem, *not* worked) for far too long.

Patients Are Intimidated by the Complexity of Costs and Coverage

It's much more complicated for patients now. Knowing that you *have* coverage isn't enough. Now, to avoid billing surprises, engaged patients need to know who their insurer is, which of those insurer's various plans they're covered under, what their covered benefits are, what their deductible is, which providers are in their network and which aren't, etc.

These two factors—a patient's separation from the actual cost of their care, and the increasing complexity of insurance coverage—have contributed to disengagement. Patients frequently don't understand their own benefits. They often cannot—or will not—give providers correct information about their insurance eligibility and coverage. They don't understand (or sometimes can intentionally misrepresent) their eligibility for care, and they don't understand their OOP costs. The assumption of insurance covering the majority of your care is ancient history for most—rules and copayments have put the nail in that coffin.

Providers Haven't Been in a Position to Help Sort Things Out

It's not just patients who are overwhelmed by the complexity of the system. Providers are overwhelmed, too. Providers struggle to give valid, front-end, OOP cost estimates to patients, which contributes to the perception of a lack of transparency in the industry. Like the food expert in the fancy restaurant, they're ordering for you from a menu with no prices listed.

The concept of transparency (or the T-word) has been tossed around in the healthcare industry for some time, but most efforts at implementing any kind of transparency have failed miserably. In August 2018, CMS attempted to clarify the Affordable Care Act's (ACA) provisions around transparency and proposed rules changing the requirements for providers around price transparency. CMS stated:

> … we are concerned that challenges
> continue to exist for patients due to insufficient
> price transparency … Therefore, as one step to

further improve the public accessibility of charge information, effective January 1, 2019 we announced the update to our guidelines to required hospitals to make available a list of their current standard charges via the internet in a machine-readable format and to update this information at least annually, or more often as appropriate. This could be in the form of the chargemaster itself or another form of the hospital's choice, as long as the information is in machine readable format.[74]

The new transparency guidelines were greeted with a tsunami of backlash. CMS summarized their critics' concerns in the Response to Comments section of the final rule. Concerns expressed to CMS included:

- The information contained in the chargemaster would not be useful to patients and would only increase confusion, as it would not inform them of their out-of-pocket costs for a particular service
- The chargemaster contains terms that are difficult for patients to understand, does not depict negotiated discounts with insurers, and lacks contextual information
- Payer-specific charge information is proprietary and confidential, and publication could undermine competition
- Patients may forgo needed care if they were informed of the charges in advance
- Price information in the absence of quality information can mislead the patient[75]

AHA (as well as many other prominent organizations—HFMA, AHIP, FAH, AMA and others) indicated,

"This approach would confuse—not help—patients in understanding their potential out-of-pocket cost obligations, would severely disrupt private contract negotiations between providers and health plans, and exceeds the Administration's legal authority."[76] CMS responded to these concerns with the following message: "After consideration of the public comments we received, we currently do not believe there is a need to further update our guidelines beyond the updated guidelines that we previously announced would be effective January 1, 2019 ..."[77]

In other words, live with it. The industry and yours truly have asserted a law requiring a public display of prices will only cause confusion if *not* coupled with actual OOP costs to the patient. Seven months later, in November of 2019, CMS finalized the rule, which will be effective in 2021 as of this writing.[78] The final rule requires hospitals to "make public" not only "gross charges" but also "payer-specific negotiated charges."[79]

The finalized rule makes the first rule look like kindergarten. CMS basically said, "OK, fine. If publishing the gross charges isn't useful, then show me what will be useful to your patients." That is—payer-specific negotiated charges. And they put some teeth in it by establishing penalties and fines for noncompliance. I applaud CMS. The industry is at odds with these incremental changes and rules, but think big picture, gang. When we look back at this, each of these steps is critical. Display the charge, allowable amount, patient benefits and the cost to the patient. We have to crawl before we walk, and walk before we run. Breathe deep, the T-word is a marathon, not a sprint. The T-word may become a four-letter word very soon for the industry, but in the long term I believe it will lead to better results for our patients and provider collection efforts.

I agree with CMS on their overall approach: they're trying to move the transparency needle. They're thinking big picture. These incremental changes can, indeed, be scary in the short term, but the market needs guidance, leadership and courage to summit the healthcare transparency peak. Right now, we are a bunch of scared chickens in the henhouse, with the CMS fox lurking. During a session on transparency at a Becker's Hospital Review conference last year, the audience was hostile toward the panel, with comments like "It's not possible for providers to comply with this new rule," and "We can't accurately predict the cost of care without the patient being within the hospital walls." We have to stop with this "transparency isn't possible in healthcare" excuse fest. Indeed, this is a complex issue, but we've fixed harder things. Remember when diagnoses-related groups (DRGs) came out? How about the latest version of the International Statistical Classification of Diseases and Related Health Problems (ICD-10)? We are sophisticated, brilliant people in this market, but are frankly too scared to fix this for our patients. It's time to stop treating transparency like a four-letter word. We need to be bold.

The truth is, we *can* estimate the cost of care: for most things, we can get to a very accurate estimate. For example, for routine, common diagnostic testing and routine prescriptions, we can get really accurate and close. And from a volume standpoint, routine services make up more than 60 percent of everything performed.[80] On everything else, I argue, we can get close enough, even if only to collect a deposit. For common surgeries, like knees and backs, we can collect within a range and still do OK. When predicting costs, healthcare is an art—not a science—and it will always be harder to estimate the cost of things like less-common surgeries and inpatient care, but we can get close. CMS gets this … the new rule lists 300 procedures, and the 70 of them chosen by CMS just so happen to be the most common. The other 230 can be chosen by the provider to specialize the offering. Collaboration and flexibility … I love this country.

In every other industry, an estimate (or better yet, the exact price) for services can be provided—airlines, retail, food services, car mechanics, contractors, etc. Why does it have to be so hard for healthcare? Is there really that much variability in cost that's outside a predictable range? Have you been to the pharmacy lately? They provide an instant estimate *all* day for every script. I acknowledge there is variability in delivery and cost—but we're just too scared to take the leap. Get close on what you can, and don't throw the baby out with the bath water.

We have the ability to do accurate estimates, and just as important, patients want this. Providers can estimate OOP costs, collect deposits, initial payments, establish payment plans, etc. The key will be leveraging analytics to ensure accuracy. The tools are available. We just need to start using them instead of throwing up our hands and saying, "It can't be done." We better figure it out, gang, or the government is going to figure it out for us.

When we focus on what's *not* possible, patient experience suffers, as does revenue cycle management (RCM). Complex, unanticipated bills and poor explanations lead to poor payments. One recent survey found the patient's financial experience is highly correlated with their payment behavior. Over 75 percent of patients pay their bills—either in full or in stages when they are happy with their billing experience—but only about 50 percent pay their bills if they have a poor billing experience.[81]

53

Poor billing practices—including a lack of transparency up front—lead to unhappy patients. Unhappy and confused patients aren't in a hurry to pay their bills. The complexity of the system has overwhelmed patients, and providers haven't leveraged the tools available today to support the patient financial experience to make it more transparent and frictionless.

The Consumer Is Entitled

U.S. consumers seem to bring a "have it your way" mentality to most of the goods and services they purchase, including healthcare. Our society tends to want everything, all the time, all paid for, and they want it *now*. Look at package delivery services. Two-day delivery was once considered fast. Not anymore. *Same-day* delivery is now the fastest growing expedited delivery option, according to a recent consumer survey.[82] The survey also found consumers are willing to pay for faster delivery—especially Millennials, with 54 percent saying they'd paid extra for faster delivery in the past 12 months.[83]

The "have it your way, get it fast" mentality may work for fast food and retail delivery services, but it doesn't work for healthcare. It only leads to inefficient care and higher costs for everyone. When we get care fast and are disengaged, we are sitting blindfolded at that fancy restaurant—eating too much food at too high of a cost, and it becomes unaffordable.

All of these factors contribute to why we have a sick-care system in the U.S. instead of a true healthcare system. To sum up, the current system is ineffective, inefficient and expensive. In the next chapter, I will explain how every stakeholder—from patient to provider to payer to employer—is sinking under the weight of the healthcare system's unsustainable spending.

CHAPTER 3

HEALTHCARE BANKRUPTCY

At least 13 hospitals filed for bankruptcy in the first 6 months of 2019.[84] Patients aren't faring better. Medical issues are the number one cause of bankruptcy, representing 66.5 percent of all personal bankruptcy filings (figure 3.1). Think we have an unaffordability problem? The current U.S. healthcare spending rate is increasing at an unsustainable pace. We can't go on like this.

Figure 3.1 Causes of Personal Bankruptcy

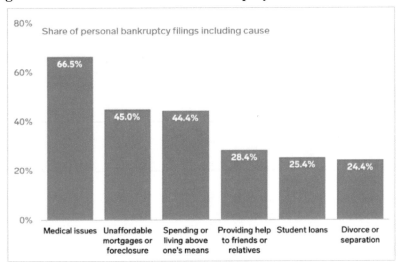

Source: Hillary Hoffower. "Staggering medical bills are the biggest driver of personal bankruptcies in the US." Business Insider. June 25, 2019. Accessed Aug. 9, 2019.
https://www.businessinsider.com/causes-personal-bankruptcy-medical-bills-mortgages-student-loan-debt-2019-6

One way to quantify the situation is to look at health consumption expenditures as a percent of the gross domestic product (GDP) compared to other countries. In 1970, health expenditures totaled only 6 percent of the U.S. GDP, but over the last 50 years, that number has grown to 17 percent (figure 3.2). For those who don't like percentages (like me), that is $3.5 trillion, or $10,739 per person.[85]

Figure 3.2 Health Consumption Expenditures as Percent of GDP, 1970–2017

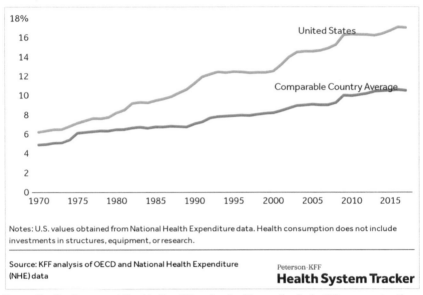

Notes: U.S. values obtained from National Health Expenditure data. Health consumption does not include investments in structures, equipment, or research.

Source: KFF analysis of OECD and National Health Expenditure (NHE) data

Peterson-KFF
Health System Tracker

Source: Bradley Sawyer and Cynthia Cox. "How does health spending in the U.S. compare to other countries?" Peterson Center on Healthcare and Kaiser Family Foundation. Peterson-KFF Health System Tracker. December 7, 2018. Accessed December 12, 2019. https://www.healthsystemtracker.org/chart-collection/health-spending-u-s-compare-countries/

Centers for Medicare & Medicaid Services (CMS) projects that health spending will continue to grow faster than the GDP over the next 10 years, and that healthcare's share of the GDP will reach 19.4 percent by 2027.[86] As alarming as that trajectory is, "percent of GDP" is still a rather abstract concept. Look at it this way: almost $1 in every $5 spent will be on healthcare.

Do you think it's OK to spend that much on your healthcare?

As of the writing of this text, the national GDP was $21 trillion.[87] Twenty percent of the U.S. GDP is roughly $4.2 trillion. That's trillion with a "T." Just for the sake of sanity, let's quantify the estimated incremental increase between that and the current GDP. By my math, this represents roughly a mere $700 billion (with a "B"). That means if I stacked Benjamins (each $100 bill), it would be enough for me to build a staircase to the International Space Station … and back (figure 3.3).

Figure 3.3 How Much Is a Billion Dollars?

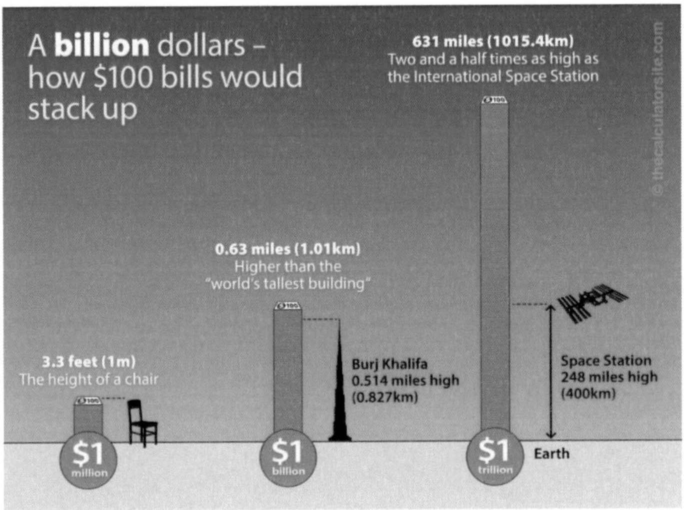

Source: Becky Kleanthous. "How Much is a Billion?" The Calculator Site. December 30, 2019. Accessed January 5, 2020. https://www.thecalculatorsite.com/articles/finance/how-big-is-a-billion.php

I know it's hard to wrap our heads around billions of dollars and stairways to heaven stacked with $100 bills, but if we zoom in on what this looks like at the household level, the impact of rising healthcare costs becomes more obvious. For example, according to the 2019 Milliman Medical Index, the cost of healthcare for a typical American family of four, covered by an average employer-sponsored preferred provider organization (PPO) plan, is $28,386, including the premium share paid by employers and employees and out-of-pocket expenses including deductibles and copays.[88] Almost 29 grand! That's a nice car these days. But instead, it's spent on healthcare, and probably represents one of the larger line items in the average American's household budget. Many American's monthly healthcare spending rivals that of their mortgage payment.[89]

If we go deeper and look at how this increased healthcare spending impacts each of the stakeholders in the system—patients, providers, payers and employers—it becomes even more clear our healthcare system is headed for bankruptcy.

Unsustainable for Patients

Patients are feeling the impact of already high—and getting higher—healthcare costs the most. That's due to the fact that while healthcare costs are rising for *all* stakeholders, an increasing *share* of those costs is shifting to patients.

Payer and employer strategies for curbing costs—such as increasing deductibles, copays and coinsurance—are hitting patients in the pocketbook. Ironically, patients arguably have the least capacity of any of the stakeholders in the system to absorb these price increases. A recent Federal Reserve report pointed out 4 out of 10 adults would either borrow or sell something or not be able to pay at all if faced with an unexpected expense of $400.[90] Four hundred dollars is a sneeze in an emergency room! It takes very little to reach that amount of out-of-pocket patient liability in a hospital.

The Federal Reserve report also found one in five adults experienced a major, unexpected medical bill in 2018, with the median expense between $1,000 and $4,999.[91] Among adults with medical expenses, 4 out of 10 reported having unpaid debt as a result of those bills.[92] Furthermore, one in four adults skipped medical care in 2018 due to an inability to pay. This is going the wrong direction.

To add fuel to the fire, patients with less disposable income forgo care more often. In households with an income below $40,000, more than one-third (36 percent) reported deferring medical treatment due to costs. For households with incomes between $40,000 and $100,000, one-quarter (24 percent) went without medical care; for households with incomes above $100,000, 8 percent reported going without medical care due to costs.[93] As you consider the income levels above, note the cap for most financial aid benefits at hospitals is in the $35,000 to $75,000 range, or approximately 135 to 300 percent of the 2019 Federal Poverty Level (FPL) for a family of four. Beyond this "cap," individuals are often out of income for financial assistance per the hospital's policy, meaning the bill will be entirely the patient's responsibility to bear. As a result, patients aren't going to the doctor because they fear what will happen when it comes time to pay the bill.

If it's not fear that's motivating action (or inaction in this case) then patients feel care is too expensive anyway. A recent West Health/Gallup survey found three out of four Americans believe they pay "too much" for healthcare relative to the quality of care they receive.[94] The same survey found Americans borrowed $88 billion to pay for healthcare costs in 2018.[95] Patients are taking out loans and borrowing on credit to pay for the very same healthcare they feel is too expensive in the first place—and are subsequently stuck in an unaffordable cycle of bills and medical debt—ultimately leading to bankruptcy. In fact, 45 percent of Americans worry a major health event could end in personal bankruptcy.[96] Each year, 530,000 families experience bankruptcies linked to illness or medical bills.[97]

All of this unpleasant news may drive one to ask the question, "What role does health insurance play in this equation?" The most recent data from the Kaiser Family Foundation shows the following distribution of health insurance coverage (figure 3.4):

Figure 3.4 Health Insurance Coverage of the Total Population, 2018

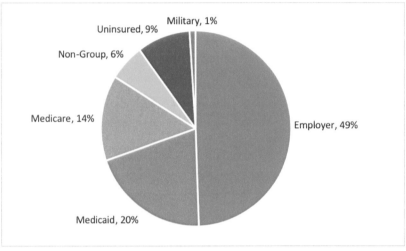

Source: Based on data from the Kaiser Family Foundation, "Health Insurance Coverage of the Total Population." 2018. State Health Facts. https://www.kff.org/2fdbf6d/

Almost half of Americans receive their health insurance through their employer—and this percentage is actually decreasing over time. Trended data show the percentage of Americans receiving health insurance through their employer has dropped from 54 percent in 2008 to 49 percent in 2017.[98] At the same time, the percentage receiving Medicaid has increased from 13 percent in 2008 to 21 percent in 2017, due largely to the Medicaid expansion provision included in the Affordable Care Act (ACA). The percent of the population covered by Medicare increased from 11 percent in 2008 to 14 percent in 2017, which makes sense with the "silver tsunami" of the aging population. This has had a detrimental impact on hospital revenue by diluting the payer mix for providers. There are fewer commercially insured patients and more covered by governmental insurance, meaning providers are seeing the same or more patients with less reimbursement.

At the same time, the number of *uninsured* is on the rise. A recent Gallup report indicated the uninsured rate has climbed to a four-year high.[99] The report notes, "The U.S. adult uninsured rate stood at 13.7 percent in the 4th quarter of 2018 … well above the low point of 10.9 percent reached in 2016."[100] Wrong direction, again.

Skyrocketing costs combined with the trend of cost shifting to patients is also accelerating the percentage of patients who are *underinsured*. Basically, being underinsured is like a bait and switch. That is, I bought insurance and thought I was well-covered but it turns out this insurance doesn't cover anything affordable, due to high-deductible health plans (HDHP) and cost sharing. The Commonwealth Fund has established the following definition of underinsurance:

- Someone who is insured all year whose out-of-pocket costs, excluding premiums, over the prior 12 months, equals or exceeds 10 percent of the household income (this measure is used if a person uses his or her plan);
- Or, whose out-of-pocket costs, excluding premiums, are equal to 5 percent or more of the household income if the income is under 200 percent of the Federal Poverty Level (this measure is used if a person uses his or her plan);
- Or, whose healthcare plan deductible represents 5 percent or more of the household income.[101]

The percentage of *underinsured* adults in the U.S. has risen dramatically in the last 15 years, from 12 percent in 2003 (the first year the measure was used in the Commonwealth Fund's Biennial

Health Insurance Survey) to 29 percent in 2018 (figure 3.5). Almost a third of Americans have "insurance" that leaves them with unaffordable copays, deductibles or coinsurance for healthcare services.

Figure 3.5 Percent of Underinsured Adults, 2003–2018

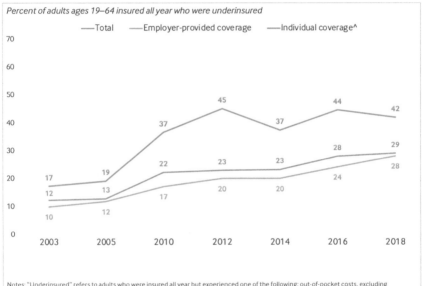

Notes: "Underinsured" refers to adults who were insured all year but experienced one of the following: out-of-pocket costs, excluding premiums, equaled 10% or more of income; out-of-pocket costs, excluding premiums, equaled 5% or more of income if low-income (<200% of poverty); or deductibles equaled 5% or more of income. Total includes adults with coverage through Medicaid and Medicare. Respondents may have had another type of coverage at some point during the year, but had coverage for the entire previous 12 months. ^ For 2014 and 2016, includes those who get their individual coverage through the marketplace and outside of the marketplace.

Data: Commonwealth Fund Biennial Health Insurance Surveys (2003, 2005, 2010, 2012, 2014, 2016, 2018).

Source: Sara R. Collins, Herman K. Bhupal and Michelle M. Doty. "Health Insurance Coverage Eight Years After the ACA: Fewer Uninsured Americans and Shorter Coverage Gaps, but More Underinsured." The Commonwealth Fund, Survey Brief. February 2019. Accessed July 24, 2019. https://www.commonwealthfund.org/sites/default/files/2019-02/EMBARGOED_Collins_hlt_ins_coverage_8_years_after_ACA_2018_biennial_survey_sb_v4.pdf

This trend holds true even for patients who have insurance through their employer. Due to cost-shifting strategies, such as the increased use of HDHPs, the percentage of adults who are considered underinsured even though they have insurance coverage through their employer has risen from 10 percent in 2003 to 28 percent in 2018.[102]

In other words, insured or not, Americans are having a hard time paying for healthcare. Recent headlines highlight the pain:

- "Americans can't afford to get sick—and limited plans could make things worse (*The Hill*, November 1, 2018)[103]
- "Health insurance deductibles soar, leaving Americans with unaffordable bills" (*Los Angeles Times*, May 2, 2019)[104]
- "'We're Drowning': Financially Crippled Americans Are Reaching a Breaking Point as Health Insurance Drains Their Savings" (*Kaiser Health News*, May 3, 2019)[105]
- "Washington Couple Dies in a Murder-Suicide Over Angst About Medical Expenses" (*USA Today*, August 10, 2019)[106]

Unsustainable for Employers

You can't blame employers for trying to get a handle on healthcare costs. With employers still providing health insurance for almost half (49 percent) of the U.S. insured population (see figure 3.4), they are in the health insurance business whether they like it or not. And they are paying for it. Employers share of medical costs represent almost 60 percent of the spend (figure 3.6).

Figure 3.6 Relative Proportions of 2019 Medical Costs

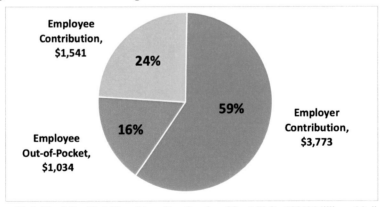

Source: Chris Girod, Sue Hart, Dave Liner, Tom Snook and Scott Weltz. "2019 Milliman Medical Index." Milliman Research Report. Figure 7. Relative Proportions of 2019 Medical Costs. July 2019. Accessed July 26, 2019. http://assets.milliman.com/ektron/2019-milliman-medical-index.pdf

Employers want to be able to offer a competitive benefit package so they can retain—and add—employees as they grow their businesses. At the same time, increases in health insurance premium costs are constraining business growth by diverting revenue from employee wage increases or business growth initiatives. One survey estimated companies spend an average of 7.6 percent of their operating budgets on employee healthcare.[107] That's more than most margins in healthcare.

The Move Toward High-Deductible Health Plans

Employers are trying to keep their healthcare spending as low as possible by managing their premium and claim costs. One of the primary strategies employers can use to keep premiums low and control healthcare spending is to shift costs to employees via HDHP and high-coinsurance plans. These plans shift employer costs to the employee by reducing the total cost of the premiums employers negotiate with health insurance providers. Lower premium costs save money for both employers and employees—on the front end anyway.

Theoretically, these plans also reduce claims costs by encouraging employees to make smarter choices about how, when and from whom they access healthcare. As we already saw in chapter 1, it doesn't really work that way, but employers have been moving to these cost-sharing plans anyway as a way to control healthcare costs. Thus, my mantra, death to the deductible.

But the beat goes on, and HDHP is still the plan *du jour* for most employers. In just the past 10 years, the number of adults with employment-based coverage enrolled in a traditional plan decreased from 85.1 percent in 2007 to 56.6 percent in 2017 (figure 3.7). Over the same time period, the percentage of adults enrolled in HDHPs increased from 14.8 percent to 43.4 percent.[108]

Figure 3.7 Percentage of Adults Aged 18–64 With Employment-Based Coverage, by Type of Private Coverage and Year: United States, 2007–2017

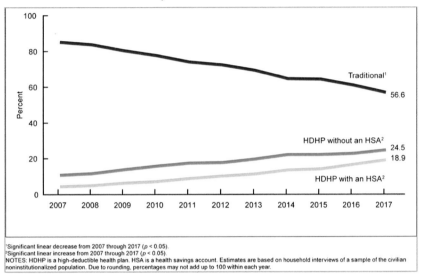

[1]Significant linear decrease from 2007 through 2017 ($p < 0.05$).
[2]Significant linear increase from 2007 through 2017 ($p < 0.05$).
NOTES: HDHP is a high-deductible health plan. HSA is a health savings account. Estimates are based on household interviews of a sample of the civilian noninstitutionalized population. Due to rounding, percentages may not add up to 100 within each year.

Source: Robin A. Cohen, Ph.D. and Emily P. Zammitti, M.P.H. "High-deductible health plan enrollment among adults aged 18–64 with employment-based insurance coverage." NCHS Data Brief, No. 317. Hyattsville, MD: National Center for Health Statistics. August 2018. https://www.cdc.gov/nchs/data/databriefs/db317.pdf

Where did the idea for high-deductible plans come from in the first place? You guessed it: The government. Bloomberg did a piece on HDHPs:

> How the U.S. insurance system came to stick its customers with increasingly onerous medical bills is a 15-year-long story of miscalculations and missed opportunities. It started in 2003 when President George W. Bush and congressional Republicans passed a change to the tax code that encouraged employers to experiment with high-deductible plans, which ask patients to pay out of pocket for care—sometimes thousands of dollars—before insurance coverage kicks in. The trend got a push

when the financial crisis hit: as the economy stalled and employers shed nearly 9 million jobs over 3 years, companies desperate to slash costs turned to high-deductible plans to save money. The next wave came with the arrival of Obamacare in 2010. Millions who were previously uninsured could now get coverage, but many of them took on deductibles of $1,000 or higher.[109]

The Escalating Deductible

Not only has the percentage of employees enrolled in HDHPs grown, but the size of those deductibles has grown as well (figure 3.8). It's a bad idea to put a high, unaffordable amount out there, applied *after* everything is done, on things no one can pinpoint the cost of, and let patients choose where they should go and the type of care they need. Again, death to the deductible.

Figure 3.8 Deductibles in Private Health Plans Have Grown Over the Past Decade

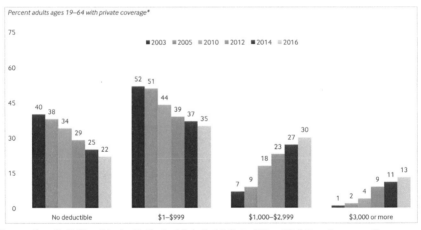

Source: Sara R. Collins, Munira Z. Gunja, Michelle M. Doty. "How Well Does Insurance Coverage Protect Consumers from Health Care Costs?" Findings from the Commonwealth Fund Biennial Health Insurance Survey, 2016. The Commonwealth Fund, Issue Brief. October 2017. Accessed July 25, 2019.
https://www.commonwealthfund.org/sites/default/files/documents/___media_files_publications_issu e_brief_2017_oct_collins_underinsured_biennial_ib.pdf

Health Savings Accounts Aren't Really Helping

Health savings accounts (HSAs) were conceived as one way to mitigate the OOP impact of HDHPs. The idea was patients could set aside money in tax-advantaged savings accounts to pay for OOP healthcare expenses. However, HSAs haven't really caught on with patients.

Research by EBRI shows enrollment in HSAs grew considerably after introduction in 2004 but growth has slowed in recent years (figure 3.9).

Figure 3.9 Average Growth Rates in Health Savings Account-Eligible Health Plan Enrollment, by Select Time Periods

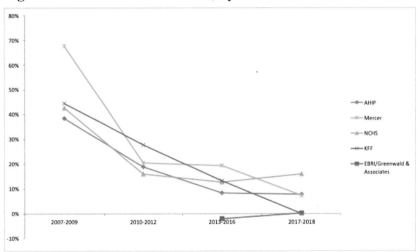

Source: Paul Fronstin, Ph.D. "Enrollment in HSA-Eligible Health Plans: Slow and Steady Growth Continued into 2018." Employee Benefit Research Institute (EBRI) Issue Brief. March 28, 2019, No. 478. Accessed August 9, 2019. https://www.ebri.org/docs/default-source/ebri-issue-brief/ebri_ib_478_hsaenrollment-28mar19.pdf?sfvrsn=e86b3f2f_4

The bottom line on HSAs, however, is they are most helpful to people who have disposable income available to save in the first place. That's not most Americans. Studies show only 13 percent of HSA account holders contributed the maximum amount to their HSA accounts.[110] Bankrate.com concluded:

… a few super-savers, presumably with more
disposable income, are the real winners from the
HSA experiment. If you have a substantial
emergency fund sitting in a savings account, save at
least 10 percent of your income in a retirement
account, and are pretty healthy, an HSA is
something to consider. Everyone else, though,
needs to shore up their finances.[111]

Ultimately, employer and payer cost-control strategies,
such as the use of HDHPs, places the burden on the patient.
Despite the fact patients can't afford those high deductibles; those
plans are encouraging patients to defer medical care rather than
make better choices; and HSAs aren't being used in the manner
intended (per the points above), it unfortunately seems to be the
best solution the industry can come up with at this time.

Given the cost burden to employers and employees to fund
healthcare coverage, it's no surprise many employers would like to
get out of the health insurance business altogether. They are stuck
in the middle of paying for unsustainable spending. But there is
some light at the end of the tunnel. Some of them are finding
creative ways change the game, by cutting commercial payers out
altogether by either turning to self-funded plans or making direct-
to-provider arrangements (see chapter 7 for more about direct-to-
provider contracting).

Unsustainable for Government Payers

The U.S. government is still the largest payer in the U.S.
healthcare system. National health expenditure data from CMS
shows private health insurance had a 34 percent share of health
spending in 2017, compared to the 37 percent share of Medicare

(20 percent) and Medicaid (17 percent) combined.[112] As the largest payer in the system, the government is also severely impacted by rising healthcare costs. In 2018, Medicare made up 15 percent of the total federal budget; spending on Medicaid, the ACA and the Children's Health Insurance Program (CHIP), claimed another 11 percent of the budget (figure 3.10). This means that more than one in four of all government dollars are allocated to healthcare. That's more than Social Security, more than the defense budget and, in fact, more than any other line item in the federal budget.

Figure 3.10 Medicare as a Share of the Federal Budget, 2018

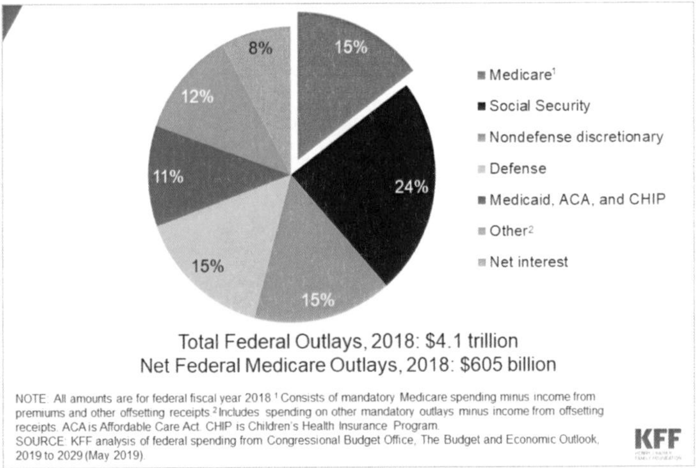
15%
24%
15%
15%
11%
12%
8%
Medicare1
Social Security
Nondefense discretionary
Defense
Medicaid, ACA, and CHIP
Other2
Net interest
Total Federal Outlays, 2018: $4.1 trillion
Net Federal Medicare Outlays, 2018: $605 billion
NOTE: All amounts are for federal fiscal year 2018. 1 Consists of mandatory Medicare spending minus income from premiums and other offsetting receipts. 2 Includes spending on other mandatory outlays minus income from offsetting receipts. ACA is Affordable Care Act. CHIP is Children's Health Insurance Program.
SOURCE: KFF analysis of federal spending from Congressional Budget Office, The Budget and Economic Outlook, 2019 to 2029 (May 2019).
KFF

Source: Juliette Cubanski, Tricia Neuman and Meredith Freed. "The Facts on Medicare Spending and Financing." Kaiser Family Foundation. Issue Brief. August 20, 2019. Accessed September 26, 2019. https://www.kff.org/medicare/issue-brief/the-facts-on-medicare-spending-and-financing/

Medicare benefit payments totaled $702 billion in 2017, up from $425 billion in 2007.[113] At the current rate of increase, Medicare spending is projected to rise to 18 percent of total federal spending by 2028.[114] That is, if Medicare is still around in 2028—current projections show the Medicare Hospital Insurance (Part A) trust fund will be insolvent by 2026.[115] Medicare is funded from general revenues (41 percent), payroll taxes (37 percent), and beneficiary premiums (14 percent).[116]

The problem is healthcare costs are rising faster than revenue for the Medicare program. This is textbook negative cash flow, and *that* isn't sustainable for the long term. There are a number of reasons behind Medicare's looming fiscal crisis. Part of it is due to simple demographics: the U.S. population is aging (the "silver tsunami"). That means more Medicare beneficiaries are using the benefits—and there are fewer workers per beneficiary to make the payroll tax contributions to pay for silver surfers.[117]

As a result, the government is looking at doing some serious belt-tightening in the near future. As of this writing, President Trump's proposed 2020 budget includes billions of dollars in cuts to Medicare. Depending upon who is doing the calculating, those cuts amount to between $515 billion and $845 billion for the Medicare program over the next decade.[118]

One analysis estimates 85 percent of the savings in the proposed budget will come from reductions in provider payments, rather than cuts that directly impact beneficiaries.[119] This may be reassuring news for Medicare beneficiaries; not so much for providers. Getting paid from CMS is going to get harder, not easier, in the coming decade. Will these cuts to Medicare be realized? I believe these cuts are going to happen but a lot may hinge upon which administration takes over after the next election in 2020.

If that doesn't depress you, here's some more sad news: President Trump's proposed budget also includes reform and cuts to Medicaid. Proposed reforms include adding work requirements and repealing the Medicaid expansion facilitated by the ACA.[120]

The budget proposes changing Medicaid to a block grant program, with states awarded a capped, lump-sum fund payment, instead of the current matching system.[121] Depending on how you calculate the cost of these changes, the Medicaid cuts will equal somewhere between $777 billion and $1.5 trillion over the next 10 years.[122] Last I checked, Medicaid was not covering the cost of care in the first place, and now Uncle Sam has plans to take more money out of provider's pockets.

Unsustainable for Commercial Payers

Payers have an important role to play in the healthcare system. The job of payers, or managed care, is to ensure enough providers are there to provide care in a network, and to "manage the care." Managing the care includes basing payments on effective, evidence-based treatments and implementing cost controls to keep utilization and premiums in check.

As noted above, HDHPs have been the market's idea of a silver bullet to manage costs and utilization from patients. Payers have implemented these strategies and put deductibles into orbit at the employer's request (as employers try to manage costs). Payers have increased copays and coinsurance. They've narrowed networks. They've pulled about every lever there is to keep premiums as low as they can, but there's not much more they can do besides reducing plan benefits. The resulting imminent—and apocalyptic—scenario is payers aren't going to be able to provide an affordable insurance product in an unaffordable healthcare system.

While the ACA has been in effect, there has been a floor as to how far plans can legally reduce benefits. However, President Trump's administration recently put into effect regulations allowing for "short-term health insurance plans" that don't have to comply with ACA minimum plan benefits.[123] These plans are now available in the marketplace—however: buyer beware. Even though the plans can be cheaper than ACA-compliant plans available in the marketplace, that affordability comes at a cost. The new plans don't meet the "minimum essential coverage" specified by the ACA. The new plans offer varying levels of coverage and benefits, but they control costs by introducing unexpected restrictions. Some have benefit caps, some have very narrow networks, and some have restrictions such as excluding coverage for preexisting conditions. One short-term policy even excludes coverage "for hospital room and board and nursing services if admitted on a Friday or Saturday, unless for an emergency, or for medically necessary surgery that is scheduled for the next day."[124] Apparently you cannot be an inpatient on a weekend with this plan.

These short-term plans have the potential to cause many problems related to insufficient coverage and patient debt. Less expensive plans with fewer benefits may increase the affordability of insurance premiums, but they may also increase the problem of underinsurance.

In the meantime, if payers can't increase premiums any faster (premium increases have already outpaced wage increases in each of the last 10 years), and if they can't reduce benefits any further due to regulation, what can they do to reduce costs?[125] There is only one other lever—the cost of the care provided, in the form of claims. Payers can just not pay the claims. They can manipulate the claims to reduce the number and volume of claims they pay out. It's a simple math problem—if there isn't enough revenue, let's cut the claims cost. By implementing and enforcing thousands of pages of policy rules about everything from pre-authorizations to medical necessity, payers can lower claim costs by simply not paying them because of a rule. Who bears the brunt of these rules? Patients and providers.

Unsustainable for Providers

Commercial payers, the government and employers are shifting costs to patients; but as we saw at the beginning of this

72

chapter, patients often can't afford those increased costs. At the same time, payers are trying every trick in the book to make it harder for providers to get paid. So who is left holding the bag in this unsustainable healthcare system? You already know the answer: providers. When payers won't pay and patients can't pay, providers are stuck in the middle. Alarming trends in a number of areas—including underpayments, denials and uncompensated care—suggest today's healthcare status quo is unsustainable for providers as well.

Underpayments

It's well known providers can't sustain their operations based on the rates government payers—like Medicare and Medicaid—provide. This is due to aggregate payments for Medicare and Medicaid beneficiaries that are consistently *lower* than the cost of providing care (i.e., underpayments).[126] The commercial payers then fill that gap, by "subsidizing" the underpayments from governmental payers.

The Rand Corporation recently produced a study revealing the reimbursement from commercial payers is almost two-and-a-half times that of Medicare.[127] Here's a news flash, gang: The commercial payers aren't going to fill this underpayment gap in perpetuity. This topic was front and center at a conference I recently attended when payers put providers on notice by directly stating "get your house in order."

How bad are the underpayments? The American Hospital Association (AHA) collects and reports on the aggregate impact of underpayments each year. The AHA's findings for 2017 included the following:

- Combined underpayments were $76.8 billion in 2017. This includes a shortfall of $53.9 billion for Medicare and $22.9 billion for Medicaid.

73

- For Medicare, hospitals received payment of only 87 cents for every dollar spent by hospitals caring for Medicare patients in 2017.
- For Medicaid, hospitals received payment of only 87 cents for every dollar spent by hospitals caring for Medicaid patients in 2017.
- In 2017, 66 percent of hospitals received Medicare payments less than cost, while 62 percent of hospitals received Medicaid payments less than cost.[128]

By way of comparison, 10 years earlier, in 2007, the AHA calculated that combined underpayments totaled $32 billion.[129] That means the aggregate impact of underpayments has more than doubled in the past 10 years. Almost $77 billion went unpaid to providers, with a big "B," and no one from Medicare is picking up the phone to say, "Hello, we're sorry we didn't pay you enough— here is your missing money." Providers have to get it and defend it themselves, adding more to the administrative costs of care.

Denials

Based on my conversations with providers across the country, denials are the number one issue plaguing providers right now. As payers have implemented tighter rules to control costs, claims denials have increased.

Per an Advisory Board study, in 2017, 1 in 10 claims were denied at an average 350-bed hospital, representing an increase of more than $3 million in adjustments (a 79 percent increase) since 2011 (figure 3.11). Denial write-off adjustments average 3 percent to 4 percent of net revenue, which equates to $262 billion in initially denied claims for healthcare providers annually.[130] Lots of "Bs" going out the door because a payer rule was not clearly delivered or followed.

Figure 3.11 Denials Are Not Getting Any Better …

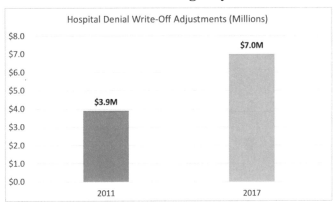

Source: Eric Fontana and Lulis Navarro. "Our 2017 revenue cycle benchmarks are out. How do you stack up?" Advisory Board. December 14, 2017. Accessed July 30, 2019. https://www.advisory.com/research/Revenue-Cycle-Advancement-Center/at-the-margins/2017/12/revenue-cycle-benchmarks

Alongside the increase in volume of denials, the appeal overturn rate is getting worse. The commercial overturn rate is down 11 percent over the past two years; the Medicaid overturn rate dropped by 10 percent in the same time period (figure 3.12). Not only is it harder to manage a denial, when you are "right" and are fighting to get your money, you are also losing more often.

Figure 3.12 Hospitals Are Also Losing on Appeal

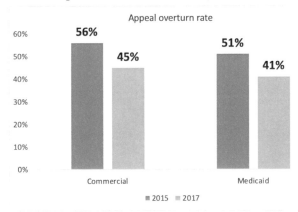

Source: "Hospital Revenue Cycles Showing Strength but Risks Include Denials." Biennial Revenue Cycle Survey. Advisory Board. https://www.prnewswire.com/news-releases/hospital-revenue-cycles-showing-strength-but-risks-include-denials-300555731.html

Uncompensated Care

Uncompensated care is calculated as the total of the financial assistance provided by a hospital plus a hospital's bad debt. According to the AHA, in 2017, uncompensated care costs totaled $38.4 billion across Americas hospitals (n = 5,262). In total since 2000, hospitals have provided more than $620 billion in uncompensated care to patients. This figure does not include other unfunded costs of care, such as underpayments from Medicare and Medicaid (figure 3.13). Interestingly, uncompensated care ticked down in 2015 with Medicaid expansion and other ACA efforts, but it is climbing back up.[131] I anticipate it may surpass the pre-ACA days and top $45 billion before 2025.

Wrong direction again, gang.

Figure 3.13 Uncompensated Care Versus Uninsured Rate

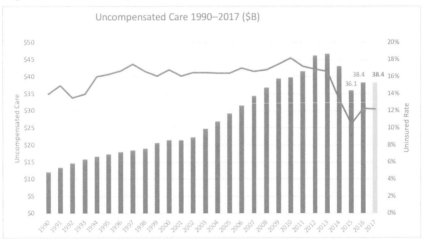

Source: "Uncompensated Hospital Care Cost Fact Sheet." American Hospital Association. January 2019. Accessed July 31, 2019. https://www.aha.org/system/files/2019-01/uncompensated-care-fact-sheet-jan-2019.pdf

Between underpayments, increasing denials and higher levels of uncompensated care, many hospitals are struggling to survive. Profit margins are squeezed to the point that (for many hospitals) long-term sustainability is in question. Profit margins at not-for-profit hospitals have been steadily slipping per a report from Fitch Ratings (figure 3.14). There's been a plummet in operating margin from 3.5 percent in 2015 to 1.9 percent in 2017, and Fitch has kept not-for-profit hospitals in a "negative" outlook.

Figure 3.14 Operating Risk

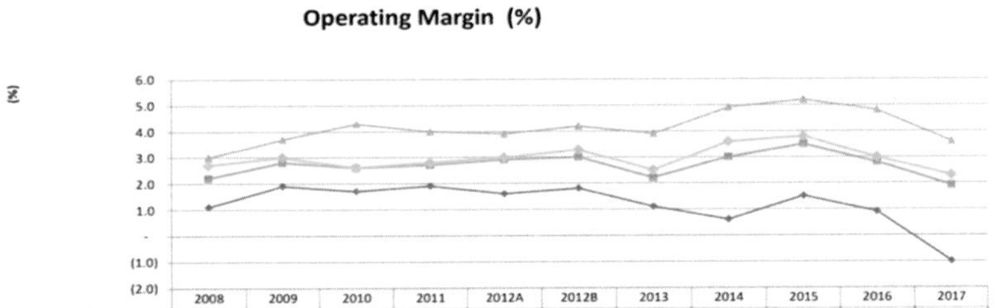

Operating Margin (%)

	2008	2009	2010	2011	2012A	2012B	2013	2014	2015	2016	2017
Overall	2.2	2.8	2.6	2.7	2.9	3.0	2.2	3.0	3.5	2.8	1.9
AA	3.0	3.7	4.3	4.0	3.9	4.2	3.9	4.9	5.2	4.8	3.6
A	2.7	3.0	2.6	2.8	3.0	3.3	2.5	3.6	3.8	3.0	2.3
BBB	1.1	1.9	1.7	1.9	1.6	1.8	1.1	0.6	1.5	0.9	(1.0)

2012A - Reflects median prior to bad debt reclass
2012B - Reflects median after bad debt reclass

Source: Kevin Holloran. "2019 Healthcare Market Outlook." [From J. Wiik resources, presented at 2019 HFMA Annual Conference]

Rural hospitals are also struggling. A February 2019 study of rural hospitals' financial risk found 21 percent of rural hospitals—430 hospitals across 43 states—are at high risk of closing unless their financial situations improve. The report noted those 430 hospitals "represent 21,547 staffed beds, 707,000 annual discharges, 150,000 employees and $21.2 billion in total patient revenue." That's a whole lot of necessary healthcare that won't be available anymore unless something is done to address affordability, cost and outcomes. The closing of hospitals is sounding the alarm: Uncompensated care needs to be holistically addressed in healthcare.

Hospital bankruptcy filings are also increasing. Law firm Polsinelli publishes a quarterly Distress Indices Report detailing Chapter 11 bankruptcy filings. The firm's most recent report (May 2019) states "the Health Care [Distress] Index … has experienced record or near-record highs in each of the last eight quarters" (figure 3.15).

Figure 3.15 Polsinelli | TrBK Health Care Services Distress Index: 1st Quarter 2019

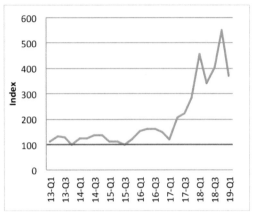

Source: Jeremy R. Johnson, Bobby Guy and Robert Dempsey. "1st Quarter 2019 Distress Indices." Polsinelli | TrBK. Accessed July 31, 2019.
https://www.distressindex.com/reports/1q2019

The report states "Health Care services [Chapter 11] filings have increased from 1.13 percent in 2010 to 8.99 percent last quarter" and notes this reflects "a significant upward trend in general filing levels since 2010." In contrast, the firm's general Chapter 11 Distress Research Index has decreased 53 percent from the benchmark period of the 4th quarter of 2010, "reflecting the significant downward trend in general filing levels since 2010."

Hospitals are declaring bankruptcy? I never thought I would see the day, but the inefficiencies in delivery and the complexities in reimbursement have finally reached an impasse. Ultimately, what does all this mean? Patients are going broke; providers are going bankrupt. The spending is unsustainable. Maybe insurance can help bridge this spending gap with some other plan and coverage innovations. "No way" you say? Let's find out in chapter 4.

SECTION TWO

WHY IS THIS SO HARD?

CHAPTER 4

INSURANCE—WHY DO WE NEED IT?

Health insurance wasn't always a part of the healthcare system, although it may seem that way now. From the time this country was founded, up until the early 1900s, the patient was the only payer and there wasn't a third party to step in and help pay for healthcare services.[132] As I explained in my first book, health insurance didn't come on the scene until the late 1920s. And the government didn't get involved in the health insurance business until Medicare and Medicaid were established in 1965.

Today everyone blames healthcare insurers—especially commercial insurers—for healthcare's unaffordability problem. But would today's healthcare system work if healthcare insurance didn't exist? Let's find out together, shall we?

Commercial Insurers

Insurance boils down to a math problem (a.k.a. actuarial science). This is true whether you're talking about auto insurance, homeowner's insurance or health insurance. It's all about managing risk. How much financial risk are you willing to take on with respect to potentially negative or catastrophic events? How much financial risk can you afford to take on?

Theoretically, Americans are no longer required to buy health insurance. The ACA, which became law in 2010, required most Americans to carry a basic level of health insurance coverage. This requirement was known as the "individual mandate" and was enforced with a tax penalty for those who could not document the required health insurance coverage. However, the Tax Cuts and Jobs Act of 2017 eliminated the individual mandate penalty.[133] So, now, Americans can skip purchasing health insurance. Per the National Center for Health Statistics, 30.4 million people, of all ages, were uninsured in 2018.[134]

Why Are People Going Without Insurance?

It's true—for many reasons—some Americans still don't have health insurance coverage. As I noted in chapter 3, depending on who's doing the measuring, the uninsured rate in the U.S. is currently around 14 percent.[135] Reasons for lack of health insurance vary, but studies suggest almost half (45 percent) of the uninsured population state they can't afford the cost of health insurance.[136]

But the question becomes, in today's U.S. healthcare market, can anyone really afford *not* to have health insurance? The short answer is: You need insurance if you want access to healthcare. Studies show lack of health insurance impacts access to care and leads to negative health outcomes:

> People without insurance coverage have worse access to care than people who are insured. One in five uninsured adults in 2017 went without needed medical care due to cost. Studies repeatedly demonstrate that the uninsured are less likely than those with insurance to receive preventive care and services for major health conditions and chronic diseases.[137]

Health Insurance Increases Healthcare Access by Pooling Risk

Health insurance increases access to healthcare services by pooling risk across populations—whether that's a population of employees in an organization (employer-provided health insurance coverage) or individuals buying coverage on the health insurance exchange. The actuarial science underlying health insurance premium calculations has become increasingly sophisticated. As healthcare has gone digital, an exponentially increasing volume of data (big data) is at the disposal of actuaries and medical underwriters in the health insurance industry. In addition, the advent of new technology tools (a.k.a. "insurtech") holds the promise of increasing savings and efficiency in the insurance industry by providing more precise risk analysis.[138]

When I worked in the insurance industry (just a few years ago), the science of calculating risk across populations was already extremely precise. We could effectively calculate to the *penny* any impact on premium cost if including or excluding any coverage benefit.

I once visited the actuarial floor and said, "Hey, a major employer in California is looking at the impact of smoking and gender on per-member-per-month premiums (PMPM). What impact will that have?" They responded, "Well, it depends. Do you want it by age, too? Or how about employment status?" I was amazed. It took them a week or so to get back to me, but they had those numbers sliced and diced down to the PMPM penny. These calculations can be done with even more precision today.

Health insurance spreads the risk out and makes it affordable by using data to calculate the likelihood of care utilization and claims occurring. For example, according to Centers for Disease Control and Prevention (CDC) data, 7.6 percent of the population experienced an overnight hospital stay in 2017.[139] Hospitalization is included in the essential benefits defined by the Affordable Care Act (ACA)—even though, theoretically, less than 10 percent of the population will use those benefits.

Spreading the risk—and cost—of hospitalization across the insured population makes it possible for individuals to access inpatient care when hospitalization is required.

Insurance also acts as a cost containment mechanism. Imagine if health insurance didn't exist, and each person had to negotiate their own rates with their doctor or the hospital. For example, if you come to the hospital with symptoms of appendicitis, you're not likely going to want to take time to negotiate rates before you get the care you need. FYI, the average price of a laparoscopic appendectomy in large employer plans in 2016 was $20,192, with the range between $7,528 at the lower end and $35,308 at the high end.[140] It's a little challenging for average patients to come up with that sum on their own.

How Sharing the Risk Translates at the Employer Level

As I noted in chapter 3, nearly half of Americans currently get their health insurance through their employer.[141] The concept behind insurance—shared risk—explains why all employer plans are not created equal, even if they all meet the Minimum Essential Coverage Standards specified by the ACA. A single employer with a large, young population of employees is going to have a lower risk—and therefore, a lower claims cost—than an employer with a small or older population of employees. For example, think of information technology companies. Florida-based Ultimate Software, ranked number eight on *Fortune's* 100 Best Companies to Work For, still pays 100 percent of health coverage for employees and also offers health insurance coverage for part-timers.[142]

Presumably, large companies with young employees working desk jobs have a lower claims risk than small companies and/or companies with an older demographic in construction. As a consequence, the larger company can afford to be more generous with respect to both plan benefits and the employee's share of premium costs. On the other hand, a small mom-and-pop shop, where the only employees are Mom (age 68) and Pop (age 72) is going to have a much higher claims risk. Reason being, the older you are the more likely you are to deal with health problems; and second, Mom and Pop's shared risk pool is two, instead of the hundreds or thousands found in a larger company.

That's why there's so much variance in the employee's share of premium cost and plan benefits, even among all employer-based insurance plans. Besides the size of the pool, and the age of the participants, other factors that can impact claims risk include the riskiness of the industry (construction workers may submit more healthcare claims than those with desk jobs); lifestyle factors (e.g., number of smokers in the population); geographic factors (residents of some geographic regions are more likely to be in good health than residents of other areas); etc.

Profitability

Most commercial insurance companies are doing pretty well. They don't take losses. After all, they're in the business of calculating and managing risk so they know perfectly well what the numbers are.

The 2019 Fortune 500 company list shows UnitedHealth Group saw a 12.5 percent increase in revenue between the current year and the previous year, and a 13.5 percent increase in profits. Cigna saw a 16.9 percent increase in revenue, and a 17.9 percent increase in profits. And Anthem saw a 2.3 percent increase in revenue and a decline in profits of 2.4 percent.[143]

As of Q2 2019, UnitedHealth Group reported 8 percent year-over-year revenue growth.[144] An analysis of 2019 Q2 revenue by *HealthLeaders* showed the following figures:

- UnitedHealth Group "achieved total quarterly revenues once again north of $60 billion"
- Cigna achieved "nearly $39 billion in total revenues and shareholders' net income of $1.4 billion, an increase of $600 million year-over-year"
- Centene Corp "posted revenues of $18.4 billion, a 29 percent year-over-year increase" [145]

You might be saying, "But wait, they had to pay claims, right? That's just the top line." Correct, grasshopper. But don't go get the party balloons yet. If you take the UnitedHealth Group example above, their net income (after costs) *doubled* in one quarter in 2016 to $3.6 billion, and surpassed $10 billion (10.6 billion to be precise, with a "B") in 2017, which was up 50.5 percent over the prior year.[146]

The individual insurance exchanges have not had the same yellow brick road. Profitability in the individual insurance market was initially impacted by implementation of the ACA. Immediately after the ACA was implemented in 2014, insurer financial performance as defined by medical loss ratios (MLR) declined. (Note: In health insurance, MLR refers to the proportion of premium revenues spent on clinical services and quality improvement, as opposed to other costs, such as administrative overhead and marketing. The ACA requires health insurance companies to issue rebates to consumers if their MLR percentage does not meet minimum standards.) However, according to the Kaiser Family Foundation,

"loss ratios began to decline in 2016, suggesting improved financial performance."[147]

The fact is, we all need health insurance. And without pushback from insurers to providers, prices might be even higher than they are. But should commercial insurers be as profitable as they are? The bottom line is we live in the United States—a capitalistic society. In the context of capitalism, you don't necessarily want to restrict profitability or attack a company that's doing well. It makes no more sense to attack an insurer's profits than it does to attack Microsoft or Walmart for doing well. We pay insurance premiums to keep healthcare costs in check. Insurance is a necessary buffer against skyrocketing healthcare costs. No matter who is paying those premiums—ourselves, the government or our employers—healthcare wouldn't be accessible without the bridge insurance provides.

Government Insurers

Before the 1960s, the government had almost no role in providing healthcare. The government got into the health insurance business after the Social Security Administration conducted a "Survey of the Aged" and found families headed by persons aged 65 or older made up one-third of all families in poverty.[148] Furthermore, the survey found only half of the elderly had health insurance coverage.[149]

Medicare was created to address that exact gap. Today Medicare covers more than 40 million Americans.[150] The latest statistics show more than 10,000 people enroll in Medicare *each day*.[151] As of 2017, Medicare accounted for nearly 15 percent of total federal spending (see figure 3.4) and 20 percent of total national health spending.[152] Medicare's role providing healthcare access for the elderly is becoming more critical as the population ages. Nearly 50 years ago, in 1970, the median age of the U.S. population was 28.1; by 2018 the median age had risen to 38.2.[153]

That may not seem like much of a shift, but by 2030, the U.S. Census Bureau projects one of every five U.S. residents will be of retirement age. Those people are going to need health insurance. And for many of them, their employers (or past employers) are no longer going to be the source of that insurance. As the Kaiser Family Foundation has noted:

> Employer-sponsored insurance provided retiree health coverage to 3 in 10 (30 percent) of traditional Medicare beneficiaries in 2016. Over time, however, fewer beneficiaries are expected to have this type of coverage, since the share of large firms offering retiree health benefits to their employees has dropped from 66 percent in 1988 to 18 percent in 2018.[154]

So the need for coverage for the elderly is increasing, even as the government tries to find ways to reduce costs to keep the Medicare program sustainable. Similarly, Medicaid was created to ensure those in poverty have access to healthcare through government-provided health insurance. The ACA Medicaid expansion provisions significantly increased the number of Medicaid beneficiaries in the U.S.

As of April 2019, 72.4 million individuals were enrolled in either Medicaid or the Children's Health Insurance Program (CHIP).[155] In all, total Medicaid enrollment has increased 26.1 percent over the 2013 (pre-ACA) baseline.[156] Again, as we saw in the last chapter, even as enrollment in Medicaid grows, the government is searching for ways to reduce the cost of the program.

Government plays an important role in providing access to healthcare for vulnerable populations (the elderly, the poor). Granted, the government pays less than cost to providers; however, without the government's assistance, the elderly and poor would fall entirely into the self-pay or charity care buckets for providers.

As mentioned in the last chapter, the payer mix is diluting—there are more government insurance enrollees and less commercial insurance, and thus, the private payers subsidize the Medicare payments. Figure 4.1, below, shows the payer mix at a typical hospital and how much the commercial insurers must make up to bridge the gap, while uncompensated care is offset by Medicare and Medicaid.

Figure 4.1 2019 Payer Mix at U.S. Hospitals

Hospitals are paid 34 percent more than Medicare rates, on average
Synthesis of rates by payer relative to Medicare rates

Payer	Payer share of hospital costs	Payment relative to Medicare
Medicare	40.8%	100%
Medicaid	18.5%	78%, 106%
Private payers	33.4%	189%, 241%
Uncompensated care	4.2%	0%
Average		**134%**

Note: The average among payers is weighted according to the American Health Association's reported share of patient costs by payer. CAP used the midpoints between the estimates for private insurance and for Medicaid payment ratios. Data points in the table come from multiple sources and do not all cover the same time period.
Sources: CAP analysis of American Hospital Association, "Trendwatch Chartbook 2018: Table 4.4: Aggregate Hospital Payment-to-cost Ratios for Private Payers, Medicare, and Medicaid, 1995 – 2016" (Chicago: 2018), available at https://www.aha.org/system/files/2018-05/2018-chartbook-table-4-4.pdf; Peter Cunningham and others, "Understanding Medicaid Hospital Payments and the Impact of Recent Policy Changes" (San Francisco: Henry J. Kaiser Family Foundation, 2016), available at https://www.kff.org/report-section/understanding-medicaid-hospital-payments-and-the-impact-of-recent-policy-changes-issue-brief/; Jared Lane Maeda and Lyle Nelson, "An Analysis of Hospital Prices for Commercial and Medicare Advantage Plans: 2017 Annual Research Meeting AcademyHealth" (Washington: U.S. Congressional Budget Office, 2017), available at https://www.cbo.gov/system/files/115th-congress-2017-2018/presentation/52819-presentation.pdf; Chapin White and Christopher Whaley, "Prices Paid to Hospitals by Private Health Plans Are High Relative to Medicare and Vary Widely" (Santa Monica, CA: RAND Corp., 2019), available at https://www.rand.org/pubs/research_reports/RR3033.html.

CAP

Source: Emily Gee. "The High Price of Hospital Care." Center for American Progress. June 26, 2019. Accessed September 1, 2019. https://www.americanprogress.org/issues/healthcare/reports/2019/06/26/471464/high-price-hospital-care/

Insurance Reform

As patients, providers, payers and employers have wrestled with the healthcare unaffordability problem, various legislation has been proposed and implemented to reform healthcare and contain escalating healthcare costs. Two aspects of insurance reform with the greatest impact on providers right now are the ACA and the establishment of exchanges with cost-sharing reductions.

The Affordable Care Act Debacle

While the ACA didn't solve America's healthcare unaffordability problem, it did put in place a few things that were net positive for providers. It decreased the overall uninsured rate, in part by increasing Medicaid enrollment. But even though Medicaid doesn't pay for the cost of care, Medicaid enrollees offer providers some form of reimbursement, rather than none.

In 2016, when Republicans took control of the presidency, the Senate and the House, repealing and replacing the ACA (a.k.a. Obamacare) was a priority. After several failed attempts (OK, five, but who's counting?), they were unable to accomplish repeal and replace. But they have been successful at chipping away at the ACA and destabilizing it.

PwC summarized the Trump administrations changes to the ACA as follows:

> The administration's efforts to chip away at the
> ACA can be seen around the law's edges through
> softening individual and employer mandates,
> expanding access to health insurance plans that
> don't conform to ACA rules, reducing operational
> and financial support for individual exchanges,
> dialing back on Medicaid spending and expanding
> the use of health savings accounts.[157]

Consumers are feeling the effects of this chipping away. An analysis by the Kaiser Family Foundation estimated 2019 health insurance premiums were 16 percent higher due to legislative change designed to undermine the ACA, as illustrated in the following chart (figure 4.2).

Figure 4.2 Premium Impacts From Legislative and Policy Changes to the ACA

Premium Impacts From Legislative and Policy Changes to the ACA

+16%

+10%

+6%

Current

Current

Current

Individual mandate penalty repeal
Expansion of AHP / STLD plans

Loss of CSR payments*

Combined Impact*

* Silver Exchange Plan Premiums

SOURCE: Kaiser Family Foundation analysis of insurer rate filings to state regulators, state insurance regulators, and ratereview.healthcare.gov. Premium impact due to CSR loss is from Congressional Budget Office (CBO) estimate.

NOTES: Premium changes represent the change in premiums before accounting for the premium tax credit. How each premium impact relates to other impacts depends on how each insurer calculates rate impacts. We conservatively assume the rates are additive (6% + 10% = 16%), as opposed to multiplicative (1.06 x 1.1 = 1.166, or 16.6%). *The CBO estimate of the loss of CSR payments' effect was specifically for silver exchange premiums. However, some insurers also applied a CSR load onto other metal levels and/or off-exchange premiums.

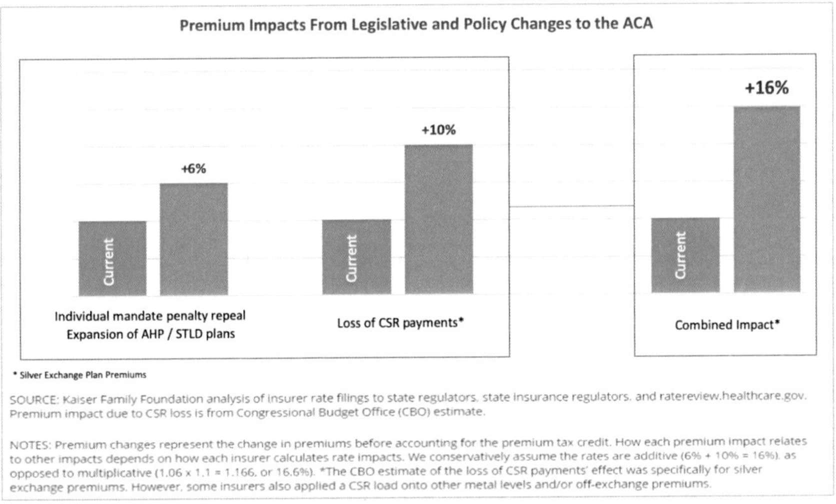

Source: Rabah Kamal, Cynthia Cox, Rachel Fehr, Marco Ramirez, Katherine Horstman and Larry Levitt. "How Repeal of the Individual Mandate and Expansion of Loosely Regulated Plans are Affecting 2019 Premiums." Kaiser Family Foundation. October 26, 2018. Accessed August 12, 2019. https://www.kff.org/cdd3526/

Providers are feeling the effects as well. Fitch Ratings recently stated,

> "Taken together in aggregate, these efforts to defund the ACA reduce healthcare coverage and pressure not-for-profit hospitals, which provide care to a large proportion of uninsured and Medicaid patients. Of a hospital's revenue sources, self-pay and Medicaid pose the highest risk to revenue sufficiency to recover costs. The less people that are covered, even by Medicaid, the higher a hospital's exposure to self-pay patients, and the greater stress on its operating margin."[158]

Public sentiment toward the ACA remains somewhat divided, with the most recent numbers suggesting 52 percent hold a favorable view of the ACA compared to 41 percent holding an unfavorable view (figure 4.3).

Figure 4.3 The Public Is Divided on the Affordable Care Act

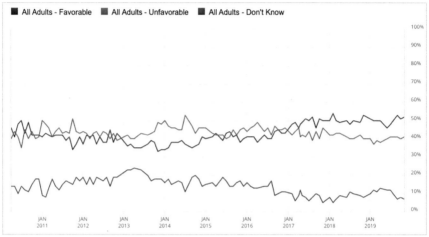

Note: The margin of sampling error including the design effect for the full tracking poll sample is typically plus or minus 3 percentage points. For results based on subgroups, the margin of sampling error may be higher.

Source: "KFF Health Tracking Poll: The Public's Views on the ACA." Kaiser Family Foundation. November 20, 2019. Accessed December 12, 2019. https://www.kff.org/interactive/kff-health-tracking-poll-the-publics-views-on-the-aca/#?response=Favorable--Unfavorable--Don't%2520Know&aRange=all

Although views are mixed on the ACA overall, there are certain provisions of the ACA Americans feel very strongly about. Interestingly, the least popular provision was the individual mandate, which is no longer in effect. Hello?! Remember the point about spreading out risk? The individual mandate is what ensured both healthy and sick people would be purchasing health insurance, thereby spreading out the risk and keeping premiums lower across the board.

Exchanges and Cost-Sharing Reduction

Private health insurance exchanges—where individual consumers or employers could shop for health insurance—existed before the ACA was implemented. What the ACA did was to require every state to set up a public health insurance exchange, where consumers could buy individual or family plans compliant with ACA requirements. Since implementation of the ACA, each state has a marketplace, although the types of marketplaces vary (figure 4.4).

Figure 4.4 State Health Insurance Marketplace Types, 2020

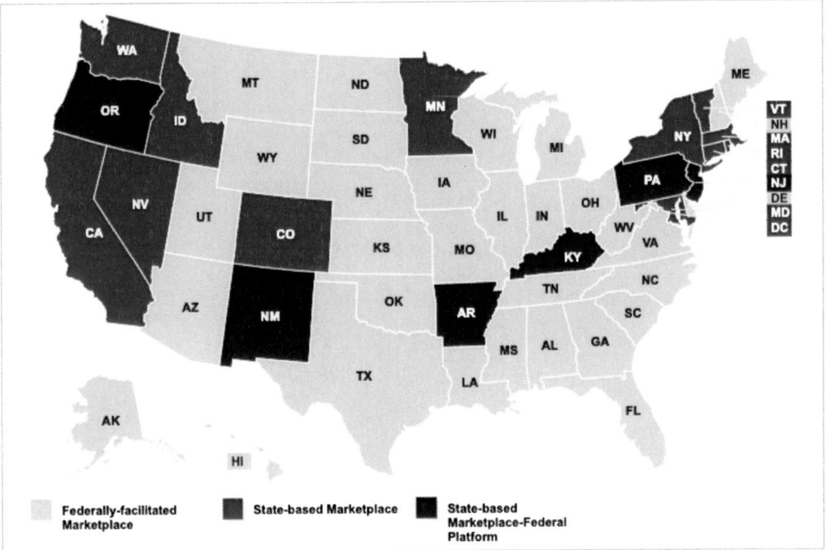

Source: "State Health Insurance Marketplace Types, 2020." Kaiser Family Foundation. KFF State Health Facts. (n.d.) https://www.kff.org/ed168d3/

Regardless of what type of marketplace the state provides, the role of the marketplace (a.k.a. exchange) is the same: it provides consumers with the opportunity to shop for ACA-qualified health insurance plans. The exchanges are also the *only* place consumers have access to the premium subsidies and cost-sharing subsidies established by the ACA. Both of these subsidies work to reduce premiums and out-of-pocket costs for eligible enrollees.

The premium subsidy is an income-scaled subsidy that can either be applied to reduce monthly premiums or be taken in a lump sum as a tax credit at the end of the year. Eligibility for the premium subsidy is based upon household income; household income must be less than 400 percent of the Federal Poverty Level (FPL) in order to qualify.[159]

The cost-sharing subsidy, a.k.a. the cost sharing reduction (CSR), is a discount designed to lower a consumers' share of deductibles, copayments and coinsurance.[160] Eligibility for the cost-sharing subsidy is based on household income; in addition, to qualify, enrollees *also* have to enroll in a "silver" level plan. A silver health plan generally falls in the middle on the exchanges— lower premiums and out-of-pocket (OOP) costs than a platinum or gold plan, but higher premiums and OOP costs than a bronze plan.[161] The deductible is also significantly larger—in the couple-of-thousand-dollar range to start (figure 4.5).

Figure 4.5 Deductible Size Varies by Plan Type

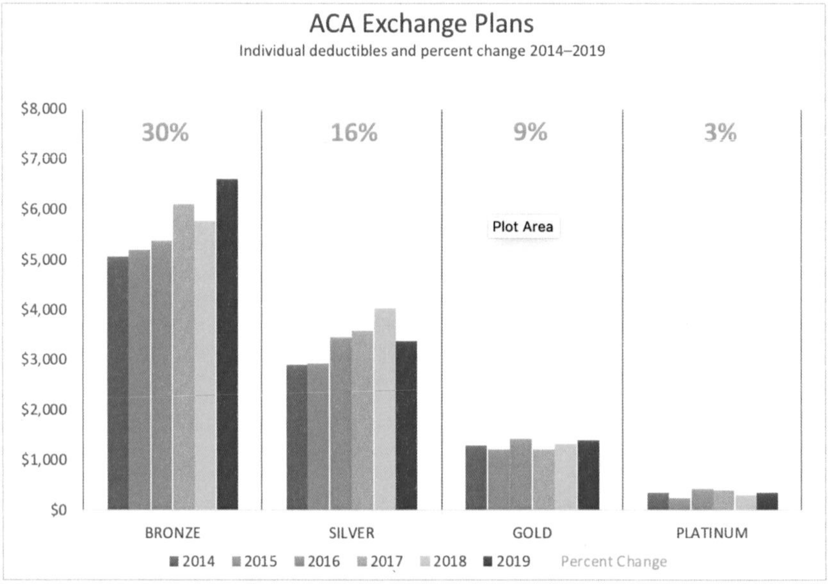

Source: Averages aggregated from multiple sources. HealthPocket (2017, 2018); Kaiser Family Foundation (2019).[162]

As originally established by the ACA, CSR subsidies were paid to insurance companies to reduce OOP costs for consumers and keep premium costs low on the exchanges. The Trump administration stopped reimbursing insurers for these subsidies in 2017.[163] A recent article offers perspective:

> Despite the fact that the Trump administration has cut off funding for CSR, nothing has changed about eligibility for CSR or premium subsidies. Both continue to be available to all eligible exchange enrollees. The funding cut was announced on October 12, 2017, but insurers in the majority of the states had already based their 2018 premiums on the assumption that funding was going to be cut. And insurers in some other states were given a short window during which they could refile rates with the cost of CSR added to the premiums. This helped to prevent insurers from exiting the market, since they could offset the lack of federal CSR funding with higher premiums, most of which are covered by larger premium subsidies.[164]

As noted, CSR benefits are still available to exchange enrollees despite the fact insurers are no longer being reimbursed. This has impacted premiums, although the impact has varied by state, according to how each state handled the elimination of federal funding for CSRs.[165]

The long-term impact of eliminating CSR subsidies is a raise in premiums for plans available on health insurance exchanges. The Kaiser Family Foundation reported, "... in response to policy decisions by the Trump administration to eliminate payments to insurers for required cost-sharing subsidies and reduce funding for outreach and enrollment assistance in the marketplaces, along with uncertainty over the future of the individual mandate, insurers responded by increasing average benchmark premiums by 33 percent for 2018."[166]

More changes to CSR may be in our future, as the Trump administration continues to make changes to the ACA.

Election Pressures on Healthcare Reform

A 2019 survey of American voters found the number one area of concern is healthcare (figure 4.6). That—combined with election year pressures—pretty much guarantees healthcare reform is going to be at the top of the political agenda.

Figure 4.6 What Is the Top Issue Facing America Today?

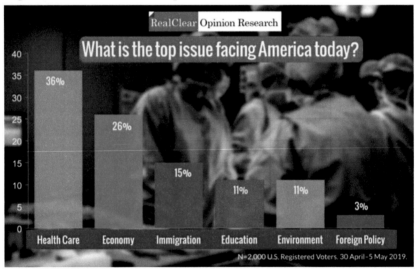

Source: Carl M. Cannon. "'Medicare for All' Support is High … But Complicated." RealClear Opinion Research. May 15, 2019. Accessed August 10, 2019. https://www.realclearpolitics.com/real_clear_opinion_research/new_poll_shows_health_care_i s_voters_top_concern.html

Many different types of reform are being proposed and discussed, but a few of the more significant ones are single-payer, "Medicare for All" and compulsory health insurance.

Single-Payer

A single-payer healthcare system is one in which there is one payer for all citizens. In this scenario, private insurers would disappear. A single payer—most likely the government—would provide health insurance for everyone. "Single payer" refers to a means of financing healthcare, not a means of delivering it. Medicare itself is an example of a single-payer system.

In a recent Wharton podcast, the question was asked, "Could a national health insurance program work for the United States?"

> The answer to that question "depends on what you mean by work," said Mark Pauly, Wharton professor of healthcare management and professor of business economics and public policy. "If we woke up tomorrow morning and we had single-payer Medicare for all, people wouldn't be dying in the streets; healthcare would get provided and paid for," he said. "The question is whether it will work better than either what we currently have, which is not a very high bar, or whether it will work better than some other alternatives."[167]

Medicare for All

Medicare is already the largest payer in the world. It covers the most people, has the highest spend and the most dollars, and the most claims go through it. There's something to be said for expanding it, since it already occupies the most real estate. But most hospitals could not sustain their operations on a Medicare-only fee schedule, simply because Medicare payments don't cover the cost of care—something to ponder as we evaluate single-payer as well. For it to work, there will have to be significant tightening of the belt—most hospitals cannot sustain an operational model on straight government (Medicare) payment.

There are many examples of this, including many high technology services that may be used for the treatment of the patient and result in good outcomes, but they aren't covered as part of Medicare's benefit package. Many of the exclusions are technology related. Technology has outpaced funding with Medicare, and Medicare won't ever catch up because we are so innovative in this country. The tax base can't fund technology at the rate we would like it to, and we have a major chronic disease problem (as detailed in my first book). Medicare doesn't fund provider costs of care, so there's a huge underpayment issue involved in Medicare for All.

Yet, Medicare for All is a huge rallying cry right now, especially among Democrats. Various versions of Medicare for All have been introduced in Congress as far back as the early 2000s. Various versions of H.R. 676, the Expanded & Improved Medicare for All Act, were introduced in 2003–2004, 2005–2006, 2007–2008, 2009–2010, 2011–2012, 2013–2014, 2015–2016 and January of 2017.[168] The 116th Congress (2019–2020) saw a new spate of Medicare for All legislation being introduced, including H.R. 1384 Medicare for All Act of 2019, introduced in February of 2019 (117 cosponsors); Senate Bill 1129 Medicare for All Act of 2019, introduced by Senator Bernie Sanders in April of 2019 (14 cosponsors); and H.R. 2452 Medicare for America Act of 2019 introduced in May 2019 (23 cosponsors), among others.[169]

Medicare for All means different things to different people. Essentially, there are many variations on the theme of expanding the role of public programs in healthcare being considered in Congress which reflect these varying points of view.

As of May 2019, the Kaiser Family Foundation summarized the various plans being considered under five general categories, as follows:

- Medicare for All, a single national health insurance program for all U.S. residents:
  - o Medicare for All Act of 2019 by Rep. Jayapal, H.R. 1384
  - o Medicare for All Act of 2019 by Sen. Sanders, S. 1129
- A new national health insurance program for all U.S. residents with an opt out for qualified coverage:
  - o Medicare for America Act of 2019 by Rep. DeLauro and Rep. Schakowsky, H.R. 2452
- A new public plan option that would be offered to individuals through the ACA marketplace:
  - o Keeping Health Insurance Affordable Act of 2019 by Sen. Cardin, S. 3
  - o Choose Medicare Act by Sen. Merkley, S. 1261 and Rep. Richmond, H.R. 2463
  - o Medicare-X Choice Act of 2019 by Sen. Bennet and Sen. Kaine, S. 981 and Rep. Delgado, H.R. 2000
  - o The CHOICE Act by Rep. Schakowsky, H.R. 2085 and Sen. Whitehouse, S. 1033
- A Medicare buy-in option for older individuals not yet eligible for the current Medicare program:
  - o Medicare at 50 Act by Sen. Stabenow, S. 470
  - o Medicare Buy-In and Health Care Stabilization Act of 2019 by Rep. Higgins, H.R. 1346
- A Medicaid buy-in option that states can elect to offer to individuals through the ACA marketplace:
  - o State Public Option Act by Sen. Schatz, S. 489 and Rep. Luján, H.R. 1277.[170]

Got all that straight? I can't believe there are so many versions. These are very complex pieces of legislation, consisting of hundreds of pages each. The American public generally won't research all the necessary information—but will likely rely on the media to interpret—and base their vote on the short-form description and the candidates' platforms. What I'm saying is—we need to do our homework. Will this new plan expand coverage, improve outcomes *and* lower costs? If not, who's paying and who's impacted? *Vox* analyzed nine Democratic healthcare proposals and compared how the different proposals would impact coverage, private insurance, premiums, taxes and government regulation of healthcare prices (figure 4.7).

Figure 4.7 Comparison of Democratic Healthcare Plans

	Do ALL AMERICANS gain coverage?	Do Americans still get INSURANCE AT WORK?	Do public plan enrollees pay PREMIUMS?	Does it require a TAX INCREASE?	Does the GOVERNMENT REGULATE health care prices?
Jayapal (D-WA) and the House Progressive Caucus's **Medicare-for-all bill**	✓	✗	✗	✓	✓
Sanders's **Medicare-for-all bill**	✓	✗	✗	✓	✓
DeLauro (D-CT) and Schakowsky's (D-IL) **Medicare for America bill**	✓	✓	✓	✓	✓
Merkley (D-OR) and Murphy's (D-CT) **Medicare buy-in bill**	✗	✓	✓	✗	✓
Schakowsky (D-IL) and Whitehouse's (D-RI) **Medicare buy-in bill**	✗	✓	✓	✗	✓
Bennet (D-CO), Higgins's (D-NY) and Kaine (D-VA) **Medicare buy-in bill**	✗	✓	✓	✗	✓
Schatz (D-HI) and Lujan's (D-NM) **Medicaid buy-in bill**	✗	✓	✓	✗	✓
Stabenow (D-MI) **Medicare-at-50 bill**	✗	✓	✓	✗	✓
The Urban Institute's **Healthy America proposal**	✗	✓	✓	✓	✓

Source: Vox analysis

Vox

Source: Sarah Kliff and Dylan Scott. "We read 9 Democratic plans for expanding health care. Here's how they work." June 21, 2019. Accessed August 14, 2019. https://www.vox.com/2018/12/13/18103087/medicare-for-all-explained-single-payer-health-care-sanders-jayapal

The catch is paying for it. Many people who say they support Medicare for All aren't looking at the price tag. *Vox* notes, "Most Democrats have focused their energy on figuring out what exactly an expanded Medicare program looks like. Legislators have given significantly less attention to how to pay for these expansions."[171] Four of the proposals *Vox* analyzed, including Senator Sanders Medicare for All bill, would require tax increases to implement. Is that palatable to our country's tax base?

The Committee for a Responsible Federal Budget analyzed the cost of a number of variations of Medicare for All plans, and came up with estimates ranging from $13.8 trillion to $36-plus trillion over 10 years (figure 4.8). Those are big dollars with very large "T"s, people. How big is the "T" in taxes to pay for it? To put this in perspective, we spent about $3.7 trillion per year on healthcare in 2018, 4.4 percent more than 2017, outpacing the 1.6 percent inflation rate.[172]

These Medicare for All plans outline a spend of $36 trillion over 10 years, or $3.6 trillion per year. That's on pace with what we spent for everything, but pay attention, grasshopper … the cost is shared differently. Employers, patients and Uncle Sam split the costs, depending on the plans. In the Medicare for All model, Uncle Sam funds it all through our taxes (most of the plans have tax implications). The math gets a little fuzzy when insured folks stop paying premiums through their employer and start paying Uncle Sam—I might need an accountant. But let me ask you this: When have we seen the government keep to a budget or a plan? Remember the unsustainable spending described in chapter 3?! Are we saving costs and making better outcomes, or are we trying to cover everything, for everyone, and we'll just figure out how to pay for it later? This has been one of the large shortfalls of the ACA, and these plans—thus far—have very scary spending projections, on which no right-minded Chief Financial Officer (CFO) would sign off.

Figure 4.8 Potential Cost of Medicare for All

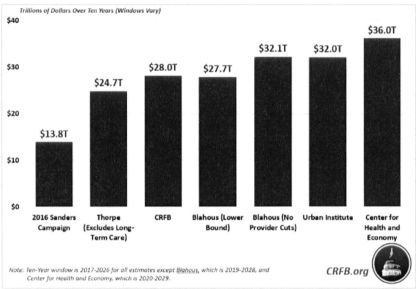

Source: "How Much Will Medicare for All Cost?" Committee for a Responsible Federal Budget. February 27, 2019. Accessed August 15, 2019. https://www.crfb.org/blogs/how-much-will-medicare-all-cost

The bottom line is although Medicare for All and other single-payer plans may increase access, they aren't healthcare cost-control mechanisms. The money to cover escalating healthcare costs has to come from somewhere, and I don't think people have the appetite for the tax increases that would go along with a Medicare for All plan. In the end, the political viability of those costs is what is going to matter.

According to *Vox* journalist Dylan Scott, it's not the specific numbers, but the context that matters:

It doesn't matter whether one think tank's score of a particular single-payer bill that will never become law shows $50 trillion in new spending or $5 trillion in savings. The pertinent questions for Medicare for All are whether the tax increases necessary to fund a single-payer program are politically tenable and how much providers would be paid under this new system.[173]

In my humble opinion, if the Democrats only offer a Medicare for All or single-payer option, they're going to lose. If the Republicans focus on the ACA "repeal and replace," they're going to lose. That's my prediction. The topic of healthcare is currently monopolizing the U.S. election process. But the problems we need to solve are about our country's healthcare for the long term—into 2050 and beyond—not just for the next election cycle. Any new healthcare legislation needs to reflect that long-term perspective, rather than focusing on what is going to win an election. Our country must address cost and make some hard decisions on coverage if we are ever going to get to affordable coverage. Right now, one can't have affordable coverage for an unaffordable product. And, I know what you're thinking—it's easy for the dude writing this book to outline what's broken with no solutions ... well, let's look at the fine state of Massachusetts and see if I gain any credibility, shall we?

Compulsory Insurance

The ACA's national individual mandate is gone, but some states have been, or are experimenting with, state-level compulsory health insurance. Since the bigger the risk pool the lower the premium cost, the assumption is that if you have a statewide risk pool (a) premiums will be affordable and (b) premium revenue will be adequate to cover claims.

The state of Massachusetts passed a compulsory health insurance law more than a decade ago. The law went into effect July 1, 2007, and requires that "most residents over 18 who can afford health insurance have coverage for the entire year, or pay a penalty through their tax returns."[174] The law defines "Minimum Creditable Coverage (MCC)" that residents must have to be considered insured and avoid tax penalties. Among other requirements, the plan must be comprehensive, cover preventative doctor visits without a deductible and cap annual deductibles at $2,000 for an individual and $4,000 for a family.[175] Residents whose incomes are below 150 percent of the FPL are exempt from the requirement.[176]

Well done, Massachusetts. I find it interesting almost every state (except for Virginia and New Hampshire) requires car insurance coverage, but so few states require health insurance.[177] You can't drive a car unless you have auto insurance, but you can live your whole life without health insurance. That seems out of alignment.

How has the compulsory insurance law affected health coverage in Massachusetts? Kaiser Family Foundation data from 2017 shows Massachusetts has the lowest uninsured rate (3 percent) among all 50 states.[178] I am intrigued by this—a low single-digit uninsured rate is basically unheard of anywhere else— but it has worked here. But how is the plan doing? Well, a 2018 *U.S. News & World Report* ranking of healthcare access by state ranked Massachusetts in the number two spot, behind Connecticut.[179] A 2019 *WalletHub* analysis ranked Massachusetts number one in healthcare outcomes, number two for lowest average monthly insurance premium and number one for lowest infant mortality rate.[180] I'm starting to like this.

Spending trend data also seems to indicate that what Massachusetts is doing is working. I'm starting to *really* like this. A 2018 cost trends report by the state notes:

- The Massachusetts growth rate of 1.6 percent in 2017 was below the national growth rate of 3.1 percent, continuing a consecutive eight-year trend of spending growth below the U.S. rate.

- Growth in commercial healthcare spending was also below the national rate for the fifth consecutive year. Cumulatively between 2012 and 2017, this lower growth rate amounts to commercial spending that was $5.5 billion lower over this time period than would have been the case if growth rates matched the national average.[181]

Would this plan work in other states? Massachusetts has some unique characteristics that may be helping this plan work. According to U.S. Census data, Massachusetts' population represents about 2 percent of the total U.S. population. Could the same plan work if rolled out to the other 98 percent of the U.S. population? Massachusetts has a highly educated population (42 percent with a bachelor's degree or higher versus the U.S. average of 31 percent) and a wealthier population (Massachusetts had a median household income of $74,167 in 2017 versus the U.S. median household income of $57,651).[182] Other factors making a difference for Massachusetts are the urbanization of the population and the number of teaching hospitals in the state. Numerous studies have documented poorer health outcomes for rural populations.[183] As of the last decennial census, 92 percent of Massachusetts' population lived in urban areas.[184] Compare that to the state of Tennessee, which has a population (6.8 million) similar to Massachusetts (6.9 million).[185] But in Tennessee, only 66 percent of the population lives in an urban area.[186]

Massachusetts also has a large number of teaching hospitals. This matters because teaching hospitals typically provide more free care to the poor and uninsured than other hospitals do.[187] At last count, Massachusetts boasted 37 teaching hospitals, while Tennessee, its closest peer with respect to population, has only 16 teaching hospitals.[188] These unique characteristics may or may not impact the success of its healthcare model. But the possibility of replicating the Massachusetts model in other states is still worth evaluating.

A handful of other states are following in Massachusetts' wise footsteps. New Jersey signed a compulsory health insurance bill into law in 2018, becoming the second state in the U.S. to do so.[189] The District of Columbia put an individual mandate in place beginning in 2019; Vermont put an individual mandate in place beginning in 2020 and Maryland is looking at similar legislation.[190] Now I'm *loving* this. We should follow this closely, gang—we have a state with improved access and lowered costs that is paying on outcomes. Now *that's* something to ponder further.

Will We Need Insurance in 50 Years?

I've heard people say, "We don't have a healthcare system in America—we have healthcare *payment* systems." It's true we have a complex system: we have Medicare, Medicaid, TRICARE, the U.S. Department of Veterans Affairs (VA) system, commercial private insurance, workers compensation, etc.

And if we could go back in time, I don't think anyone would intentionally create as many systems as we have now. "Hey, let's have hundreds of different payers who all pay different rates, and let's have the government pay a lot, and employers pay a lot, and patients pay a lot; and let's base payment on coding and utilization instead of outcomes, then throw it all out there for consumers to figure out and see how it goes." *How is it going?*

Until something better—and more affordable—comes along, this is the system we are stuck with. In this myriad of healthcare systems, providers are struggling to figure out how to manage costs in order to survive. Buyers of healthcare (employers, government and patients) have frankly *had it*. They're done with the excuses and inefficiencies. They want to know the costs, they want to know that costs are monitored, and ultimately, they want to *choose* when and how they will obtain and pay for care. Providers are going to need to be creative and accommodating to the new healthcare consumer or they will lose.

Insurance itself isn't the problem. Insurance exists to solve the healthcare unaffordability problem caused by various factors that drive rising cost. Insurance is a *bridge*, not a destination. In chapter 5, we will look at three significant factors contributing to high costs and unaffordability: fraud, waste and abuse.

CHAPTER 5

NO LINE OF SIGHT TO COSTS

Now you see it, now you don't. Leaked revenue can manifest itself in many ways, and that indirectly impacts healthcare cost. It's complex enough to manage the costs you *can* see, so imagine how challenging it can be to manage the invisible costs. I'm talking about fraud, waste and abuse (a.k.a. FWA). FWA is particularly challenging as a cost driver because it's hard to identify and can be difficult to manage. Without visibility into these indirect drivers of cost in the U.S. healthcare system, they can be very difficult to address.

Fraud

It's been estimated healthcare fraud costs the U.S. somewhere between $68 billion on the low end to $230 billion on the high end, each year. That's the equivalent of about 3–10 percent of the total annual spending on healthcare in the U.S.[191] Fraud happens at every level of the system, ranging from corporate malfeasance to individual cases of patient identity theft. It angers me that so much healthcare is stolen, right under our noses.

Medicare/Medicaid Fraud

As the numbers of patients enrolled in government health insurance (Medicare, Medicaid, etc.) have increased, the instances of health insurance fraud have increased as well. The government has become more "attractive" to bad guys as their share of the patient pool has increased. These criminal architects have come up with all kinds of tricks, from submitting claims on deceased

Medicare beneficiaries using the obituaries as their guide, to setting up shell practices and billing actual patients for services they never had.

The Office of the Inspector General (OIG) of the U.S. Department of Health and Human Services (HHS) is responsible for detecting and eliminating fraud in federal healthcare programs.[192] The dollars lost to fraud are staggering—especially considering the people who are actually caught committing fraud represent just the tip of the iceberg.

In 2007, the U.S. launched its first Health Care Fraud Strike Force in South Florida to combat escalating fraud. The Strike Force model integrates the resources of investigators and prosecutors across governmental agencies to identify and prosecute fraud in regions with high occurrences of fraud.[193] According to the U.S. Department of Justice (DOJ):

> The Strike Force uses advanced data analysis techniques to identify aberrant billing levels in healthcare fraud "hot spots"—cities with high levels of billing fraud—and target suspicious billing patterns as well as emerging schemes and schemes that migrate from one community to another.[194]

Since 2007, the Strike Force—which operates nationally in 10 different states—has charged almost 4,000 defendants who collectively billed the Medicare program for more than $14 billion.[195] The government making progress ... I love it.

In 2018 alone, the U.S. DOJ recovered $2.5 billion in settlements and judgements related to healthcare industry fraud, including drug and medical device manufacturers, managed care providers, hospitals, pharmacies, hospice organizations, laboratories and physicians.[196] This marks the ninth consecutive year the department's civil healthcare fraud settlements and judgements have exceeded $2 billion.[197]

Fraud is being committed at all levels of the industry—from large corporations to small physician offices. One of the largest civil fraud settlements of 2018 was against drug wholesaler AmerisourceBergen.[198] AmerisourceBergen Specialty Group, a wholly owned subsidiary, was found to be taking manufacturers' drug vials—including overfill—emptying them into another container and repackaging them.[199] By emptying the overfill into the plastic container, the company created more doses than it purchased from the manufacturer. The scheme enabled the company to bill multiple healthcare providers for the same vial of drug, which caused Medicare and Medicaid to pay for the same drug twice.[200]

A former chief operating officer at the company—who was terminated after he spoke up internally—was the whistleblower in the AmerisourceBergen case.[201] In another 2018 case, a man was sentenced to 46 months in prison for a scheme in which he fraudulently billed Medicare for $8.3 million in durable medical equipment that was not medically necessary.[202]

Fraud and the Opioid Crisis

Recent anti-fraud efforts have included a special emphasis on the opioid crisis, since illegal opioid prescriptions have played a major rule in fueling the nation's current opioid crisis. It's been estimated the opioid crisis caused more than 470,000 deaths between 1999 and 2017.[203] What does Medicare fraud have to do with the opioid epidemic? More than you might think, since nearly one in three Medicare Part D beneficiaries received at least one opioid prescription (figure 5.1).

Figure 5.1 Medicare and the Opioid Epidemic

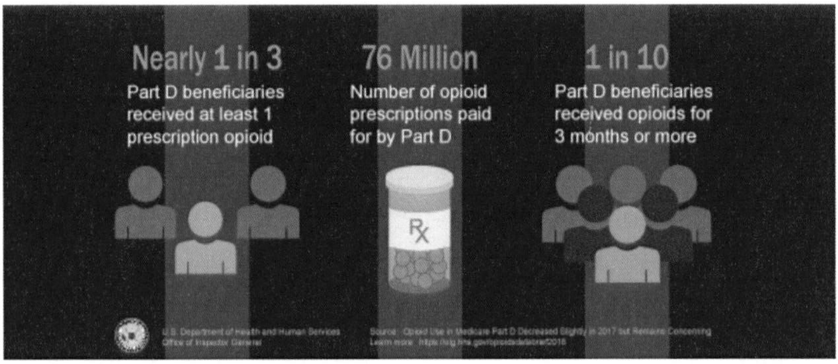

Source: "Combatting the Opioid Epidemic." Office of the Inspector General. U.S. Department of Health and Human Services. (n.d.) Accessed August 19, 2019. https://oig.hhs.gov/reports-and-publications/featured-topics/opioids/

In the spring of 2019, the HHS OIG conducted the largest ever prescription opioid law enforcement operation.[204] Called the Appalachian Regional Prescription Opioid Surge Takedown, the operation resulted in charges against 53 medical professionals for participating in the illegal prescription and distribution of opioids and other narcotics and for healthcare fraud.[205] Data analytics helped identify the Appalachian region as a problem hot spot:

> Thirty-six percent of Part D beneficiaries in five States in the Appalachian region received a prescription opioid in 2017; these States are Alabama, Kentucky, Ohio, Tennessee and West Virginia. Almost 49,000 beneficiaries in these states received high amounts of opioids, far exceeding levels the Centers for Disease Control and Prevention (CDC) says to avoid.[206]

According to the CDC, more than 130 people in the U.S. die each day of an opioid overdose.[207] The total economic burden caused by opioid misuse is estimated to exceed $78.5 billion per year, including healthcare costs, lost productivity, addiction treatment and criminal justice involvement.[208] You might be thinking: "That doesn't have a direct impact on my healthcare costs. I don't have a prescription for opioids, nor does anyone I know." Think again. Our tax dollars fund Medicare and Medicaid—so these expenses come right out of our wallets.

Medical Identity Theft

Fraud happens at the patient level as well. As healthcare costs have risen, so have occurrences of medical identity theft, which are estimated to cost U.S. consumers tens of billions of dollars annually, according to the Ponemon Institute, a research center dedicated to privacy, data protection and information security policy.[209] Medical identity theft occurs when a patient uses Medicare or health insurance information that belongs to someone else to receive treatment, prescriptions, medical devices or other health benefits.

Medical identity theft is a particularly destructive form of theft, with far-reaching consequences for patients:

- It can cost far more than purely financial identity theft. Federal law generally limits consumers' liability for fraudulent credit card charges to $50, but there are no such protections for a stolen medical identity. Among victims of medical ID theft, those who lost money spent an average of $13,500 to resolve the problem, including legal as well as medical costs, according to the same Ponemon survey mentioned above.[210]
- It's considerably harder to undo the damage. Financial and personal complications "can endure for years," the World Privacy Forum said in a 2017 report, with many victims suffering "long term problems with aggressive medical debt collection" and severely impaired credit

113

due to phony bills. Some have even faced prosecution because thieves used their identities to stockpile prescription drugs.

- It can harm your health as well as your finances, potentially causing treatment delays, incorrect prescriptions and misdiagnoses. As the Federal Trade Commission (FTC) notes, "If a scammer gets treatment in your name, that person's health problems could become a part of your medical record. It could affect your ability to get medical care and insurance benefits, and could even affect decisions made by doctors treating you later on."[211]

In addition to creating a nightmare for patients, medical identity theft impacts providers as well. Once the fraud has been discovered, payers don't pay fraudulent claims. "This isn't our patient? Why are you billing us for this?" Subsequently, the provider is left holding the bag—having just provided somebody with free care. The situation becomes even more intricate if the provider has turned the patient over to collections before discovering the medical identity fraud. The patient is then double-victimized—initially by the thief, and then by the provider, who is trying to collect on the debt after the payer denies the claim.

Numbers on the annual financial impact of medical identity theft are hard to come by, but it is a fast-growing form of fraud. The most recent available statistics indicate the number of cases of medical identity theft increased by almost 22 percent, impacting nearly half a million people in a single year.[212] Medical identity theft is a form of fraud that providers can be proactive in minimizing, preventing harm to patients and to their bottom line— I'll have more to say about that in chapter 8.

Waste

It's been estimated more than 30 percent of U.S. healthcare spending—exceeding $1 trillion annually—is wasted.[213] The authors of one study suggested the U.S. healthcare system is more prone to waste than other industries because of a lack of aligned incentives:

> Inefficiencies persist within the healthcare system because—in contrast to other economic sectors in which competition and other economic incentives act to reduce the level of waste—none of the healthcare system's players have strong incentives to economize. Although it is necessary for protection against the potentially catastrophic costs of treatment, generous health insurance coverage insulates patients from the true cost of medical care … Fee-for-service providers are paid for all services, whether or not they are necessary. Furthermore, because physicians advise patients on what care they need and also provide that care, they lack incentives to ration. Insurance and medical uncertainties muffle price competition and, in our litigious climate, promote overscreening and overtreatment. Health insurers, chastened by the backlash against managed care, act passively in reimbursing healthcare spending and, as expenditures increase, merely pass costs along to purchasers in the form of higher premiums … Together, all these factors allow inefficiency to thrive in the U.S. healthcare system.[214]

Many different variables contribute to waste in the system, from administrative complexity to inefficient care delivery to overutilization (figure 5.2). But regardless of what term you use to describe it, it boils down to the same thing: almost $1 out of every $3 we spend on healthcare contributes to inflated costs while doing nothing to improve patient outcomes.

Figure 5.2 Causes of Waste in the U.S. Healthcare System

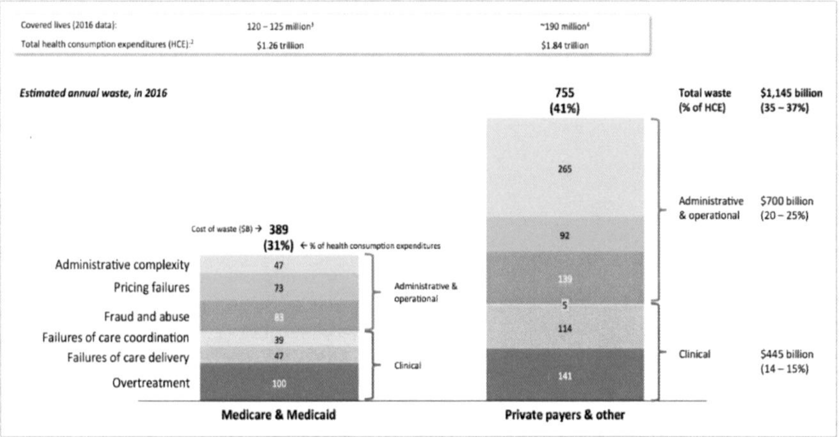

Sources: JAMA. 2012Waste categories and magnitudes based on work by Berwick DM, Hackbarth AD. Eliminating waste in US health care. JAMA. 2012;307(14):1513-6. Original estimates based on 2011 spending levels have been extrapolated to 2016 using National Health Expenditures (NHE) data.
1 Health consumption expenditures include all NHE, less investment (research, structures, and equipment) and public health outlays by federal and state governments.
2 Includes 55.4 million Medicare enrollees, 71.2 million Medicaid enrollees, and 6.5 million children covered by CHIP per the Centers for Medicare and Medicaid Services data, less 10 million lives covered by both Medicare and Medicaid in 2016, per the American Community Survey.
3 Includes 173.1 million lives covered by employer-sponsored insurance in 2016, plus 17.5 million covered by a plan purchased directly, of which the majority bought plans on an Affordable Care Act exchange. To avoid double counting, this figure excludes 7.3 million individual Medigap plans.
Source: Daniel P. O'Neill and David Scheinker. "Wasted Health Spending: Who's Picking Up The Tab?" Health Affairs Blog, DOI: 10.1377/hblog20180530.245587. May 31, 2018. Accessed August 26, 2019. https://www.healthaffairs.org/do/10.1377/hblog20180530.245587/full/

Waste occurs at all levels within the system, from the organizational level down to the individual patient level. A study in the *Milbank Quarterly* suggests that addressing waste in the system begins with conceptualizing it.[215] The study's authors categorized healthcare waste in three areas: administrative, operational and clinical. Here is what waste currently looks like in these three broad areas in the U.S. healthcare system.

Administrative Waste

Administrative waste is caused by inefficient or overly complex processes. This can lead to excessive administrative overhead. As I noted in chapter 1, there are hundreds of health insurers in the U.S. offering thousands of different plans.[216] This complexity leads to a lot of administrative overhead, as you can see in figure 5.2, above. That's not a judgment about the complexity of the U.S. system—it's just a fact. One study compared U.S. healthcare administrative costs to administrative costs in eight other countries.[217] The study found "administrative overhead consumes 25 percent of outlays in U.S. hospitals, which is far higher than in countries that don't rely on multiple private payers, with the difference due to 'the complexity of the reimbursement system.'"[218]

The administrative complexity of the U.S. healthcare system is not new. And it has long been recognized as a contributing factor to healthcare system waste.

Back in 2003, economist Henry J. Aaron published an editorial in the *New England Journal of Medicine* that described the U.S. system as "an administrative monstrosity, a truly bizarre mélange of thousands of payers with payment systems that differ for no socially beneficial reason, as well as staggeringly complex public systems with mind-boggling administered prices and other rules expressing distinctions that can only be regarded as weird."[219] Sadly, 16 years later, this description of our healthcare system still applies today.

It makes sense that in this multi-payer system, the lion's share of administrative costs are specifically related to billing and insurance-related (BIR) functions.[220] Hospitals, in particular, expend a lot of resources on the shell game known as "denials." Denials, as I pointed out in chapter 3, are a big issue for providers. And are often a big waste of time and resources as well.

I'm sure this scenario is familiar: Surgeon Smith is coming to the hospital. He's got the patient's clinicals, X-rays, etc. to document the need for the surgery. But as the provider, I've got to have a referral, and an authorization, and a precertification and a piece of parchment with a wax seal on it that says, "The payer is going to pay this claim because I am following the rules." But then you reach out to the payer and the payer says: "We can't guarantee payment of the claim until we see how it's coded and whether the procedure was medically necessary or not. And we can't make that determination until we receive the claim."

So the provider thinks, "What do I do now?!?" but goes ahead with the surgery and hopes all the t's are crossed and the i's are dotted. Too many times, claims are initially denied and then have to be appealed. And they may or may not be paid upon appeal. Either way, the back and forth of this game creates a huge administrative expense that impacts the whole system. Electronic claims processing was supposed to help ease this administrative burden, but due to a lack of standardization in claims processing, it seems electronic billing hasn't made a dent yet.[221]

Operational Waste

In chapter 2, I wrote about how current payment models can reward the wrong things. That's one way the operational waste is introduced into the system. One legacy of the fee-for-service (FFS) payment model is that "the more services I perform, the more I get paid" construct actually rewards operational inefficiency, rather than efficiency, in many cases.

Operational waste exists in many different forms, including duplication of services, inefficient processes, overly expensive inputs and errors (figure 5.3).

Figure 5.3 Types of Operational Waste

Type of Waste	Description	Health Care Examples
Duplication of services	Producing unnecessary repeated services	Tests or procedures done more frequently than clinically necessary
Inefficient processes	Poor process design that causes unnecessary movement or inventory in the production of services	Time spent waiting; unnecessary transport of people or material; useless motions; multiple stock items due to lost or misplaced supplies
Overly expensive inputs	Producing services with expensive equipment or personnel when less expensive inputs would suffice	Physicians providing services for which nurses are equally competent; use of brand drugs for patients who get equal benefit from generics
Errors	Quality defects that result in rework or scrapping	Defective medical devices; rework of tests or procedures; health and cost consequences of medical errors

Source: Tanya G.K. Bentley, Rachel M. Effros, Kartika Palar and Emmett B. Keeler. "Waste in the U.S. Health Care System: A Conceptual Framework." The Milbank Quarterly. 2008 Dec.; 86(4): 629-659. DOI: 10.1111/j.1468-0009.2008.00537.x Accessed August 28, 2019. https://www.ncbi.nlm.nih.gov/pmc/articles/PMC2690367/#

One example that comes to mind to illustrate "overly expensive inputs" is the proliferation of freestanding emergency departments (FSEDs), which I addressed in chapter 1. These are expensive access points that are popping up everywhere, like Starbucks. From an institutional growth perspective, a provider might say, "Why don't we open up a freestanding ED on the west side of town? What would the revenue projection be for that? What would the expenses be to run it?" It's the same conversation a provider might have when considering building a new wing or acquiring or merging with another hospital or health system. What is often lacking is the medical need to expand or add these facilities. Was the existing ED inadequate? Is that area underserved? More often than not, it's a market share or revenue play: "I'm going to occupy that square before the other guy."

I think hospital growth can be good in some cases, but someone is paying for all of those profuse plant costs and expansions.

These types of growth strategies have impacts across the organization: How many people would I need to hire to say "hello" to these patients? How many people would I need to add to submit the claims for services performed in the new facility? These types of conversations should include not just finance, but also revenue cycle management (RCM)—because growth and economy of scale does not always equate with cost savings; in fact, sometimes it results in higher costs. There are hospitals and freestanding emergency departments being built across the street from each other. There is most certainly not a medical play there: it's about profits, even for not-for-profit organizations.

Clinical Waste

Clinical waste is about providing care with low questionable—or even negative—value. Providing excessive services is one example. For instance, when you say the words "chest pain" in the healthcare system you are going to get the full treatment—wash, wax and dry—no matter where you enter the system. And it's great the health system will jump in and give you an EKG, a cardiac enzyme test, a chest X-ray, etc., to make sure you are not really having a heart attack. It's important to do those things because you want to make certain you capture a correct diagnosis and do what's best for the patient.

Frequently, a patient presenting with these symptoms may actually just have indigestion or a strained chest muscle from working out at the gym yesterday. A lot of resources go into ruling things out, and there's debate on the medical necessity and cost of these interventions. I'm not suggesting we use cost considerations to direct the practice of medicine, but the system often defaults to the most comprehensive or expensive treatment without any regard to efficacy or cost. As patients we'll typically comply, as we don't have other guidance—proactive or reactive—to turn to for input.

Providing duplicative services is another example of both clinical and operational waste. For example, maybe a patient had a CT scan in the morning, and then another one in the afternoon, and a third one in the evening. Why? Were the scans repeated because the technologist didn't perform the correct exam? Did the patient actually need three separate scans to stay on top of an issue? Or was it because the patient had three different doctors involved and they weren't communicating with each other? Or perhaps the issue couldn't be visualized on CT or maybe it was the wrong test in the first place, setting up a cascade of wasted resources and time? That is how clinical waste comes about.

You really can't talk about clinical waste without also talking about end-of-life care. I know this can be a (very) sensitive subject. On one side, you have a patient and their family, who may want to exhaust every medical resource to continue life for an unknown timeframe and outcome. They want the chance—and rightfully so. On the other side, you have the provider (and indirectly the insurer), who see these cases day in and day out, and know clinically there isn't a chance for an outcome that will be positive. The prognosis is very poor and no matter what resources are provided, these patients' quality of life, health status and their need to be in an acute care facility will not change. And the care is not reimbursable. The patient is "stuck."

It's important to note the majority of hospitals treat patients regardless of their ability to pay. It's part of both their mission and Conditions of Participation with Medicare. That said, hospitals also need to serve in the role of financial counselor.

End-of-life costs are exhaustive and can have little impact to patient health—that's why it's called "end of life." To ease the clinical and financial burdens, hospitals can offer palliative and hospice care in an effort to step down the care, placing the patient with experts who do this for all their patients. An ICU has a 2-to-1 nurse-to-patient ratio, 24/7 monitoring, negative pressure rooms and 4-plus physicians rounding constantly. Those resources and level of care, at end of life, require considerable consideration from a clinical, resource and cost standpoint. They're evaluated daily, regardless of the acuity of the patient.

As difficult as it is to point out, end-of-life care can represent another example of potential clinical waste—purely from a revenue cycle point of view, but also from a patient outcome perspective. A lot of care happens in the last 6 to 12 months of a patient's life that doesn't change their quality of life. Our society fears death, and our intuitions can sometimes provide a disproportionate amount of healthcare to the elderly. There's a cost to all of that care and we're all paying for the clinical waste. Maybe they lived six months longer with treatment, but were they throwing up every day? Were they mostly lying in bed sedated because they were in so much pain? This can be a touchy topic, but sometimes you have to consider, "Well, they got to live a year longer but what kind of life did they have?"

An analysis published in 2016 by the Kaiser Family Foundation found 8 of every 10 people who died in the U.S. were on Medicare, "making Medicare the largest insurer of medical care provided at the end of life."[222] Further analysis found about 25 percent of all Medicare spending is for beneficiaries age 65 or older, during the last year of their life.[223] In addition, "Among seniors in traditional Medicare who died in 2014, Medicare spending averaged $34,529 per beneficiary—almost four times higher than the average cost per capita for seniors who didn't die during the year."[224]

Medicare spending in the year of patients' death varied by age, peaking at age 73 with an average cost of $43,316 (figure 5.4). Think about these figures for a moment. According to U.S. Census data, the median household income in 2014 for householders aged 65 and older was $36,895.[225] In other words, the average Medicare spending at end of life ($34,529) was nearly equivalent to the average senior's household income. Elderly individuals on a fixed income have equitable healthcare costs paid by the government and cost-share by the patient. This care may or may not have had an impact, but it was paid.

Figure 5.4 Medicare Spending at the End of Life

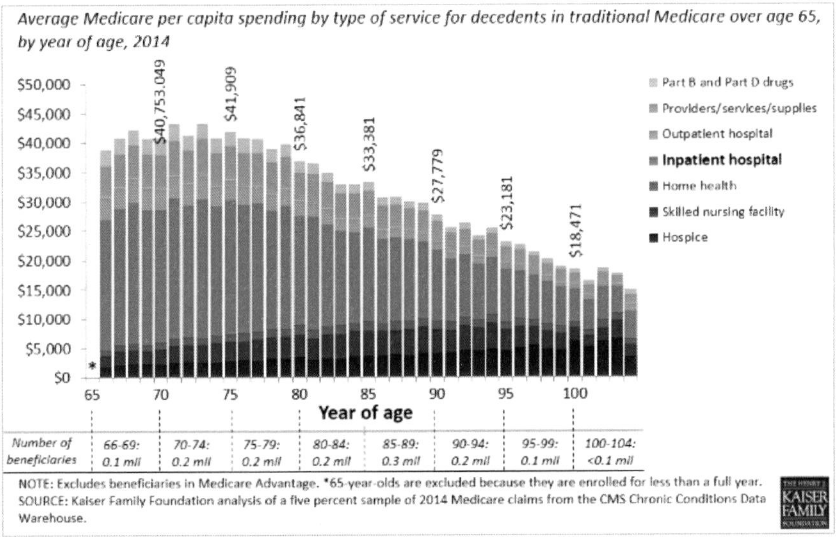
Average Medicare per capita spending by type of service for decedents in traditional Medicare over age 65, by year of age, 2014
$50,000
$45,000
$40,000
$35,000
$30,000
$25,000
$20,000
$15,000
$10,000
$5,000
$0
*
$40,753.049
$41,909
$36,841
$33,381
$27,779
$23,181
$18,471
65
70
75
80
85
90
95
100
Year of age
Part B and Part D drugs
Providers/services/supplies
Outpatient hospital
Inpatient hospital
Home health
Skilled nursing facility
Hospice
Number of beneficiaries
66-69: 0.1 mil
70-74: 0.2 mil
75-79: 0.2 mil
80-84: 0.2 mil
85-89: 0.3 mil
90-94: 0.2 mil
95-99: 0.1 mil
100-104: <0.1 mil
NOTE: Excludes beneficiaries in Medicare Advantage. *65-year-olds are excluded because they are enrolled for less than a full year.
SOURCE: Kaiser Family Foundation analysis of a five percent sample of 2014 Medicare claims from the CMS Chronic Conditions Data Warehouse.
KAISER FAMILY

Source: Juliette Cubanski, Tricia Neuman, Shannon Griffin, and Anthony Damico. "Medicare Spending at the End of Life: A Snapshot of Beneficiaries Who Died in 2014 and the Cost of Their Care." Kaiser Family Foundation. July 14, 2016. https://www.kff.org/ece99cd/

I'm not advocating withholding medical care for those at the end of their lives. As I said, our hospital (as I would argue most would), exhausted all clinical resources to accommodate patients and their families' wishes. My point here is the benefits may often not outweigh the costs. That meter is often running without anyone watching those dollars.

On a personal note, I love my grandparents dearly, who were both very ill at the end of their lives, and I'm certain they both received "too much" care in their final months and just wanted to be left alone. I also served on an ethics committee at my hospital—I was the big bad finance guy. This committee looked at patients who had an atypical length of stay in an intensive level of care, such as the intensive care unit (ICU) or a telemetry unit. For example, a patient who was on a ventilator but still in acute inpatient care rather than a long-term acute care (LTAC) facility or skilled nursing facility.

This was one of the most difficult duties I had as a chief revenue officer. I was the guy who echoed the clinical prognosis from the attending and the insurance carrier's acknowledgement. The guy who informed the family and health teams that the payer is no longer paying. This is why we had an ethics committee—it allowed for a forum to discuss the clinical and financial options to the organization and the patient. We asked tough questions: What does the patient and the family want? What can we do? How long can we do it? Who is going to pay for it? We would put these options in front of the patient and their family as a liaison between them and their insurance. It was a tough job.

I didn't like doing it, but basically, I would say, "Yep, Mr. Smith has been here 10 days since the doctor wrote his last status note and it was the same note as the last 8 times, saying, 'No prognosis, no outcome and we don't have a clear discharge plan for this patient.' It's $10,194 per day, each day. He's still here but the payer stopped paying two weeks ago." It hurts me to say it, but we need an awareness of it.

Payers are starting to push back on clinical waste by refusing to pay for things they don't feel are medically necessary, or are not reimbursable under plan rules. They are turning off the faucet for practices they feel are wasteful. Payers are asking: Was that procedure medically necessary? Could it have been done at a lower cost as an outpatient?

Medicare, for example, has begun to put rules in place to control the cost impact of duplicative practices. For example, Medicare now has a cascading reimbursement rule that basically states, "Hey, hospital, we're not going to pay you 100 percent of the charge for that CT scan of the chest, abdomen and pelvis, even though there are three different CPTs! You only had a small incremental cost on number two and number three, so we *will* pay 100 percent for the first one but only 75 percent on the second and 50 percent on the third." If the *same* one happened in the same day, there would be only one payment. Rules like that are helping to curb some of the waste. Payers are not there to clean up providers' inefficiencies.

Abuse

A variation of fraud and waste may be more accurately characterized as abuse of the payment system. Instead of submitting outright fraudulent claims, this is when providers prepare claims in a specific—but unjustified—way in order to maximize payment. One common term for this is "upcoding" (i.e., assigning an inaccurate billing code to increase reimbursement). This might involve assigning a higher-level service or procedure code than was actually performed, or reporting a more complex diagnosis than is supported by the provider's documentation.

An example of this kind of abuse is the $270 million settlement between the U.S. Department of Justice and Medicare Advantage Organization (MAO) HealthCare Partners Holdings, LLC, which was announced in late 2018.[226] Medicare Advantage Organizations are paid a fixed, monthly amount to provide healthcare to beneficiaries enrolled in their Medicare Advantage plans.[227] This amount is subject to "risk adjustment" based on the health status of the beneficiaries. In HealthCare Partners' case, the organization engaged in several types of practices intended to inflate Medicare reimbursement. For example, HealthCare Partners "disseminated improper medical coding guidance instructing its physicians to use an improper diagnosis code for a particular spinal condition that yielded increased reimbursement from Centers for Medicare & Medicaid Services (CMS)."[228]

According to a whistleblower in the HealthCare Partners case:

> HealthCare Partners engaged in "one-way" chart reviews in which it scoured its patients' medical records for diagnoses its providers may have failed to record. It then submitted these "missed" diagnoses to MAOs to be used by them in obtaining increased Medicare payments. At the same time, it ignored inaccurate diagnosis codes that should have been deleted and that would have decreased Medicare reimbursement or required the MAOs to repay money to Medicare.[229]

The increase in upcoding and related practices can correlate with the adoption of electronic medical records. It's easier to have upcoding and inflated charges in an electronic health record (EHR) versus a paper process. Automated billing processes allow providers to implement rules like: "Whenever you bill for 'A,' add 'B,' 'C' and 'D' as well." A good example of this is an imaging-guided biopsy. The CT biopsy imaging study "A" should always have the needle guidance charge "B," and sometimes there is sedation "C" and pathology "D." What if, in a particular case "B" and "C" happened, but "D" didn't? With electronic records, we don't necessarily have the same checks and balances against these kinds of errors as we did when all billing was done by hand.

Technically, the case I just described (billing for "A," "B" and "C" but not "D") is a false claim—it's fraud—because it shouldn't have been billed that way. But in this case, it's an artifact of the automated billing system, which is designed to make the billing process more efficient but not necessarily error-proof. The government penalizes you on the fact that you knowingly billed this claim without verifying it—looking at every claim is hard in an automated system, and here we are.

It's hard to assign a number to this kind of system abuse. While some mistakes may be unintentional (the coding system can be fairly complicated), others are systematic and committed with the specific intent of fraudulently increasing reimbursement. A recent article on Medicare fraud and abuse explained:

> During the 2016 fiscal year, the Medicare fee-for-service improper payment rate reached an estimated 11 percent, or roughly $40.4 billion. This improper payment rate does not measure fraud, but rather payments that did not meet Medicare coverage, coding or billing rules … While Medicare fraud contributes to improper payments, not all improper payments constitute Medicare fraud. While

Medicare fraud is done intentionally, erroneous billing results in the same consequences—overpayment—even though unintentional.[230]

Just like with other cases of fraud, "big data" and data analytics is helping government investigators identify and crack down on patterns of abuse. Data analysts look for suspect patterns that can indicate abuse, such as providers that use expensive billing codes at a higher rate than their peers, providers that seem to use a particular billing code more often than their peers, or any other pattern in which the billing codes indicate an outlier.[231]

On the Medicare side, increasing attention is being paid to the integrity of coding, billing and documentation on the part of providers. CMS understands, however, that not all "abuse" is intentional. That's why CMS supports a number of compliance projects designed to help providers identify and address services with a high probability of improper payment.[232]

One such initiative is the Programs to Evaluate Payment Patterns Electronic Report (PEPPER). Per CMS:

PEPPER is an electronic report that provides provider-specific Medicare data statistics for discharges/services vulnerable to improper payments. PEPPER cannot be used to identify the presence of payment errors, but it can be used as a guide for auditing and monitoring efforts to help providers identify and prevent payment errors. PEPPERs are sent to facilities such as Short-Term Hospitals, Long-Term Hospitals, Critical Access Hospitals, Hospices, Inpatient Rehabilitation Facilities, Partial Hospitalization Programs, Skilled

Nursing Facilities, Inpatient Psychiatric Facilities
and Home Health Agencies.[233]

By supplying provider-specific Medicare data and statistics about discharges and services, the PEPPER report can support providers' compliance efforts.[234] The reports show providers areas in which they are an outlier in comparison to peers. This data can be used internally to identify trouble spots where improper payments may be occurring.[235] Looking at the PEPPER can help providers identify whether they are an outlier in a specific area. In one of the hospitals I worked at, we reviewed our PEPPER report on a quarterly basis. I loved our PEPPER meetings, as I am a big data nerd, and it always had interesting findings. As an example, if you looked at your PEPPER report and saw your facility was an outlier for pneumonia codes compared to regional peers, that's something you might want to look into. "Say, we're coding a lot of pneumonia but all our peers are coding respiratory illness, not pneumonia. Why? Is something special happening here that's not happening somewhere else?" We would meet with the medical coders and pulmonologists to ensure we didn't have an internal, behavioral practice that wasn't aligned with Medicare standards.

Like HHS's Medicare Fraud Strike Force, the PEPPER is another way the U.S. government is trying to address costs associated with fraud, waste and abuse. Fraud, waste and abuse all contribute to the healthcare unaffordability problem. These issues also challenge providers by making it harder to get a line of sight to costs. But even if the system was able to minimize—or eradicate—cost inflation due to ineffective utilization, fraud, waste and abuse, managing healthcare costs would still be a game of risk. And that's what chapter 6 is all about: Risk.

CHAPTER 6

A GAME OF RISK

The healthcare payment system boils down to a game of risk. Each stakeholder—patient, provider, payer and employer—is trying to drive down their own risk. And in order to do that, they may have to shift the risk to somebody else. Each stakeholder has different considerations when it comes to risk and different strategies for managing it. At the same time, emerging payment models are shifting risk in nontraditional ways. Most of these new models involve shifting risk away from employers and payers and back to consumers and providers.

Risk Considerations by Stakeholder

Patients

It only makes sense for consumers of healthcare to share some of the financial risk. For one thing, they are the ultimate beneficiary of the care. For another, as I've pointed out previously, patient behavior has a huge impact on health outcomes. So why not have patients assume some of the financial risk as well?

In some ways, this is already happening. Higher deductibles and overall higher out-of-pocket expenses definitely shift financial risk to patients. The problem is the risk-shifting that occurs with higher deductibles doesn't necessarily decrease healthcare costs over the long-term, it just discourages patients from getting early care when they need it, and it leaves providers with a lot of uncollectable debt. Another way to shift risk to consumers is to tie premium costs to patient behaviors. One example of this is "tobacco rating." The Affordable Care Act (ACA) prevents insurers from using health, medical history or gender to differentiate health insurance premiums. On the other hand, it does allow insurance companies to consider age and location to some extent as factors influencing premiums.[236] And it also allows insurance companies to charge tobacco users up to 50 percent more than people who don't use tobacco—a practice known as tobacco rating.[237]

Numerous studies have documented increased per capita healthcare expenditures for smokers over nonsmokers.[238] So why not have the smokers themselves shoulder some of that risk via higher health insurance premiums? Of course, there are no silver bullets—one study found smokers faced with tobacco-rated premiums were likely to skip purchasing insurance altogether rather than purchase insurance with a higher premium.[239] Other consumers simply lie about their tobacco use.[240] Still, the concept has appeal. A number of payers are using health-reward programs, where patients have the opportunity to earn incentives for healthy behaviors.

For example, Cigna's Healthy Rewards program offers discounts on health products and programs (e.g., a 30 percent discount on Jenny Craig weight management program; discounts on hearing exams and hearing aids; and discounts on alternative medicine like acupuncture, massage, etc.).[241] And Aetna's Healthy Rewards program offers gift cards to patients who complete their annual exams, get flu shots, and participate in proactive check-ups like breast cancer screenings and the like.[242]

Neither of these programs directly shift financial risk to patients but they do incentivize healthy behaviors with rewards. Could these programs be modified to actually shift risk to patients for risky behaviors?

For example, maybe if you weigh 10 pounds less at the end of the year, the insurance company (or employer) will cut your premium by 10 percent. Or if you quit smoking, or get so many daily steps in or bring your cholesterol down—the reward would be a discount on your premium.

Conversely, if you chose to smoke or gained unhealthy weight should your health insurance premium go up or down based on those choices? There isn't a lot of that happening right now, but imagine if incentives and penalties were in place based on how the patient lived their life? It would drive healthcare costs down if there were dollars attached to behaviors. Risks and rewards would be shared equally through premium adjustments, affording the payer and employers some leverage in plan design, risk and ultimately, affordability.

For example, wearables are growing significantly in healthcare, and for good reason. According to a report from Accenture, U.S. consumer use of wearables increased from 9 percent in 2014 to 33 percent in 2018.[243] UnitedHealthcare is leveraging the popularity of wearables to incentivize members to exercise.[244] UnitedHealthcare members participating in the UnitedHealthcare Motion program can earn as much as $1,095 annually toward their health savings accounts by logging 10,000 steps each day.[245] UnitedHealthcare even subsidizes the cost of purchasing a smart watch or activity tracker.

According to UnitedHealthcare, members who participate in the Motion program cost an average of $222 less than members who don't participate in the program.[246] This seems like a great model for health plans and employers: associates sign up for the program and monitor their lifestyle; employers incentivize behaviors like exercising or seeing the doctor, and there you have it—lower risk and lower costs.

Employers

Employers are motivated to hire and retain employees with a competitive benefits package, while managing claims costs, but shouldn't go bankrupt from healthcare expenses. Healthcare costs can thwart company growth by tying up resources that could otherwise be invested back in the company, so employers keep a very close eye on their healthcare spending each year. Most employers want to do what's best for their employees. They want to manage their employee base in a way that drives health, so their employees can be at work and not ill, stuck at home. The healthier their employees are, the more productive they are at work and the better the company performs. Thus, there are a lot of aligned incentives as far as employers being invested in good health outcomes for their employees. With respect to financial risk—employers are in the position of carrying a significant share of employee healthcare costs, whether they want to be in that position or not. Healthcare costs per employee have risen faster than salaries (figure 6.1).

Figure 6.1 Healthcare Cost per Employee Versus Salary Cost

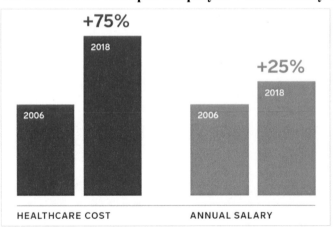

Source: Ali Diab. "American employers are in the healthcare business." Collective Health. February 28, 2018. Accessed September 4, 2019. https://blog.collectivehealth.com/employer-driven-healthcare-270bfb7ee8c7

Per a 2019 survey conducted by the National Business Group on Health (NBGH), large companies are estimating the total cost of healthcare, including premiums and out-of-pocket costs for employees and dependents, will equal $15,375 per employee in 2020 (an increase of 5 percent over 2019).[247] In 2020, large employers will cover 70 percent of these costs, with employees paying about 30 percent.[248] Given these numbers, it's no surprise employers are very highly motivated to find alternative ways to shift financial risk away from their organizations toward patients, providers and payers.

Insurers

Insurers have a different relationship with risk because they understand how behaviors impact the actuarial value. They have very good data on what a population of employees—or an individual—is likely to generate in claims costs. They have to be good at that. If they didn't manage that risk well, they would be out of business. If the insurance company overestimates the risk for a particular group, their premium costs will be too high and misaligned with the market. But if they underestimate risks, they will incur losses. This is why actuaries are in demand—and paid very well. According to the Bureau of Labor Statistics Occupational Outlook Handbook, the 2018 median pay for actuaries was $102,880 (more than 2.5 times the median annual wage for all workers).[249] At the same time, the job outlook for actuaries is stellar, with an anticipated employment growth rate of 20 percent between 2018 and 2028.[250]

In addition to pricing premiums competitively for the market, insurers also have to pay attention to their medical loss ratio (MLR), per ACA requirements. Before the passage of the ACA, insurance company MLRs were not regulated at the federal level.[251] After the ACA was passed in 2010, however, the ACA legislation and accompanying regulations imposed a federal minimum MLR requirement on fully funded health plans (self-funded plans are not subject to the same insurance regulations).[252] The MLR requirement now covers all licensed health insurers, "including commercial insurers, Blue Cross and Blue Shield plans and health maintenance organizations."[253]

CMS explained the need for MLR controls by saying, "Many insurance companies spend a substantial portion of consumers' premium dollars on administrative costs and profits, including executive salaries, overhead and marketing."[254] The ACA's MLR requirement is 80 percent for plans that cover individuals and small businesses and 85 percent for large group plans.[255]

So not only do insurers have to hit the sweet spot that balances claims costs against revenues from premiums, they also have to calculate costs accurately in order to comply with federal limits on MLR. In layman's terms, this means for every dollar spent on healthcare only 15 to 20 cents of that dollar can go back to the health plan for administration and profits. If it goes above that, the carrier must give the policy holders a "rebate" of the difference.[256]

Even with these constraints, insurers are in the best position of any of the healthcare system stakeholders to manage risks. Insurers have two advantages over the other stakeholders: they have access to the most accurate actuarial data and they have the largest risk pools. A 2017 McKinsey & Company analysis showed that in select metropolitan statistical areas (MSA), the leading insurers far outranked leading providers in terms of number of covered lives and number of inpatient days (figure 6.2). Based on this data, McKinsey concluded health insurers are best positioned to change payment models.

Figure 6.2 Insurer and Provider Concentrations in Select Metropolitan Statistical Areas

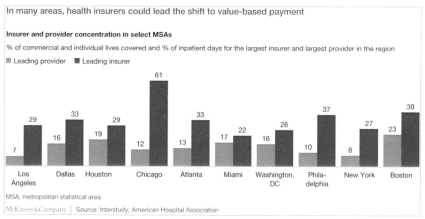

In many areas, health insurers could lead the shift to value-based payment

Insurer and provider concentration in select MSAs

% of commercial and individual lives covered and % of inpatient days for the largest insurer and largest provider in the region

■ Leading provider   ■ Leading insurer

MSA, metropolitan statistical area.

McKinsey&Company | Source: Interstudy; American Hospital Association

Source: Dan Fields, Brian Latko, Tom Latkovic and Tim Ward. "US health insurers: An endangered species?" McKinsey & Company. May 2017. Accessed September 4, 2019. https://healthcare.mckinsey.com/us-health-insurers-endangered-species

Providers

As a provider, you don't have much choice in accepting risk. You see who comes through your door, but you would like to have some predictability about getting paid for services provided. You would also like to use the most efficient technologies available, but because payment systems tend to lag behind technology innovations, you risk not getting paid if you use technology that has outpaced reimbursement.

An example is pacemakers. The first pacemaker implantation was performed in Sweden in 1958.[257] It took some time for the technology to be refined enough to be consistently effective, but by the early 1960s, implanted permanent cardiac pacemakers were being used to treat bradycardia in the U.S.[258] It took a bit longer—until roughly 1965—before pacemakers were generally accepted in the United States (figure 6.3).

Coincidentally, that also was the year Medicare and Medicaid were born.[259] But implantable device coverage was new to Medicare. Medicare covered Part A (hospital) and Part B (outpatient care), but did not get into the details of implantables.

Enter the Health Care Financing Administration (HCFA, now known as CMS), which promulgated rules to help Medicare beneficiaries fund the $300–$500 cost of the implantable, and engaged the Food and Drug Administration (FDA) and the Department of Health and Human Services (HHS) to publish coverage guidelines for pacemaker implantation in 1979.[260] This was shortly followed by a decision memorandum from Medicare which clearly defined cardiac pacemakers as a covered benefit.[261]

Figure 6.3 Rate of Adoption for Innovations in Cardiac Pacing

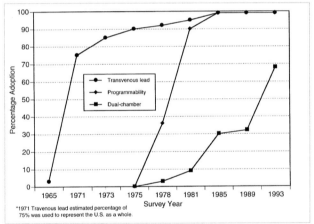

Source: Kirk Jeffrey and Victor Parsonnet. "Cardiac pacing, 1960–1985: A Quarter Century of Medical and Industrial Innovation." Circulation. Vol. 97. (pg. 1978–1991). Figure 5. May 19, 1998. Accessed September 17, 2019. https://www.ahajournals.org/doi/10.1161/01.CIR.97.19.1978

So for almost 20 years, there were patients who needed and could significantly benefit from a pacemaker, but HCFA (CMS) didn't pay for it. Patients paid cash for the pacemaker, and HCFA paid for the procedure to install it at the hospital. The hospitals were then left deciding whether they apply the best intervention with the pacemaker for "free," or provide substandard care and get paid. This still happens today as technology continues to outpace payment. Indirectly, it represents a cost control on the payer side. CMS needs to review clinical evidence before determining whether or not a particular procedure or device will be covered; if the decision is positive, CMS issues strict guidelines on indications that warrant use of the covered device or procedure. But until CMS makes a determination, providers risk forfeiting payment if they use unapproved technologies. The point is providers are already in a position of risk—with ethical implications—in the treatment decisions they make every day. And now with these new value-based payment models, even more risk is directed to providers.

Changing Payment Models

The federal government, as the biggest purchaser of healthcare in the nation, often leads the way in driving healthcare innovation. By sheer force of size, CMS policy initiatives not only impact provider practices, but also the larger market, like commercial insurer payment policies. CMS has taken the lead in moving away from paying providers for the quantity of services provided (the fee-for-service model) and toward value-based care programs, which reward healthcare providers for the *quality* of care they provide. The CMS emphasis on value-based programs aligns with CMS's take on healthcare's Triple Aim:

- Better care for individuals
- Better health for populations
- Lower cost[262]

Due to pressure from CMS and marketplace forces, the FFS model may become less relevant over time. Change Healthcare estimated by 2021 only 25 percent of the healthcare industry's business will be aligned with a pure FFS model (figure 6.4).

Figure 6.4 Decline of Pure Fee-for-Service Accelerates

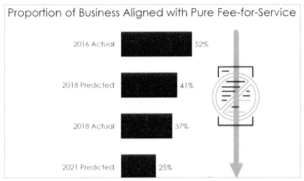

Source: Susan Sebelsky and Andrei Gonzales. Finding the Value in Value-Based Care: The State of Value Based Care in 2018 [Slide 11]. Change Healthcare. June 2018. [Wiik resources, presented: 2018 AHIP Conference]

Over 2,000 healthcare industry stakeholders shared their primary uses of a dozen value-based reimbursement models, with "risk sharing" and "pay-for-performance leading" (figure 6.5).

Figure 6.5 Use of Value-Based Reimbursement Models

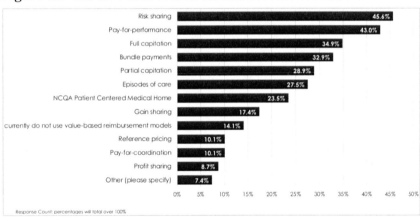

Source: "The 8th Annual Industry Pulse Report." Use of Value-Based Reimbursement (Figure 8). Change Healthcare. 2018. Accessed September 5, 2019.
https://www.changehealthcare.com/blog/wp-content/uploads/change_healthcare_industry_pulse_report_2018.pdf

These new value-based initiatives exist under many different names—value-based programs, value-based care, value-based reimbursement, value-based purchasing, value-based payment models, pay-for-performance—but no matter what you call them, the focus is the same: tie payment to quality outcomes rather than provision of services.

Value-Based Care

As I pointed out in chapter 2, the adoption of value-based care models is slowly growing. As of late 2018, the Health Care Payment Learning and Action Network (LAN) estimated 34 percent of all healthcare payments were tied to value-based care, up from 23 percent in 2015.[263]

How much financial risk are providers really taking on? It depends on who's doing the counting. A 2019 report by Numerof & Associates turned up a more conservative number than the LAN, estimating "the median percentage of revenue in models with either upside or downside financial risk has remained at 10 percent for three years in a row."[264] The report went on to state:

> Most organizations are still experimenting with risk-based contracts. As in our last survey, over three-quarters of respondents reported some experience with an alternative payment contract, but for most (66 percent), less than 20 percent of revenue was involved. Among those who claimed experience with an alternative payment contract, a substantial portion (31 percent) didn't risk actual loss. Their risk was upside only—not receiving a "bonus" if targets weren't achieved.[265] In addition, nearly a quarter of respondents cited "the threat of financial loss as the primary barrier to moving to a risk-based model."[266]

In spite of provider hesitancy toward shouldering more financial risk (than they already do), CMS continues to move ahead with value-based programs, seeking to find the right balance between risk and reward that'll move the needle on healthcare costs. Providers, if all things were equal, would be happy to receive FFS payments in perpetuity. A *Forbes* article (written by a medical doctor) stated, "only 7 percent of practicing physicians express enthusiasm for eliminating fee-for-service payment models … Physicians are hesitant, if not unequivocally opposed, to taking bold steps to re-engineer incentives in the system."[267]

Frankly, an FFS model simply is not affordable or sustainable in the long term. One type of value-based care model initiated by CMS to meet providers in the middle is the Accountable Care Organization (ACO) model. The ACO model was born out of the ACA.[268] In the ACO model, a group of providers work together to coordinate care, provide chronic disease management and improve the quality of patient care. CMS's payment to ACO is linked to healthcare quality goals and patient outcomes that result in cost savings.[269] As of July 1, 2019, there were 518 ACOs in the U.S., serving 10.9 million beneficiaries.[270]

ACOs typically comprise physicians, hospitals, Federally Qualified Health Centers (FQHC), rural access hospitals, critical access hospitals and affiliated skilled nursing facilities—in other words, a combination of providers specializing in different levels of care.[271] ACOs, like many other value-based care models, require providers to enroll, track and manage patient care across affiliated facilities.

The idea is better care coordination—especially across transitions of care—will reduce duplication of services, lower costs and improve patient outcomes. Since 2012, when Pioneer ACOs were initiated, Medicare has rolled out a number of different types of ACO models, building on lessons learned from earlier models. In order to achieve performance goals, risk is shared across the providers in the ACO. Risk is shared differently, depending on the ACO model used:

- *Advance Payment ACOs* (ended in 2015)—Provided upfront payments to ACOs to help small, rural providers move to ACO model. Provided monthly population-based payments, with the potential to share in savings after CMS recovered the advance.
- *Pioneer ACOs* (ended in 2016)—Included both financial risk and reward for participating ACOs.
- *Next Generation ACOs*—Offers several different models, which all require participation in both upside and downside financial risk.
- *ACO Investment Model (AIM)*—Provides upfront pre-payments; designed to increase ACO participation for small and/or rural providers.
- *Medicare Shared Savings Program (MSSP) ACOs* (permanent ACO program)—Provides financial incentives for meeting/ exceeding savings targets and quality goals. Different tracks (Track 1, Track 1+, Track 2, Track 3) allow ACOs to choose between sharing in both savings and losses, or just savings.[272]

The financial risk arrangements of each MSSP track are described in figure 6.6.

Figure 6.6 Each Track of the Shared Savings Program

Track	Financial Risk Arrangement	Description
1	One-sided	Track 1 ACOs do not assume shared losses if they do not lower growth in Medicare expenditures.
Track 1+ Model	Two-sided	Track 1+ Model ACOs assume limited downside risk (less than Track 2 or Track 3).
2	Two-sided	Track 2 ACOs may share in savings or repay Medicare losses depending on performance. Track 2 ACOs may share in a greater portion of savings than Track 1 ACOs.
3	Two-sided	Track 3 ACOs may share in savings or repay Medicare losses depending on performance. Track 3 ACOs take on the greatest amount of risk, but may share in the greatest portion of savings if successful.

Source: 2018 Quality Performance Category Scoring for Alternative Payment Models (Table 3.1). Quality Payment Program. Centers for Medicare & Medicaid Services. Accessed September 6, 2019. https://www.cms.gov/Medicare/Medicare-Fee-for-Service-Payment/sharedsavingsprogram/program-guidance-and-specifications

When performance goals are achieved, participating providers receive reimbursements based on the shared savings, while in other tracks, providers repay losses. I like this—there is skin in the game for all stakeholders. The most recent available data from CMS reported just under $800 billion in total earned shared savings for Performance Year 2017.[273]

It's amazing the progress that can be achieved when there are shared risks toward a common goal. Aggregate CMS data indicates cost savings are being achieved across the various ACO models (figure 6.7).

Figure 6.7 Risk-Bearing ACO Models Generated Net Medicare Savings Relative to Benchmarks, 2016

Type of ACO	No. of ACOs	At-Risk for Shared Losses?	Gross Medicare Spending on Services (in millions)	Medicare Payments to ACOs for Shared Savings (in millions)	ACO Payments to Medicare for Shared Losses (in millions)	Net Medicare Spending (in millions)
All MSSP ACOs	432	—	-$652	$701	-$9	+$40
MSSP Track 1	410	No	-$541	$61	n/a	+$72
MSSP Track 2	6	Yes	-$42	$24	$0	-$18
MSSP Track 3	16	Yes	-$69	$64	-$9	-$14
Pioneer	8	Yes	-$61	$37	$0	-$24
Next Generation	18	Yes	-$48	$58	-$20	-$63*
All ACOs	458	—	-$761 million	$796 million	-$29 million	-$47 million

NOTE: (-) Reduced spending (Medicare savings); (+) Increased spending (Medicare costs); *Incorporates $53 million in discounted benchmarks, plus $10 million in Medicare's share of savings. Analysis excludes the Comprehensive ESRD Care Model.

SOURCE: Kaiser Family Foundation analysis of 2016 public use files for MSSP, Pioneer, and Next Generation ACOs, and unpublished CMS data.

Source: "Q3: What is the evidence on savings for Medicare ACO models?" Medicare Delivery System Reform: The Evidence Link. Kaiser Family Foundation. (n.d.) Accessed September 5, 2019. https://www.kff.org/faqs-medicare-accountable-care-organization-aco-models/

MACRA/MIPS/APMS

MACRA, MIPS and APMs are another variation on the same theme of CMS programs that link payment to the quality of care. The Medicare Access & CHIP Reauthorization Act of 2015 (MACRA) is legislation that replaced previous Medicare reimbursement programs with a new payment framework focused on rewarding clinicians for quality and value rather than services.[274] The quality payment programs established under MACRA come in two flavors: MIPS and APMs.[275]

- *Merit-Based Incentive Payment System (MIPS)*. Under this program, individual and eligible groups of clinicians (practices) are subject to performance-based payment adjustments based on four weighted performance categories (2019):
  - o Quality: 45 percent
  - o Improvement activities: 15 percent
  - o Promoting interoperability: 25 percent
  - o Cost: 15 percent[276]
- *Alternative Payment Model (APM)*. Under the APM program, individual clinicians and eligible groups of clinicians (practices) may earn Medicare incentive payments based upon performance in three weighted categories (2019):
  - o Quality: 50 percent
  - o Improvement activities: 20 percent
  - o Promoting interoperability: 30 percent[277]

Clinicians and group practices have to report metrics on a number of different measures related to these weighted categories. For example, CMS defines "quality measures" across four domains: patient/caregiver experience, care coordination/patient safety, preventive health and at-risk populations.[278] The MIPS 101 Guide for 2019 indicates there are more than 250 quality measures for MIPS participants to choose from; the number of quality measures a clinician or practice needs to submit is based upon variables including the size of the practice, whether or not it is a specialty practice and the data collection type.[279] Examples of quality measures for family practices include:

- Depression remission at 12 months in adolescent patients 12 to 17 years of age

- Optimal asthma control
- Pain brought under control within 48 hours of admission to palliative care services[280]

CMS has identified 118 activities as "improvement activities," each weighted as "high," "medium" or "none." To receive points for improvement activities, participants must perform the activities for at least 90 continuous days during 2019. Examples include:

- Completing all of the modules of the Centers for Disease Control and Prevention (CDC) course "Applying CDC's Guideline for Prescribing Opioids"
- Glycemic management services
- Engagement of new Medicaid patients and timely follow-up[281]

The "promoting interoperability" took over initiatives previously incentivized under the CMS electronic health record (EHR) Incentive Payment Program, under the banner of meaningful use. Among the 39 measures of "promoting interoperability" are:

- Provide patients electronic access to their health information
- Support electronic referral loops by sending a summary of care record for a transition of care or referral
- Support electronic referral loops by receiving and incorporating health information from a summary of care record (e.g., clinical information reconciliation for medication, medication allergy and current problem list)[282]

The "cost" category (applicable to regular MIPS but not to APMs) does not require data submission by participants, but is evaluated automatically through administrative claims data.[283]

Reporting for both the regular MIPS program and the APMs is really complicated—the requirements are complicated and the reporting is complicated. Although studies are showing cost improvements, physicians are burdened by the reporting requirements. They don't like it. But the government is essentially saying, "We are open to hearing feedback on the burden, but the rule is not changing. We like this new payment model, and it seems to be driving costs down, so we need to work together to figure out a way to report on it if you want access to these dollars."

Pay for Performance

The Pay for Performance (P4P) model is another variation of value-based care. In fact, some people use P4P synonymously with value-based care. But I refer to P4P as the nongovernmental version of value-based care—in other words, P4P is how value-based care plays out in the commercial payer market.

In a commercial P4P scenario, a health insurance company might say to a provider, "We're going to compare you to all of the other hospitals of your size in which we have members. We are going to compare you on things like readmissions, referrals to specialists, use of high-cost imaging, length of hospital stays, number of infections, percentage of C-sections versus vaginal deliveries, etc. "If you score above your other provider peers, we'll give you more money. We'll pay you for your performance. If you score below your peers, we will give you less money. If you score as well as everyone else does, we will give you what you contracted for."

Both sides—the provider and the payer—have to agree to this, but even though there is an upside and a downside, it makes sense from a risk standpoint. In my experience, P4P plans also open up an opportunity for payer/provider collaboration that can lead to improvements in the system. P4P benchmarks help to put hospitals in touch with other hospitals that might have a lower mortality rate or a shorter length of stay or a lower infection rate; it opens up a way for hospitals to compare themselves to, and learn from, their peers.

In P4P plans, the insurance is not managing the providers differently: they are just reviewing claims data and pointing out variances in the data. They are showing these variances to the providers and saying, "Hey, do you want to get better? Because we will pay you more to do a better job." Because it is in both the providers, and the insurers, best interest to improve: claims costs will go down and hospital outcomes will be better, so it's a win-win. I like these as they invite collaboration between payer and provider, a relationship that seems to have a lot of friction these days.

P4P plans make sense from a revenue cycle perspective, and they can also motivate providers to make changes that increase patient financial engagement, which can directly impact outcomes. P4P plans emphasize accountability, so it's important to get the details right: Do you have the right patient? Do you have the right date of birth and the right name? Because if you don't, medications could go to the wrong patient, or the wrong information could get entered in the medical record.

Do you have the right contact information? The right phone number and email, so you can contact the patient and remind them of their next appointment or their follow-up care? Can they afford the follow-up care you have recommended? Because one of the big deterrents for patient adherence to medication regimens or treatment plans is cost. If you haven't financially engaged that patient at the front end, financial barriers may throw that patient off track, and then you aren't going to hit your P4P outcomes.

Notification requirements are another control you will sometimes find in P4P plans. The hospital signs an agreement with the payer to tell them within 24 hours that one of their beneficiaries was admitted to the emergency department. That sounds easy, but it's actually quite hard to let a payer know every time just because it's not all payers. It's only that specific payer's enrollees. So you have to know the patient is associated with that payer, and then that patient has to show up on a list and then you must notify the payer right then and there that the patient was admitted.

As an example, let's say "John Doe" (alias used for patients without known identification) showed up in the ED today. He's getting admitted here this afternoon. The hospital has no idea John Doe has insurance. Once this is known (hopefully within 24 hours), the insurance company would have to know that John Doe is being admitted and that he's at this hospital. We would say, "He's one of your members and I'm letting you know now." And that payer notification has to be time and date stamped. If it was 24 hours and 1 minute, it doesn't count. You may have a chance on appeal or a peer-to-peer to win this, but it's administratively burdensome. So hospitals are measured on a percentage of the percent of payers notified within 24 hours of admission, and if they hit the benchmark they are paid a bonus.

In my experience, payer notification benchmarks can be hard to hit. You might have the wrong patient name. You might have the wrong payer associated with the patient. The patient might not have their health insurance card on them. There are lots of possible failure modes. But the payer has a good reason for wanting that notification: They want to manage the care as early as possible. The payer wants to get in touch with the case manager on the floor and talk through possible evidence-based interventions.

Payers don't like it when they're notified late. "Hey, we've had John Doe here in the hospital for six days." Payers are likely to respond, "We weren't involved in that admission, so now we're within our rights to deny the inpatient claim. I also need to understand why the length of stay is six days, when it should've only been three days. That's how long most patients with that diagnosis stay in the hospital. What's the clinical reason for three extra days? We didn't have an opportunity to manage the care or to transfer the patient elsewhere. We're not paying for any of it now."

From an accountability perspective, P4P plans can help hospitals and payers work together to drive toward improvements in the industry. There are people in the industry who have concerns about P4P-type plans, however. The primary concern is that P4P plans might intensify existing disparities in healthcare:

> Studies and actual cases have indicated that they
> [Pay for Performance plans] harm and reduce
> access for socioeconomically disadvantaged
> populations because, despite risk adjustments,
> providers who treat a larger share of low-income
> patients will not perform as well on P4P measures
> and therefore are incentivized to avoid treating
> them. Poorer patients struggle to pay for
> medications, follow-up care and transportation and
> often engage in behaviors or unhealthy coping
> mechanisms that are detrimental to their health.[284]

Critics point to the administrative costs of collecting metrics data—especially when that data isn't standardized but is specific to each of the individual payers the provider works with.

Critics also question whether patient outcome metrics can legitimately be attributed to the performance of the provider, given that so many other factors—social determinants of health (SDOH), interactions with other providers, etc.—influence outcomes.[285]

Still, just like other value-based care programs and initiatives, P4P plans show promise for improving quality outcomes and decreasing costs overall. Unlike fee-for-service plans, P4P plans align reimbursement with the real goal of the healthcare system—providing quality patient care. And change can only happen when the incentives are properly aligned.

Value-Based Purchasing

Value-based purchasing (VBP) shows how employers are purchasing their health plans and starting to put value provisions in their contracts to allow for outcomes. Like the other models I've discussed, VBP is a model that links provider payments to improved performance by healthcare providers.[286] And, like the other models it involves greater tracking of metrics on the part of providers, for example—readmissions, hospital acquired conditions, upcharging, downcharging, upcoding, downcoding, denials, patient adherence—all kinds of different numbers that may or may not directly impact the revenue cycle but serve as measures of patient outcomes.

Employers are driving a lot of VBP because they're on the hook for insurance costs. VBP puts a fence around the patient population: "Let's take this patient population, establish what the costs *should* be compared to other organizations that do this, and try to get closer to that benchmark." An example of VBP on the employer side is the use of direct-to-provider contracts. Direct-to-provider contracts cut the middleman —commercial insurance— out. They represent a deal directly between the employer and the provider. The dialogue goes something like this: "Hey, provider, our company spent $10 million in claims with you last year. So we're going to give you $10 million this year, not a penny more, to take care of our employees. And you can keep whatever you save."

It's that simple and a pretty interesting model. The meter starts running on day one. The question is: will the patient who's covered under a direct-to-provider contract be managed differently than a patient who's managed under a traditional contract? I don't know—but now the provider is 100 percent at risk for the patient population for that specific employer. It puts the provider on notice from the employer, "We don't have a never-ending, bottomless wallet to pay for our employees' care. We've allocated funds to spend on our employees' healthcare costs, and we want to work together. Providers—you seem to have escalating costs with no end in sight. We're going to cap how much we spend on you based on what we spent last year and see how that works."

Some large companies are contracting directly with ACOs, as well as with Centers of Excellence. Both types of direct contracting have had significant gains over the last year, according to research by the National Business Group on Health (figure 6.8).

Figure 6.8 Increase in Direct Contracting for Health Services

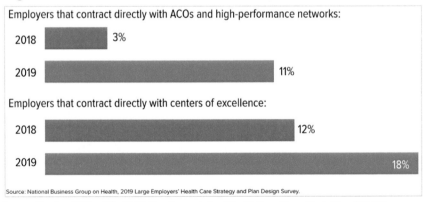

Source: National Business Group on Health, 2019 Large Employers' Health Care Strategy and Plan Design Survey.

Source: Stephen Miller. "For 2019, Employers Adjust Health Benefits as Costs Near $15,000 per Employee." The Society for Human Resource Management (SHRM). August 13, 2018. Accessed September 6, 2019. https://www.shrm.org/resourcesandtools/hr-topics/benefits/pages/employers-adjust-health-benefits-for-2019.aspx

Direct contracting is yet another strategy for focusing on outcomes, rather than providing an infinite supply of services. I'll have more to say about direct-to-provider contracts in chapter 7, where I go into detail on innovation and disruption in payment models in the industry.

The shift to value-based care is happening across the system. CMS may be leading the way, but commercial payers and employers are not far behind. I believe if U.S. healthcare had adopted this idea earlier in its history—the model of paying on patient outcomes, rather than services—we would be in a very different position now with respect to healthcare costs.

But enough about the flaws and weaknesses of the U.S. healthcare system. What you really want to know is: How do I—as a provider—get paid? That's what Section III is all about.

SECTION THREE

HOW DO I GET PAID?

CHAPTER 7

INNOVATION AND DISRUPTION

The healthcare of today is *not* the healthcare of tomorrow. There are a lot of movers and shakers and healthcare delivery is shifting to nontraditional spaces. I believe disruption is healthy. We continue to see disruption in many different industries: airlines, automobiles, grocery stores, etc.

And yet, many hospitals have continued to stick to traditional paradigms for care, delivery and payment for some time, like it was in 1985. Providers are starting to realize they can't survive that way. By 2030, we will have a different kind of hospital than we have today. Below are some of the ways the industry is beginning to change right now.

Technology and Patient Experience

Patient engagement, patient consumerism, transparency and the digital front door are the future of healthcare. Right now, these trends are disruptive, but in the future, they will be standard practice. Every other industry has seen consumerism change it fundamentally. Some fun examples: Blockbuster to Netflix, taxis to Uber/Lyft, Kodak to Shutterfly, brick-and-mortar retail to Amazon for, well, everything!

Patients as consumers are beginning to understand the organizations that combine technology and experience well, and those that don't. And they're choosing, when they have the option, to go with providers that make healthcare delivery flexible, mobile, digital and accessible—like every other industry.

Why Hasn't Healthcare Evolved?

Other industries have evolved to take advantage of the digital age. Kroger, Safeway and even Walmart now offer services to buy your groceries online and then drive to the store (you don't even have to get out of the car) to pick them up, or have them delivered to your home. And it's generally pretty inexpensive.

Healthcare is not even close to this. OK, I hear you, a hospital can't pick up its foundation and waddle to your house. Most hospitals are for short-term acute care (STAC) by definition, and were designed to resolve acute conditions. They have a purpose in treating quickly stabilize and the patients in their community. My point is not that they should be replaced, but that they need to evolve. As they become broader in treatment scope (whether appropriate or not), they haven't invested in patient-centered digital innovation, leading to inefficiencies in both care and payment, and little hope for improvement. Hospitals can do better, can't they? Think telemedicine, app-enabled software for remote monitoring and do-it-yourself lab kits through Amazon. Hospitals could do a lot of things remotely, and it could change the way patients get healthcare, just like how it has changed the way consumers shop (what did you buy from Amazon last week?).

But how is healthcare *not* like retail? Well, compared to retail, healthcare transactions lack convenient access and options. Healthcare still hasn't achieved true transparency in pricing. Imagine ordering your healthcare services online—but the prices are not listed. Healthcare billing and payment processes are also still antiquated and complicated. Consumers would *not* stand for getting a paper bill in the mail for their grocery delivery—much less getting it a couple months after they've already eaten all of those groceries.

That's where healthcare is right now.

Perhaps healthcare hasn't evolved because it's still relatively new to digitization. Consider that eBay started online auctions in 1995; Amazon started online book sales the same year, and Netflix started its streaming service in 2010. Meanwhile, back in healthcare-land, hospitals didn't really fully begin transitioning from paper to digital until 2008, when Centers for Medicare & Medicaid Services (CMS) launched its electronic health record (EHR) Incentive Payment Program.[287] Sure, hospitals may have had an order entry system or electronic medication administration, but they were pocketed systems with low adoption. There was very little use of electronics or digitized media in a holistic or integrated manner; workflows still involved some sort of paper chart or bill. Even though digitization of clinical records began in the 2000s, adoption was slow until the EHR incentive program was launched, and paper still lived on in many areas. In 2008, when the program began, only 9 percent of acute care hospitals used EHRs. It took until 2017 to get 96 percent of hospitals to use EHRs (figure 7.1).

Figure 7.1 Non-federal Acute Care Hospital Electronic Health Record Adoption, 2008–2017

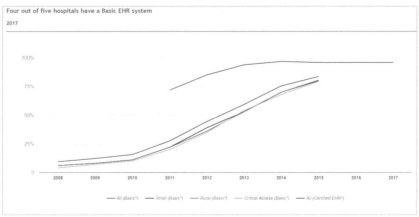

Four out of five hospitals have a Basic EHR system

2017

Source: "Non-federal Acute Care Hospital Electronic Health Record Adoption." Health IT Dashboard. The Office of the National Coordinator for Health Information Technology. (n.d.) Accessed September 27, 2019.
https://dashboard.healthit.gov/quickstats/pages/FIG-Hospital-EHR-Adoption.php

It took hospitals a significant amount of time to go paperless. One of my mantras at the hospital was "death to paper." After we went live, I would scour the halls looking for workflows on paper and eliminate them—they were error-prone, misplaced and terribly inefficient. But if you ask a physician, most would have stuck to paper charting because it's just easier than standing up a new system and the change management that comes with it. But paper charting is dangerous, inefficient and siloed.

Despite those problems, the industry took a while to break the paper habit and move forward to digital records. Perhaps that's why healthcare still isn't as up-to-speed on the digital consumer experience as other industries. Healthcare transactions still involve a lot of manual processes, navigating layers of complex regulations, and fragmented data and workflow.[288]

The Digital Front Door

The patient as consumer—especially the millennial generation—is attracted to organizations in the healthcare space that not only deliver good care but also offer easy accessibility. For example, instead of *calling* a provider to make an appointment, you can access an online appointment scheduler on your phone, find a time that works for you, and schedule yourself. (Some organizations, like Kaiser Permanente, have been doing appointment scheduling via online or mobile app for a while).

A 2019 TransUnion Healthcare survey of 2,500 patients found Millennials are also paying more attention to healthcare costs.[289] And the younger the patient is, the more engaged they are in understanding costs prior to seeking treatment. For example, only 65 percent of Baby Boomers (born 1946–1964) conducted some form of research on healthcare costs compared to 85 percent of Generation Z (born 1995 or after). Likewise, only 34 percent of Baby Boomers said having clear information on out-of-pocket costs would impact their decision to use a healthcare provider compared to 65 percent of Gen Zers.[290]

Consider if the mobile services available to you were even more expansive. What if you could load your health profile on your phone, type in what you needed an appointment for, and then do some comparison shopping? For example, inputting preferences like: "I've got BlueCross BlueShield insurance of Illinois and I don't want to travel more than 15 miles from my current location to get an appointment with a provider. But if I can save $500 or more by going outside that service area, I would drive an hour to save those bucks."

Bits and pieces of this kind of information exist—for example, most commercial insurers have a way for you to search for in-network providers in your geographic area. And sites, such as MDsave (mdsave.com), let you search for procedures by price. Payers and patient navigation firms are beginning to feed content to mobile platforms to steer patients to participating organizations, resulting in savings and consumer satisfaction. But there really isn't an easy-to-use, all-in-one solution yet.

For example, what if you could create a profile, like you are able to do for the airline industry, where you can put your preferences in: "I prefer an aisle seat in the front of the plane; I typically never check baggage; I only take one carry-on; I prefer a mobile ticket to a paper one." It's all in your profile, which makes it easy to onboard you.

What if you had the same opportunity in healthcare to have all that information in your profile and accessible? "I'm Jonathan; my primary doctor is Dr. Samson; my insurance is UnitedHealthcare; this is my preferred hospital; this is my preferred imaging center; this is my preferred lab; and this is my preferred pharmacy." It could state your preference for urgent care centers over emergency departments, that you want a board-certified physician, your preferred method of payment is via credit card, you want to auto-pay the bills once they hit the account, and you prefer to wait no longer than three days for an appointment. Every piece of accessing, interacting with and paying your healthcare could be at your fingertips—through your phone.

These types of innovations are not science fiction. They are real, they are here, and they are in use right now. For example, Vanderbilt University Medical Center (VUMC) has developed a flu tool that uses a series of questions to help patients determine if they or a family member have the flu.[291] The tool has been adapted for use with Amazon's cloud-based voice service, Alexa. Patients simply say, "Alexa, open flu tool," to access the application. It then uses a decision tree, based on a series of yes/no questions, to help patients analyze their symptoms and figure out what level of care they need.[292] In a 2018 article in *My Southern Health*, Jill Austin, Chief Marketing Officer for VUMC said:

> Voice search is one of the most important trends in consumer experience right now. It is predicted that voice search will account for at least half of all online searches by 2020. The Echo Dot was the biggest selling product of all products sold on Amazon during the past holiday season. Providing health information through voice is another way we are meeting people's needs through the channel of their choice.[293]

As of early 2019, Amazon was working with a number of different healthcare companies to develop healthcare-related tools, including:

- A voice program to allow Cigna members to manage health goals and earn wellness incentives
- A tool that lets people check the status of home delivery prescriptions (Express Scripts)
- A program that enables caregivers of patients at Boston Children's Hospital to communicate with physicians post-surgery
- Voice tools that help customers search for nearby facilities, including urgent care centers, and schedule same-day appointments (Providence St. Joseph Health and Atrium Health)
- A program that helps people manage diabetes by asking about their most recent blood sugar reading and blood sugar trends (Livongo)[294]

Hospitals need to be in front of these kinds of innovations in order to compete effectively and to be able to attract, delight and retain today's consumer. If providers don't have a digital front door—and offer the services behind it in a frictionless way—patients are going to migrate to those that do. Friction in access to clinical results, payment and other important pieces of information will not be acceptable to the digitally savvy patient. If patients can simply ask their phone to make a doctor's appointment for them, or to find the most affordable urgent care center near them, why would they go anywhere else?

Hospitals have to be digitally accessible. Patients need to be able to find your location, your hours, your wait time for appointments, the cost of care, their out-of-pocket and how other consumers are rating you. If your hospital or health system doesn't exist digitally, for a lot of patients (especially Millennials and younger) you won't exist at all. Think OpenTable or Great Clips—they have apps showing where they're located, when they're open, what the costs are, and—most importantly—what the wait is and how to get ahead in line. Some hospitals are exploring this space but the industry itself is behind in terms of adoption-at-large.

Unfortunately, most hospitals are not well-positioned for delivering a meaningful digital experience. When I talk about this topic, providers get really nervous. I've seen their eyes get as big as saucers. They say, "Hmm, yeah, we haven't really thought about that … but our patients are loyal … we'll be OK." Other industries have already revolutionized the consumer experience, and yet it's just starting to become a planned strategy in healthcare.

And guess what? Unless you meet the patient as payer, they are ultimately going to tell you, "Hey, I've loved you forever but I'm going to go to the place down the street … it's just easier."

This is true especially, I believe, for the millennial generation, which isn't really attached to much of anything. They're going to go where it's easiest and most convenient for them. That's the American way now, folks. They won't have this ongoing relationship they've had with their family doctor like previous generations did.

And don't even get me started on the friction (or difficulty) involved in payment … and you want to talk about choice? Patients are going to vote with their feet when they choose a provider to go to, all based on how easy it is to set up an appointment and pay—the care is table stakes, gang. One survey found 50 percent of respondents would leave their current doctor for a better digital experience.[295] The same study found 59 percent of U.S. consumers expect their healthcare digital consumer experience to be similar to their retail experience.[296]

The aforementioned TransUnion Healthcare survey revealed some other interesting facts about how cost information and the digital experience impact patient behavior:

- Three out of four patients (75 percent) research healthcare costs, with 24 percent relying on provider information, 22 percent searching online, 18 percent using an insurance website, and 12 percent checking with family or friends
- Six out of 10 patients (62 percent) said knowing costs in advance impacted the likelihood of pursuing care
- Nearly half (49 percent) chose their healthcare provider based on cost information
- Nearly two-thirds (65 percent) said they would be more likely to make a partial payment prior to treatment if they received an estimate of expenses at the time of service[297]

The younger the patient, the more likely they were to research costs in advance, and to consider costs in deciding which provider to choose. This is why the idea of a digital front door is such a huge disruptor.

Odd Couples

Another disruptive—but not necessarily innovative— strategy for increasing revenue is to increase market share through mergers and acquisitions (M&A). Healthcare has seen historic levels of M&A activity in recent years, both in terms of numbers of deals and the value of those deals (figure 7.2). The largest amount of M&A activity was in 2017, and 2018 saw the largest deal size. Kaufman Hall, which tracks M&A activity in the healthcare space, reported the average seller size by revenue increased from a high of $409 million in 2018 to an average of $597 million in the second quarter of 2019.[298]

The impact of these megamergers means more industry consolidation, the growth of large, regional hospital systems and the expansion of even larger national healthcare systems.

Figure 7.2 Announced Hospital Consolidations, 2006–2018

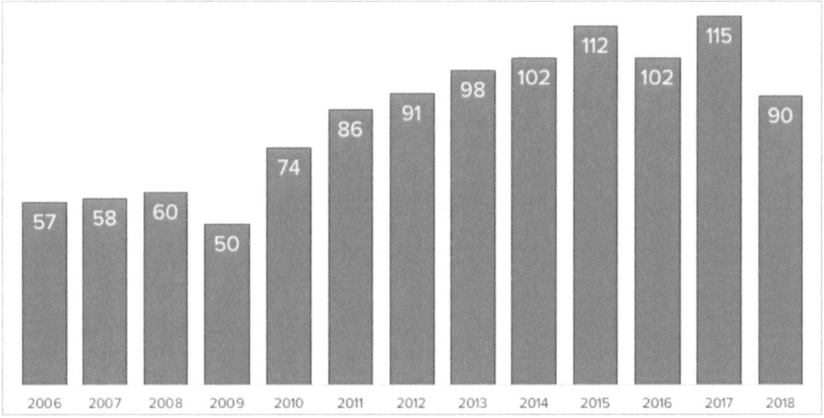

Source: "Hospital Consolidation: Trends, Impacts and Outlook." The National Institute for Health Care Management (NIHCM) Foundation. April 2019. Accessed September 18, 2019. https://www.nihcm.org/categories/hospital-consolidation-trends-impacts-outlook

There's some nuance to the activity that's happening in the acute care space as well. Census data shows the number of nonfederal, community, nonprofit hospitals decreased by 15 percent between 1975 (n = 3,339) and 2015 (n = 2,845), while the number of for-profit hospitals increased by 33 percent, from 775 in 1975 to 1,034 in 2015.[299] M&A activity is happening in both traditional and nontraditional ways. Acute care systems are merging but some unexpected partnerships are developing as well. Let's look at some of the M&A activity that's happening—and whether or not it's benefitting the U.S. healthcare system as a whole.

Acute Care Mergers and Acquisitions

There's been growing M&A activity in the acute care space. A few of the significant acute care deals over the past couple of years include:

- In April 2018, midwestern health systems Advocate Health Care (Illinois) and Aurora Health Care (Wisconsin) merged to create Advocate Aurora Health.[300] Advocate Aurora Health includes more than 500 locations, more than 8,000 physicians and 70,000 employees, making it the 10th largest, not-for-profit healthcare system in the U.S.[301]

- In November 2018, LifePoint Health and RCCH HealthCare merged under the name of LifePoint Health.[302] The combined, now privately held organization, is affiliated with regional health systems, physician practices, outpatient centers and post-acute facilities in over 80 communities across the U.S.[303]

- In February 2019, Dignity Health and Catholic Health Initiatives merged to create one megasystem—CommonSpirit Health. The resulting healthcare system is worth $29 billion, spans 21 states and includes 142 hospitals.[304]

- In March 2019, Beth Israel Deaconess and Lahey Health combined to form Beth Israel Lahey Health, now the second-largest health system in Massachusetts.[305] The new system includes 800 primary care physicians, 3,500 specialty physicians, 4 academic and teaching hospitals, 8 community hospitals, orthopedic and behavioral health specialty hospitals, and comprehensive ambulatory and urgent care centers.[306]

The irony here is all of the M&A activity hasn't necessarily been good for the revenue cycle—or for the patient/ consumer. You would *think*—if you partnered with another hospital or health system that processes and systems would become somewhat more efficient and also less expensive, and the costs of delivering care would subsequently come down, and you would ultimately realize economies of scale.

You would think one of the main considerations *driving* mergers and acquisitions would be the potential for more efficiency and the ability to control costs. You would think M&A would be a *good* thing: "Hey, we can serve more people ... we can get more volume ... we can make a bigger impact."

From a revenue cycle perspective, you would think with more infrastructure, more staff, more IT folks, you could become more efficient in billing. It would be understandable to think *that's* what would happen, and everybody would be sitting around singing "Kumbaya" and roasting marshmallows.

But that's not what's happening. In fact, I haven't seen a single study quantifying greater efficiency *has* happened. Instead, the opposite is happening. Instead, "Hospital A" merged with "Hospital B" into "System C"—and System C is charging higher prices than either Hospital A or Hospital B did. The profit margin may be going up—but the expenses aren't going down. One would think it was about survival or community but—based on the data— it appears to be about profitability and good ol'-fashioned capitalism.

An analysis conducted by the Nicholas C. Petris Center found the price of an average hospital stay increased between 11 and 54 percent in metropolitan areas with high rates of hospital consolidations (figure 7.3).

Figure 7.3 Hospital Consolidation and Rising Costs

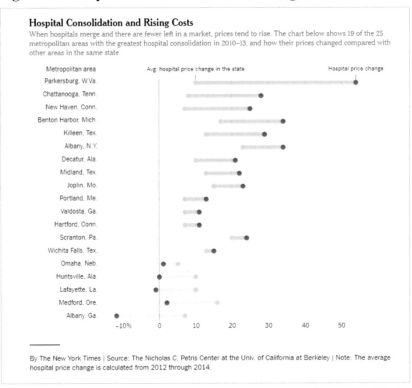

Hospital Consolidation and Rising Costs

When hospitals merge and there are fewer left in a market, prices tend to rise. The chart below shows 19 of the 25 metropolitan areas with the greatest hospital consolidation in 2010–13, and how their prices changed compared with other areas in the same state.

By The New York Times | Source: The Nicholas C. Petris Center at the Univ. of California at Berkeley | Note: The average hospital price change is calculated from 2012 through 2014.

Source: Reed Abelson. "When Hospitals Merge to Save Money, Patients Often Pay More." The New York Times. November 14, 2018. Accessed September 19, 2019. https://www.nytimes.com/2018/11/14/health/hospital-mergers-health-care-spending.html

The Health Care Cost Institute (HCCI) analyzed the concentration of hospital markets in the U.S. and the resultant impacts on healthcare prices.[307] The analysis showed M&A activity is creating larger systems and driving increased concentration in hospital markets, which, in turn, is reducing competition and driving prices up. Interestingly, areas with lower volumes (rural areas) and limited competition also saw higher prices.

A 2018 NCCI Insights review of research on consolidation came to a similar conclusion. NCCI Insights' analysis found:

- Healthcare consolidation improves integration of care and reduces duplication of clinical services. Mergers can lead to operating cost reductions of 15–30 percent for acquired hospitals.
- Reductions in hospital operating costs do not translate into price decreases. Research to date shows hospital mergers increase the average price of hospital services by 6–8 percent.[308]

So ... operating costs went down, but prices went up? Why aren't margins increasing? Help me understand *that* math. With studies like these coming out, it's no wonder the possible downsides of megamergers in the healthcare industry are starting to attract the attention of consumers, legislators and the president.

On June 24, 2019, President Trump issued the *Executive Order on Improving Price and Quality Transparency in American Healthcare to Put Patients First.*[309] Among many other directives, the executive order stated:

> Within 180 days of the date of this order, the Secretary of Health and Human Services, in consultation with the Attorney General and the Federal Trade Commission, shall issue a report describing the manners in which the Federal Government or the private sector are impeding healthcare price and quality transparency for patients, and providing recommendations for eliminating these impediments in a way that promotes competition.[310]

Because of the call for the involvement of the Federal Trade Commission (FTC), it's been suggested this directive is—in part—a response to increasing concern over provider consolidation.[311]

The regulators involved in these transactions are also starting to pay attention. When the California Department of Justice (DOJ) approved the CommonSpirit Health merger, they included a number of conditions meant to preserve the community benefit. It was like the judge was saying "I get that you are going to try to do this to make more money and better serve the community, but just to make sure, this is what you are going to have to do if your two organizations are going to become one." Many of the conditions set upon CommonSpirit Health by the California DOJ were related to preserving access to care, including:

- CommonSpirit Health is directed to create a Homeless Health Initiative in California to support delivery of treatment and services to hospitalized individuals experiencing homelessness
- The organization is directed to allocate $20 million, over six fiscal years, working with counties, cities and community-based organizations to "colocate, coordinate and integrate health, behavioral health, safety and wellness services with housing and other social services"
- Beginning in 2019, Dignity Health's California hospitals are directed to offer a 100 percent discount to patients making up to 250 percent of the federal poverty limit (financial assistance policy)[312]

In a similar fashion, when the merger of Beth Israel Deaconess and Lahey Health was approved by the Massachusetts attorney general, conditions were put in place to protect consumers. The report issued by the Massachusetts Health Policy Commission estimated the merger could potentially increase healthcare costs by up to $251 million annually.[313] To make sure that didn't happen, the Massachusetts attorney general set conditions for the newly merged system that included the following:

- A seven-year price cap (i.e., the new system's price increases are to remain below the state's annual healthcare cost growth benchmark of 3.1 percent)
- Participation in MassHealth, the state's combined Medicaid and Children's Health Insurance Program
- $71.6 million in investments supporting healthcare services for low-income and underserved communities in Massachusetts[314]

Another variation on the theme of consolidation is the story of Ballad Health. Ballad Health was formed in February 2018 by the merger of not-for-profit hospitals Wellmont Health Systems and Mountain States Health Alliance in northeastern Tennessee.[315] The merged system includes 21 hospitals spanning southwest Virginia, northeast Tennessee and parts of Kentucky and North Carolina. According to the Nashville *Tennessean*, the new system "now functions as the only hospital system for the majority of residents—about 1.2 million people—in a geographic area the size of New Jersey."[316]

Since the merger, the new health system has consolidated high-level services in Ballad Health's Johnson City, Tennessee, hospital. This has included downgrades to a hospital in Kingsport, Tennessee—the Kingsport hospital's neonatal intensive care unit has been moved to Johnson City, and the Kingsport trauma center has been downgraded.[317]

The merger was not necessarily undertaken for the purpose of increasing market share, but instead was purely a cost-savings play. The centralized facility is a 30-minute plus drive south of the Kingsport facility. Since the move was meant to lower costs by centralizing services, they figured folks would not mind the drive. Think again—the community was not pleased. The system is facing significant negative feedback surrounding "long wait times and unsafe conditions."[318]

An analysis of the situation that appeared from the Healthcare Financial Management Association (HFMA) noted:

> There's an elephant in the room. Like it or not, the provision of healthcare requires the consumption of economic resources just like the production of food, clothing or cars. Therefore, there are some inherent trade-offs that have to be made if we want lower healthcare costs. Healthcare is a high fixed and step fixed cost business . . . reducing the cost of care per unit means increasing the utilization of these fixed assets in a clinically appropriate manner. So, in the instance of the Ballad merger, the combined entity owns three hospitals in Wise County, Virginia. Two of those three hospitals had an average daily census of less than five patients per day.[319]

In Ballad Health's case, the merger was approved despite the FTC's objections due to a Tennessee law which allows a merger to bypass FTC antimonopoly rules via a "certificate of public advantage," or COPA.[320] Under the COPA law, the public benefits of the merger must outweigh the cost of the monopoly.[321] Ballad Health's COPA specifies the new system will invest $308 million in public health measures and it will not close any rural hospitals for five years.[322]

These kinds of conditions may become the new MO for healthcare megamergers. A caveat of capitalism is that monopolies are essentially bad for the market because competition is what works to drive prices down. As the healthcare industry consolidates, the market competition is disappearing, so new ways of ensuring affordability—such as conditions on mergers—may be the only way to make sure cost savings gained by providers are passed down to consumers. My point is: Pay attention people. Big business and low cost are not aligning in healthcare and we're all paying for it.

Nontraditional Mergers and Acquisitions

As the healthcare industry consolidates, other types of M&A—involving unexpected partnerships and mergers—are happening as well. In December 2018 health insurer Cigna acquired pharmacy benefits manager (PBM) Express Scripts in a $54 billion deal.[323] Cigna estimated it will realize more than $600 million in administrative savings as a result of its takeover of Express Scripts.[324] Unfortunately, given Big Pharma's track record, these savings likely end up as dividend payments to shareholders versus cost savings passed on to employers and consumers.[325] Cigna's marketing of the deal promises that together, the combined companies "are positioned to deliver better care and expanded choices and to drive down healthcare costs."[326] Only time will tell if lower costs are actually an outcome of this merger.

Meanwhile, a 2018 survey of large employers by the National Business Group on Health (NBGH) conducted prior to the Cigna-Express Scripts merger found only 1 out of 4 respondents (26 percent) was optimistic about the outcome of mergers between insurers and PBMs; 56 percent were skeptical; and 18 percent believed such mergers would lead to increased costs.[327]

Just prior to the Cigna-Express Scripts merger, CVS Health acquired Aetna for $70 billion.[328] This deal combines an insurer (Aetna) with CVS's PBM services, retail pharmacies and walk-in clinics (see more about that in the section on retail clinics, below). CVS heralded the CVS-Aetna merger as "marking the start of transforming the consumer health experience."[329] This is bizarre and unprecedented ... a retail pharmacy *buying* an insurance company?! Wow. CVS Health president and CEO Larry J. Merlo said, "By delivering the combined capabilities of our two leading organizations, we will transform the consumer health experience and build healthier communities through a new innovative healthcare model that's local, easier to use, less expensive and puts consumers at the center of their care."[330] Will Merlo's prediction of lower cost, consumer-oriented healthcare come to pass? I'd put my betting chips here versus hospital megamergers, but we'll see.

The name for this type of M&A activity, between companies in adjacent industries, is called "convergence," according to a blog post by Deloitte vice chairman of U.S. life sciences, Bill Copeland.[331] Sounds like a title to some sci-fi movie. Observing the Cigna-Express Scripts merger and similar M&A activity, Copeland goes on to say "convergence is a form of innovation only if the combined company's product or service offerings break the preexisting competitive and economic barriers

175

and constraints to offer something that has greater value to the customer for less cost and complexity."[332]

The value proposition of convergence lies in solving problems that customers can't solve for themselves, Copeland said: "For a hundred years, we thought it was enough to replace the hip, remove the cancer, fix the leaky valve, help the patient breathe or control blood-sugar levels. Alas, the consumer really wants much more."[333]

Retail Medicine

Twenty years ago it might have sounded odd to put a walk-in medical clinic in a grocery store or pharmacy. Not anymore. The number of retail clinics in the U.S. has surged over the past 10 years. A report by Accenture estimated there were only 351 retail clinics in the U.S. in 2006.[334] There are now estimated to be more than 2,800 retail healthcare clinics in the U.S. (figure 7.4).

Figure 7.4 Growth of U.S. Retail Healthcare Clinics

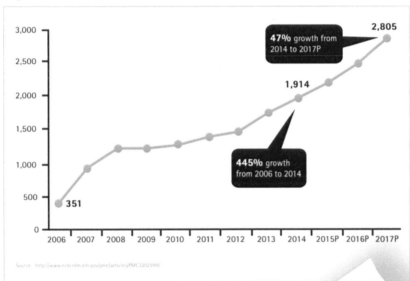

Source: "Number of U.S. Retail Health Clinics Will Surpass 2,800 by 2017." Accenture Forecasts. Accenture. November 12, 2015. Accessed September 19, 2019. https://newsroom.accenture.com/news/number-of-us-retail-health-clinics-will-surpass-2800-by-2017-accenture-forecasts.htm

Pharmacy chain CVS, for example, offers 1,100 MinuteClinic locations, focusing on low-acuity conditions such as immunizations and colds.[335] The pharmacy chain is planning a more aggressive rollout of healthcare services in the next two years: by the end of 2021, CVS intends to launch 1,500 HealthHUBs in its stores.[336] While the MinuteClinics typically have one or two exam rooms, the HealthHUBs will have three to four exam rooms and will focus on services such as chronic disease management.[337] Walgreens, with their healthcare clinics, are also in the game—between them and CVS, they have over 75 percent of the retail medicine market.[338]

It's no surprise consumers have been flocking to retail clinics. Retail clinics offer all of the conveniences traditional healthcare doesn't: seven-day-a-week accessibility, hours beyond the traditional 8 a.m. to 5 p.m., transparency in pricing, affordable care and the ability to walk in for services without a prior appointment.

How is this disruption impacting hospitals? Retail clinics (and urgent care centers) are attracting patients who might otherwise have gone to the hospital for treatment. And that's a good thing—patients selecting the right level of care, which helps lower overall costs. But the convenience of retail clinics and urgent care clinics are also drawing patients away from primary care physicians (PCP). A Health Care Cost Institute analysis found primary care physician visits decreased by 18 percent between 2012 and 2016—a change that could be due, in part, to patients taking their visits elsewhere.[339] I believe hospitals are starting to see a bleed-off, or referral leaks, to retail clinics.

A primary care physician may have had a patient for a very long time, but the referral pattern may suddenly shift because the patient is going to the grocery store, or Walgreens or CVS to get their care. And now they may only go to the hospital when they need surgery or emergency care. It's easier for the patient as well—retail clinics are convenient in care delivery and offer two very important consumer delights: access and payment. I think hospital outpatient volumes are starting to go down due to these nontraditional types of services. And hospitals are very aware of it.

That's why some hospitals are trying to protect themselves by building urgent care clinics and physician clinics as far out as they can to widen their scope. But hospitals can't afford to build 9 or 10 more clinics to keep up, from an expense standpoint. In this case, it seems the more viable solution is partnership (i.e., "if you can't beat 'em, join 'em"). By affiliating or partnering with retail clinics, hospitals and hospital systems are able to increase market share through referrals, establish more connections with consumers and experiment with nontraditional ways of delivering care.[340]

And in fact, CVS MinuteClinics do affiliate with local hospital systems in the communities CVS serves. It's a win-win partnership. CVS leverages these hospital affiliations in its marketing, which helps to establish the medical bona fides of its clinics; at the same time, hospitals and health systems benefit from the visibility and referrals the MinuteClinics generate through the increased foot traffic. As of this writing, the CVS MinuteClinic website (https://www.cvs.com/minuteclinic/why-choose-us/quality-clinical-affiliations) lists affiliations with 54 hospitals and health systems across 26 states.[341]

Direct-to-Provider Contracting

Some large, self-insured employers are attempting to curb costs by cutting out the middleman (insurance) and contracting directly with providers. When employers contract directly with providers or accountable care organizations (ACO), they have more control over the design of the health benefit plan. They also have the potential to lower the cost of care.

This arrangement can benefit providers, as well. Providers have a guaranteed group of patients and revenue they can count on (typically there are no pre-authorizations, denials, etc. to worry about), giving providers more flexibility in pursuing positive patient outcomes. In some contracts, providers can even share in the cost savings if they deliver care at a cost that's less than the employer budgeted.[342]

A 2019 survey conducted by the National Business Group on Health (NBGH) found 9 percent of large employers plan to implement directly contracted primary care models in 2020, and an additional 17 percent of large employers are considering implementing directly contracted primary care models by 2022.[343]

One interesting example of this is the direct contracting arrangement between General Motors (GM) (the automobile manufacturer) and the Henry Ford Health System (not to be confused with GM's competitor in the automotive space, the Ford Motor Company). The Henry Ford Health System announced the arrangement in August 2018. Under the agreement, GM employees can choose the ConnectedCare plan option, which gives them access to a network of more than 3,000 providers, including PCPs and specialists.

The ConnectedCare plan will offer features such as same-day or next-day appointments with PCPs; virtual visit options; regular wellness exams; monitoring of chronic conditions; and preventive screenings for conditions such as colon cancer, breast cancer and depression.[344] According to the announcement, "The health system will also help members choose the right care options, such as walk-in clinics rather than emergency rooms for minor illness and injury. In addition to monitoring member health outcomes, Henry Ford will measure overall customer satisfaction."[345]

ConnectedCare will also offer digital patient experience options, such as the ability to "access several virtual visit options at participating clinics, view test results, message their doctor, request prescription renewals and pay bills through their smartphone, tablet or personal computer."[346] This arrangement seems to have all the right pieces in place for controlling costs: a seamless provider network, a digital front door, and an emphasis on value-based care and patient satisfaction. It will be interesting to see where this goes over the next few years.

Another variation on direct-to-provider contracting is the concept of Centers of Excellence (COE). With COE, rather than contracting out primary care, a large employer will identify a number of common procedures their members have and then identify providers that offer those procedures at the lowest cost, with the best outcomes.

Walmart is one of the leaders in implementing this strategy. Walmart has identified a number of high-cost procedures and conditions and contracted with specific providers and specialists to perform those procedures. Procedures covered by Walmart's COE program, per their website, include:

- Certain heart surgeries, like cardiac bypass and valve replacements.
- Certain spine surgeries, like spinal fusions and removal of spinal discs (discectomy).
- Hip and knee joint replacements.

- Breast, lung, colorectal, prostate and blood cancers (including myeloma, lymphoma and leukemia). Patients with these diagnoses may have their medical records reviewed by Mayo Clinic specialists to evaluate the benefit of an on-site visit to a COE. If an on-site visit is recommended, the visit will be covered at 100 percent and will include a travel allowance.
- Certain weight-loss surgeries, like gastric bypass and gastric sleeve procedures.
- Organ and tissue transplants (except kidney, cornea and intestinal), ventricular assist devices (VAD) and total artificial hearts and CAR-T cell therapy.
- Outpatient radiology.[347]

Walmart partners with the high-quality providers to provide these services to enrolled Walmart employees. For example, Walmart has partnered with the Mayo Clinic in Minnesota, Florida and Arizona for transplants and cancer care, and with the Cleveland Clinic in Ohio for cardiac surgery.[348] Walmart employees enrolled in eligible plans are sent to these locations for treatment. In most cases, Walmart provides travel and lodging expenses for the patient and a companion caregiver. Why would Walmart do this? Because they realize that with a large employee base, it's worth it to send them to providers that consistently offer the best outcomes at the lowest cost. There are huge efficiencies in having patients go to a place that does 100,000 knees a year—and all they do is knees—versus a hospital that maybe does 500 knees a year. They've narrowly defined where their employees can go for these services (except in case of emergency care), but the trade-off is a better outcome, because these specialists are really good at what they do.

Consumer choice may be limited, but the outcomes and cost savings have outweighed the restricted access, according to a study published in the *Harvard Business Review* and reported by the Advisory Board:

- Of the more than 5,000 Walmart employees who had participated in the program at the time of the study, 95 percent said they were "satisfied" or "very satisfied" with the care and overall experience

- One employee said it was "the best medical experience of my life"

- Walmart employees who had spinal surgery at a COE site spent 14 percent less time in the hospital and faced a 95 percent lower risk of readmission than those treated elsewhere

- Although surgery at a COE site costs Walmart about 8 percent more than elsewhere, employees are able to return to work earlier and are less likely to be readmitted to the hospital[349]

Narrow networks—like the Walmart COE program—appear to be growing in popularity. A 2017 McKinsey analysis of the individual health insurance exchange market found the proportion of offerings featuring narrowed networks increased from 48 percent in 2014 to 53 percent in 2017.[350] I'm inclined to believe healthcare purchasers are basing their plan decisions on premium costs—not the network—and then seeing if there is any fallout. Here is a hint—there's not.

A 2018 *Kaiser Health News* article on narrow-network plans noted such plans can generate cost savings.[351] The article quoted Paul Ginsburg, a healthcare economist at the Brookings Institution as saying: "Narrow networks are a trade-off. They can be successful when done well. At a time when we need to find ways to control rising healthcare costs, narrow networks are one legitimate strategy."[352] The article also quoted Mike Kreidler, Washington state's insurance commissioner, as saying, "People have voted with their feet, moving to more affordable choices like HMOs but they won't tolerate draconian restrictions."[353]

Other Disruptors on the Horizon

Another "odd couple" disruptor on the horizon is the new joint venture between Amazon, Berkshire Hathaway and J.P. Morgan. The three partners have established a nonprofit called Haven, which is designed to improve healthcare delivery for the three organizations' combined 1.2 million employees.[354] The strategies they are going to use to improve healthcare haven't yet been completely revealed, although possibilities include a focus on employee wellness, employee steerage (steering employees to low-cost, highly effective providers and/or treatments), population health management and possible direct-to-provider contracting (see above). It's all still rather mysterious at this point, as the partners have been very close-lipped about what exactly they are up to. Per Haven's website, the organization is going to improve healthcare in the following ways:

> We are pursuing a number of commonsense fixes, as well as innovative approaches, to address issues like making primary care easier to access, insurance benefits simpler to understand and easier to use, and prescription drugs more affordable. We are also looking at new ways to use data and technology to make the overall health care system better.[355]

I believe this partnership has the potential to completely and totally revolutionize healthcare. Each partner brings something critical to the table:

- J.P. Morgan has a banking and transaction infrastructure
- Berkshire Hathaway brings a capital structure
- Amazon brings a distribution mechanism

Amazon already delivers things better than any other business in the world. They know what the consumer wants and they have completely mastered and streamlined that experience. So whatever these employees want for their healthcare, there's no better locomotive than Amazon to deliver it. And many people already trust Amazon—even to provide healthcare services they don't offer yet. A 2018 survey by LendEDU found 35.8 percent of consumers who had purchased something from Amazon in the past 30 days said they would be open to using a health insurance plan created by Amazon (Amazon does not currently offer a health insurance plan).[356] In addition, 55 percent of respondents said they would trust Amazon as their pharmacy to provide them with both over-the-counter and prescription medication.[357]

Amazon is entering the healthcare arena with a stellar reputation for delivering what the consumer wants—sometimes before the consumer even knows they want it. That's why Amazon's entry into healthcare and pharmaceuticals is making a lot of traditional healthcare organizations nervous. I anticipate Haven's future is very bright. They're going to make great strides in delivering on the Triple Aim internally, and with that achievement they will revolutionize delivery and cost to a (very) large employee base. Then they'll package it up and sell it to eager employers looking to revolutionize healthcare for their employees as well.

The nontraditional approaches to healthcare I've described in this chapter are mostly macrolevel disruptions and innovations. The examples shown have amplified significant improvements in access, quality and cost for the consumer. We're seeing consumers migrate to more convenient, lower-cost options. But where does revenue cycle management fit in this disruption? RCM professionals don't necessarily have a lot of say in whether their organization becomes part of a larger M&A deal or a partner in direct-to-provider contracting. RCM professionals are, however, able to influence how a provider manages revenue at the individual and organizational level. They have the ability to remove friction in payment from patient and payer. Managing patient as payer and protecting earned revenue from all payers is a primary, strategic objective. Chapter 8 is about new ways of doing business that RCM leadership can control—which can bring immediate results in stopping revenue leakage and collecting unrealized revenue.

CHAPTER 8

PAYMENT STRATEGIES THAT WORK

In the introduction to this book I reflected on one of my favorite sayings: "If you do what you've always done, you'll get what you've always gotten." This applies to a lot of things—from healthcare delivery models to payment models. But this saying is particularly relevant to the patient financial experience and the new state of revenue cycle management (RCM) in the healthcare industry.

When I was an RCM leader at a hospital, I was allocated a limited amount of capital and operational resources which I had to deploy in the best way I could, knowing I wasn't going to get everything. I tried to focus on the low-hanging fruit, knowing I was still probably leaving money on the table. I was constrained by limited resources, traditional processes and to some degree, lack of access to information that would have helped me do a better job— like information about how many unrealized dollars really were on the table. We did the best we could with what we had—there were solutions out there, but they were disparate in connectivity, design and delivery. They barely drove enough yield to justify the cost. That's most certainly not the case now: there are tremendous opportunities to transform the revenue cycle through cost-effective technologies. They elevate the RCM team to work effectively— like analysts, instead of processors. It is the future.

The RCM game has changed. It's no longer about yesterday's version of a biller, who spent tedious hours reviewing paper claims, making corrections to fields and resubmitting claim forms to the payer. It's not about looking at Excel spreadsheets, either. If you're still doing that, it's like driving a Pinto, circa 1985. It may get you from point A to point B, but the mileage is poor and you aren't going to get to your destination efficiently.

The old ways no longer work. The new name of the game for RCM is about leveraging data—and not just data, but big data. What is big data? You know it when you see it, right? A definition I like is "extremely large data sets that may be analyzed computationally to reveal patterns, trends and associations, especially relating to human behavior and interactions."[358]

If you work in healthcare you're familiar with big data, which has been revolutionizing clinical care for some time now. Big data enables physicians with more effective clinical decision support tools. It's behind advances in genomics and precision medicine. And it helps inform best practices for population health.

Big data has the potential to revolutionize healthcare RCM in the same way it's already revolutionized the clinical side of healthcare. It has the potential to evolve the patient financial experience and help patients become smarter consumers. It can enable providers to treat on outcome, versus presentation. It has the potential to ensure payment is frictionless from patient and payer.

Other industries are using big data to customize shopping experiences for consumers. Amazon's recommendation engine is a great example. Sign into your Amazon account and on the very first page, you'll find "recommendations for you." The recommendations are based on your purchase history, items in your cart, items you have liked or rated in the past, and items that customers with similar purchase histories to yours have purchased.[359] Think about your own experience with Amazon.

How do you feel when Amazon suggests a movie, book or other product that suits your tastes, before you even knew to look for that product yourself? It's been estimated more than 35 percent of Amazon's sales are generated by the recommendation engine,[360] which gives you an idea about how much consumers respond to and appreciate a personalized experience.

A 2016 Salesforce study found 51 percent of customers expect that by 2020, companies will anticipate their needs and make relevant suggestions.[361] The younger the consumer, the more willing they are to exchange data for personalization (figure 8.1).

Figure 8.1 Percentage of Consumers Who Are Willing to Share Personal Data

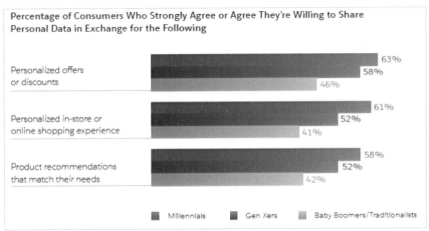

Percentage of Consumers Who Strongly Agree or Agree They're Willing to Share Personal Data in Exchange for the Following

Personalized offers or discounts: 63%, 58%, 46%

Personalized in-store or online shopping experience: 61%, 52%, 41%

Product recommendations that match their needs: 58%, 52%, 42%

■ Millennials ■ Gen Xers ■ Baby Boomers/Traditionalists

Source: Devon McGinnis. "Please Take My Data: Why Consumers Want More Personalized Marketing." Salesforce blog. December 2, 2016. Accessed October 2, 2019. https://www.salesforce.com/blog/2016/12/consumers-want-more-personalized-marketing.html

How does this apply to revenue cycle management in healthcare? Innovations in people, process and technology can ensure payer, provider and patient are empowered for frictionless payment. The clinical side of healthcare made the jump to leveraging big data years ago: RCM is well-positioned to make the same commitment.

Bottom line: If you're going to get paid in the 21st century, you're going to have to leverage big data and analytics to do it right.

In the following pages I describe three overarching strategies and a dozen specific best practices for incorporating data and analytics into your organization's RCM. It's been estimated "15 cents of every U.S. healthcare dollar goes toward revenue cycle inefficiencies."[362] Leveraging data and analytics to reduce or eliminate these inefficiencies gives hospitals and health systems the opportunity to improve the patient financial experience, improve revenue collection and reduce overall healthcare costs at the same time. It's a win-win-win for everyone involved.

The Big Picture

Before I get into the details of improving your RCM and minimizing revenue leakage, it's important to frame the strategies and best practices in the context of two overarching concepts—the three payment buckets and the patient account lifecycle.

The Three Payment Buckets

RCM is like that old carnival game, Plinko. You put the chips in at the top and they bounce through a set of pegs and end up in different buckets at the bottom. Likewise, patient payment accounts are always going to end up in one of three buckets: payment, charity or bad debt. The primary goal for RCM managers is to get as many chips in the payment bucket as possible, and second, to minimize bad debt and appropriately classify charity.

The Patient Account Lifecycle

Patient accounts have a (somewhat) predictable lifecycle (figure 8.2). In order to achieve frictionless RCM, each of the steps in the lifecycle has to be executed properly. If any of these steps aren't executed properly, the claim is not going to be paid correctly—or at all.

Figure 8.2 Patient Account Lifecycle (Commercially Insured)

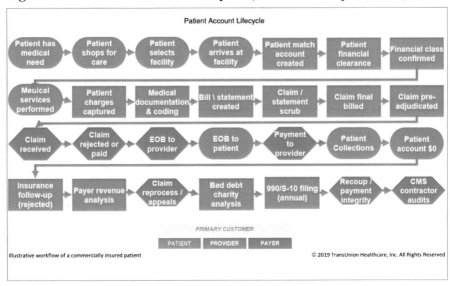

Source: Jonathan Wiik. TransUnion Healthcare. 2019.

Figure 8.2 shows what the patient payment lifecycle looks like for a patient with commercial insurance if all of the steps are executed correctly. Kind of looks like that Plinko game I mentioned, doesn't it? Every step on this chart is an opportunity for something to go wrong.

But if you can incorporate the strategies and best practices I describe in this chapter, you'll make it a lot more likely those Plinko chips will fall into the right buckets and your claims will go down the "happy path" instead of taking a turn that will affect your cash flow.

Strategy #1: Engage Patients Early

The back of the revenue cycle consistently blames the front end for errors. And the reason is the *information gathering* starts at the front end of the revenue cycle and if it's not verified correctly, can cause rework, errors and denials downstream. One in four denials directly results from errors at registration—for example, the registrar miskeying a piece of information or skipping critical data elements at registration.[363] If you get the first steps wrong, you will trip the whole rest of the way. The payment lifecycle can get really screwed up.

Not only is it important to get these first few steps right, it's also important to engage patients in the financial experience early in the revenue cycle. By engaging patients early in the process, you can identify erroneous or missing data elements early. This would result in increased patient satisfaction and point-of-service collections, as well as smoothing the way for a frictionless payment process. Before recent innovations, "matching" was the strategy. The patient would give you their ID and insurance, you would check it (hopefully in advance or before discharge) and rework what failed. Predictive analytics and real-time, mobile enrollment verification strategies exist today. Revenue cycles have the potential to meet patient and payer in the digital age and be on par with the airlines, grocery stores and giants like Amazon.

Verify the Patient's Identity and Address

The Problem: Patients don't call the hospital or the insurance company to update their personal information—ever. When they get married, move or change phone numbers, they do not pick up the phone to call the hospital and say, "Hey, for the next time I visit I want you to have the correct information." They update it when asked, at each visit to the provider. And that means the information on file is probably outdated since it's based on the patient's last visit. Compounded with the growing problem of patient identity theft it's clear patient identification errors are a significant issue requiring immediate attention.

Accurate patient identification is critical for both the clinical side and the business side of the house. A study of patient identification errors by the ECRI Institute found 9 percent of patient identification errors resulted in death or harm to the patient.[364]

Patient identification errors include both *false positives*, where two different patients' records are comingled, compromising the health data in each; and *false negatives*, where two sets of records that relate to the *same* patient are thought to relate to two *different* patients. This results in the creation of duplicate records, each of which is incomplete.[365] The consequence is compromised patient outcomes and big headaches when it comes time to file claims.

It's been estimated denied claims due to patient misidentification cost hospitals an average of $17.4 million each year.[366] This has become much more complicated with technology and disparate systems—even in the revenue cycle. The insurance company, the hospital electronic health record (EHR), the physician and another clinic may each have instances of a different spelling of a name, different policy numbers and other mismatched demographics.

The Solution: Most hospitals ask for an ID and date of birth and match from there, across many choices. It's critical to make sure you know the patient is who they say they are. You should have a robust identification process protocol in place that goes beyond two identifiers, and staff should be educated on how to better match patients to their medical record. Process audits can be helpful in verifying staff are, indeed, following identification process protocols. You can also leverage an ID solution to help you discover if the patient's name is spelled correctly, if they've moved, if they've gotten married or divorced since their last visit and other real-time demographics. An ID solution can provide information that's missing, such as a Social Security number or a mobile phone number.

An ID solution can also automate the process of ID verification—alerting staff when information changes or appears suspicious and matching patients to a Master Patient Index in a batch cleanup process. Patient-matching software can match the best instance of the data. Only the most powerful clearinghouses can see and reconcile those instances to the accuracy level required in today's digital era.

As they used to say on *The X-Files*, "the truth is out there." Only in this case, the *data* is out there. You might get tired of hearing me repeat this, but for ID verification, big data combined with analytic capabilities is a smart solution. It protects the patient and reduces downstream billing issues. It's table stakes.

Verify the Patient's Insurance Eligibility and Benefits

The Problem: Patients used to come in, give you an insurance card and say, "This is my insurance," and you would take a copy of it and hope, right? Unfortunately, a lot of things can go wrong in this scenario. The patient may not have their insurance card on them. The patient may have an old insurance card in their wallet that doesn't cover them anymore. The employer's group number or plan number may have changed, and the patient does not have the current information. Or, just as with ID verification, someone may be attempting healthcare identity theft—trying to access treatment on someone else's insurance benefits. Simply scanning an insurance card doesn't give the hospital much to fall back on when the claim is eventually denied.

Believe it or not, I still see this today: an insurance card is provided but insurance is not verified. That said, I'm inclined to believe most hospitals indeed have a very robust insurance eligibility process these days: they run eligibility and record the response. What most hospitals don't do is consistently, and more importantly, *act* on it. The information was checked, but behavior didn't change for the "schegistrar." (As I detailed in my first book, the schegistrar is a highly skilled expert in scheduling and registration. The schegistrar is key to engaging the patient in the patient financial experience at the front end for financial clearance.)

The Solution: Verification of insurance eligibility and benefits is another important piece that needs to be done right up front. I know—you're thinking "We do this already! This isn't innovative!" Yet providers waste time and resources resubmitting denied claims that weren't addressed and filed correctly. The first step in addressing this problem represents having a strong insurance verification technology in place. Second, it's mission critical to ensure staff are compliant with the standard workflow— every account, every time.

I can't overemphasize this point enough. You have invested in the technology, but is it the best? And are you leveraging it to its potential? In my health system RCM assessments, there are large gaps between what I see on paper and what I see in practice. Eligibility transactions have matured significantly in content and delivery, as have their application. Integration with the EHR, work queue development and rich, segmented, data sets can make all the difference in verifying insurance and securing accurate payment from patient and payer.

It should go without saying that best practices in this area include gathering as much insurance information as possible (electronically and seamlessly) before treatment is provided, as far in advance as you can. You have heard this and you may have directed the teams—but is it hardwired? Is it bulletproof from a people, process and technology standpoint? Can you look at *any* account in your organization and see the steps from verification to payment?

The majority of medical procedures performed are scheduled, elective procedures. I call these "no excuse patients." You know they're coming in advance. You have a choice: Verify their funding mechanisms or provide services for free. For the patients who you don't know about in advance, verification of their funding mechanism *must* happen before discharge. No excuses. Your number one cause of denials is eligibility. This means every time, for every patient, you need to capture and verify the insurance name and contact information, name of the insured (if not the patient), policy group number and patient ID number, effective start and end dates for the policy, etc. All of this information must be verified, documented and escalated as appropriate if the criteria aren't met.

The practice of capturing, verifying and documenting this information should already be in place at your organization. An innovative approach to this process builds on that foundation through implementing a data-driven, electronic healthcare insurance eligibility solution that can confirm patient eligibility, coverage and benefits information (including copays, coinsurance and deductibles) in real time, for all patients. This must be hardwired at your organization. The truth (data) about your patient's insurance coverage is out there ... you just need to deploy a solution that will let you leverage that data to improve the accuracy and consistency of your insurance eligibility and benefits-verification processes. Leveraging technology to help with this task can improve your workflow efficiencies, reduce claims denials, lower billing and collections costs, and lower uncompensated care and bad debt.

Having access to this information—and being able to verify coverage and benefits with the patient—can improve the patient financial experience. Further, having this information available to all of the hospital staff enables an empowered conversation with patients, with accurate information about their insurance benefits and payment responsibilities.

Validate Medical Necessity and Prior Authorization

The Problem: As I discussed in chapter 3, denials are one of providers' top issues right now. A recent analysis estimated around 9 percent of medical claims are initially denied, totaling $262 billion.[367] At the average hospital, more than 3 percent of net revenue is at risk due to denials.[368] Even though roughly two-thirds of those claims are recoverable, the administrative efforts associated with managing claims denials come with a cost.[369] I know, you're sick of hearing about denials. It feels like the payers are just finding a reason these days. You can't win—or can you? What if you could prevent those denials in the first place?

The Solution: Medical necessity and prior authorizations are a major factor for denials. Checking healthcare payer authorization requirements—including medical necessity and prior authorization—and ensuring the criteria are met, prior to or at the time of service, are table stakes to reduce denials.

Of course, that's easier said than done. Insurance rules have become more complicated and larger in number—it seems like the number of authorizations required increases by the thousands every day. As of 2019, the Current Procedural Terminology (CPT) manual includes 10,294 different procedure codes.[370] Multiply that by 900-plus payers, each with hundreds of different codes in play—how can you possibly stay on top of changing rules around medical necessity and prior authorization? It's simply not possible to keep up with the volume and complexity of medical necessity and prior authorization rules without leveraging big data, analytics and automation.

That's true for Medicare, as well, even though in some ways, Medicare's medical necessity rules are simpler than those for commercial payers. The Centers for Medicare & Medicaid Services (CMS) publishes a cross-walked list of ICD-10 codes and CPT codes. The list basically indicates if the patient has one of the specified ICD-10 codes, then the linked CPT code(s) are covered. It's pretty simple.

But if you don't know the rules of the game and then follow them precisely, you won't get paid. Verifying medical necessity is an often-missed but critical step in Medicare reimbursement optimization.

A data-driven authorization tool can validate procedure codes against Medicare necessity rules and determine which diagnoses would pass or fail coverage rules. In addition, the right solution can streamline and automate the process of screening for prior authorization requirements by linking to payer-published rules and also offer the option to include provider-specific custom rules.

A solution that streamlines and automates medical necessity compliance checking and prior authorization validation can stop potential claims errors before they become denials. Providers can improve the patient financial experience by helping patients understand their financial responsibilities in the context of medical necessity determinations and prior authorization requirements.

As noted earlier, if the authorization or medical necessity criterion are *not* met, the provider has a choice to either get more information or risk doing the procedure(s) for free. You need to prioritize *prevention* of denials over management of denials. Preventing a denial gets you closer to getting out of the claim game. Innovations in denial prevention include using analytics to leverage line-level detail, finding patterns in denials and, more importantly, detailing the relationship between denials and revenue. The value of each claim touch in the process must yield incremental revenue or it's a waste of time. Effective denial prevention solutions must also deliver insight into prevention, helping you remove wasteful claim touches from the workflow and identifying the upstream root cause. There are solutions that do this today. Healthcare organizations that leverage these solutions are seeing a fundamental shift from denial management to denial prevention.

Innovative providers are also negotiating themselves "out of the game." They're assuming a 1.5 percent denial rate, for example, and negotiating that in advance with their payers. Providers accept the 1.5 percent lower reimbursement, but the payer can't deny a penny more—the provider has essentially locked in their rate. Another strategy is to flip the table on the payer, granting access to the EHR for inpatient stays. All of the inpatient stays are assumed to meet criteria and are pre-certified (authorized). The burden of proof is on the payer—they (that's right, the *payer*) must tell the provider within 24 hours if the patient doesn't meet the criteria, or the bill is to be paid—according to the contract—in full. Other innovations include "gold-card programs," where payers waive authorizations for providers who have demonstrated good behavior. It's important to note all of these innovations hinge on one central concept—the providers must have data and analytics to help them determine where to focus their denial prevention efforts.

Provide the Patient with an Estimate

The Problem: Consumers are clamoring for healthcare price transparency. So is the government. But healthcare has addressed this issue inconsistently. A 2018 HIMSS Analytics survey of 1,000 patients found only 18 percent reported getting a cost estimate without asking for one.[371] Another survey found only 35 percent of consumers *with payment responsibility* indicated they had been called by the business office prior to treatment to receive an estimate.[372] A 2019 TransUnion Healthcare consumer survey of 2,500 patients revealed just under half of them received an estimate prior to care.[373]

Regardless of which number is more accurate—none are good enough to meet consumer demand. Providers have been leveraging every excuse in the book to avoid providing an estimate. They say, "We don't know what the charges will be; the deductible will change; no estimators are accurate; the patients won't want to pay anything in advance anyway." I have heard them all, and frankly I've grown tired of it. A colleague of mine recently asked for an estimate for a simple procedure—an MRI. He was told, "This is a new clinic so we don't know yet." He cancelled. Good for him!

We have to get over it, gang. We know these numbers. We may not know all of them but we can get close. Providers at least know an estimate range for the majority of services they provide. Please do not assume the American consumer can't understand or is unwilling to pay. Consumers are used to accepting estimates in any other variable service. As much as hospitals may buck the system, what's good enough for most trades—car mechanics, plumbers, contractors and more—is good enough for patients. Horseshoes, hand grenades and cigars can all get "close," and so can we.

Patients *want* to pay you and won't accept "I can't estimate it right now" anymore. Notably, a HIMSS Analytics survey reported 60 percent of patients responded they would ask for a cost estimate in the future.[374]

Providers need to stop making excuses and start financially engaging the patient. I was doing this 15 years ago at my hospital. The payers have been doing this for years, but they have no (zero) relationship with the patient. You—as providers—do. You have to make assumptions, take a risk, make mistakes and get better—for the patient. In my travels this year, I'm observing more hospitals taking this leap and their patients are thankful for it.

Even though consumers want cost estimates, they don't necessarily have a lot of confidence in the ability of hospitals to provide them. In the same TransUnion Healthcare survey mentioned earlier, only 51 percent of patients actually understood the estimate given by providers.[375] In a similar study, more than half of consumers (53 percent) trusted the insurance company to give them an accurate estimate, but only 19 percent of consumers trusted the hospital to give an accurate estimate (figure 8.3). Hospitals tied with the answer "none of the above" with respect to consumer confidence in their ability to provide an accurate estimate.

Figure 8.3 Who Is Trusted to Provide the Best Cost Estimate?

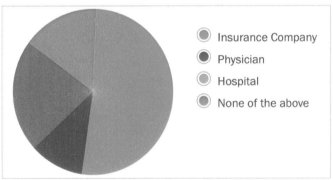

Source: "The Impact of Consumerism on Healthcare: Consumer Feedback Shows Progress on Hospital Business Office Interactions." Connance. October 2018. (Page 7). Accessed October 2, 2019. https://cdn2.hubspot.net/hubfs/634119/White%20Paper%20-%20The%20Impact%20of%20Consumerism%20on%20Healthcare%20-%20October%202018.pdf?__hssc=223962692.1.1556549010703&__hstc=223962692.ed917847dcc2518965f19e6172d4d0a9.1556549010701.1556549010701.1556549010701.1&__

The Solution: Hospitals and health systems need to enhance their ability to provide consumers with accurate, upfront estimates of the cost of care. Not only because consumers and the government are demanding it, but also because it improves revenue collection and patient satisfaction.

The practice of collecting money from patients *after* services are delivered—rather than at the point-of-service—is outdated because it makes the effort costlier in the long run. If history is any indication, the chances of being paid are a lot less likely after the patient has walked out the door.

Per the Academy of Healthcare Revenue, providers only have a 30 percent chance of collecting on medical bills once a patient has left the facility.[376] Providers' chances of collecting are 70 percent while the patient is there in front of them—this doesn't surprise me. In addition, sending bills without having a conversation around expectations and financial responsibility also has detrimental effects on patient *experience* (the envelope in the mail can't have an "awesome" conversation with the patient about their financial responsibility). And the longer a facility waits, the lower the value of the collection.

For example, at 60 days, the value drops to 75 percent of the bill; at 90 days, it plummets to 60 percent; after 180 days, 25 percent, and at 1 year it's worth just 5 percent (Figure 8.4). On the other hand, providers are 70 percent more likely to receive payment if they provide a cost estimate in advance.[377] In fact, 52 percent of people would pay from $200 to $500 or more if an estimate was given at the point of care.[378]

Providing every patient with a payment estimation prior to service or discharge is an industry best practice in driving patient payment yield and satisfaction. It's also an integral component to patient experience.

Figure 8.4 Cost of Collection Increases over Time

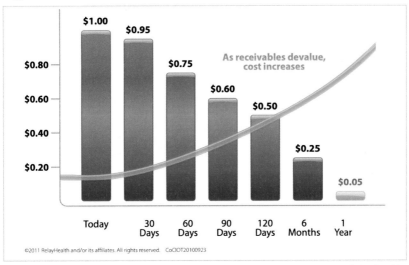

Source: "Improving Self Pay at All Points of Service." RelayHealth. 2011. Accessed October 23, 2019. https://www.ndha.org/image/cache/ImprovingSelf-PayAtAllPointsofService_RelayHealth__2_.pdf

Hospitals are catching on to the importance of offering cost estimates at the front end. CHI Health, for example, offers an online Cost Estimator (https://www.chihealth.com/en/patients-visitors/cost-estimator.html) with a disclaimer noting the estimate provided via the tool is only an estimate and is subject to change based on the variables of the procedure(s) and/or treatment(s). Other health systems have taken a more unconventional approach to estimates by actually guaranteeing the price. Memorial Healthcare System has an estimate tool (ezVerify) that calculates out-of-pocket cost information for 330 types of outpatient procedures, diagnostic services and physician visits.[379] The tool started out as a price estimator but Memorial now provides patients with a price guarantee.

In an interview with *Modern Healthcare*, Matt Muhart, Memorial's Executive Vice President and Chief Administrative Officer said, "We're not going to make our inability to be precise on a patient's out-of-pocket requirement a burden on our consumer."[380]

As more hospitals and health systems make online estimation tools available, consumers will begin expecting all of the healthcare providers they interact with to have online cost estimates available. Providers with the ability to provide accurate, out-of-pocket cost estimates for patients will increase patient satisfaction and provide a foundation for enabling point-of-service collections.

Patient Financial Clearance/Propensity to Pay

The Problem: You must understand a patient's financial situation in order to provide an effective and meaningful patient financial experience. But the patient doesn't walk in with a portfolio, right? They don't come up to the registrar's desk and say, "Here are my finances! Here is how much I make a month. Here is what my monthly bills are. Here is how much money I have in the bank right now." For other big purchases—whether you are renting an apartment, buying a car or buying a house—you have to lay your financial cards on the table. That doesn't happen (yet) in healthcare.

An analogy I like to give is that the process for obtaining financial clearance is just like what the pilot does before they take off in the plane, making sure—visually and critically—all systems are checked and double-checked prior to starting the engines and takeoff. Or think of Jiffy Lube, where they proactively review a checklist and tell you when you come in to pick up your vehicle, "Hey, we checked all this stuff—your motor oil, transmission fluid, power steering, brakes, alignment, washer fluids, etc." and then they give you your car back. And you feel good as a consumer because they have checked everything for you, communicated and thereby built trust.

The same thing could happen with the critical aspect of patient financial clearance. "We checked your insurance and your eligibility for benefits, we verified for authorizations, medical necessity, and how much you owe—everything is ready to go." That makes the patient feel good, right? But *that* scenario only happens about a third of the time.[381]

The Solution: Getting a clear picture of each patient's unique financial situation—including their ability and willingness to pay and the likelihood of them qualifying for financial assistance—can enhance the patient financial experience and improve collection efforts. Data is available to help you make these determinations for *all* of your patients. Having access to information on the patient's estimated household size and income, debt-to-income ratio, percent of federal poverty level (FPL) and residual income can help you determine which Plinko bucket each patient belongs in. And determining that in advance can help increase your point-of-service collections and streamline downstream revenue collection processes.

Having a financial clearance process can also help you determine when charity care applies. Implementing a data-driven financial clearance solution can tell you where the patient falls on the FPL chart, as well as how that value aligns with your hospital's specific financial assistance program. I'll have more to say about making a presumptive charity care determination later on in this chapter.

Separate from the patient's financial position is the patient's *willingness* to pay (a.k.a. propensity to pay). This becomes a bigger factor when the patient financial clearance results show the patient is somewhere in the middle—their income is too high to qualify for financial assistance but too low for them to pay most or all of the patient financial responsibility upfront. This is where credit score information can be helpful because it can provide insight into the patient's likelihood of paying that bill. With patient consent, credit information is especially helpful for self-pay patients because it can help your staff make informed decisions during registration and about financial counseling, billing and collections.

The healthcare market seems particularly spooked by running credit checks on patients. I understand the majority of healthcare is unplanned and often not a choice for the patient. It's frequently an unexpected expense—of which we have plenty in daily life—like an appliance or car breaking down. I'm not certain why there's trepidation on the part of providers. In any other industry, where the amounts are comparable to healthcare liabilities, credit reports are run. This is another area I believe healthcare is stuck circa 1985. Get over it! Providers are floating money like a bank so they may need to start acting like one, too. In fact, one in five hospitals are establishing loans with patients.[382]

For example, check a patient's credit to see where they are on your sliding scale, and then match them to an appropriate funding mechanism based on their unique financial position. If there's still concern, it doesn't necessarily have to be credit data— there are a myriad of alternative, noncredit data sets to predict likelihood of payment, based on where you live, what you own and other factors. Innovative revenue cycles have hardwired this piece by stratifying their patients into payment buckets across two axes— ability to pay and willingness to pay.
Create Tailored Payment Strategies
The Problem: Even if you work for one of the hospitals that actually performs financial clearance, one of the gaps is being able

to provide tailored payment strategies or options for patients once you've estimated their costs and determined their financial status.

The Solution: After you say to the patient, "Here's what we think you're going to owe," you need to also be able to say, "I want you to feel comfortable paying it, so I have created a payment plan tailored for you. We have backed it up with financial assistance (if you need it) and provided a discount based on your unique financial position." In that scenario everyone is happy, because patients not only know how much they are going to owe, but also how they are going to pay it. And providers know they're going to have a much better chance of getting paid, because patients are engaged.

Because hospitals aren't necessarily banks, it can be helpful to work with a partner who can help meet patients' needs in an innovative way, beyond the functionality of the legacy EHR. For example, if a patient is expecting a $20,000 bill, the account could be flagged for a follow-up conversation about loans. If you have the right tools and partners in place, you can tell the patient, "Hey, here's a plan with no interest. Here's a plan *with* interest. Here's a plan with 6 months of payments or perhaps a 12-month plan. Here's what the payments look like." Just like if you were evaluating different financing options for your car. As much as it's talked about, two-thirds of providers are *not* doing it. Why? I'm inclined to think legacy technology and processes haven't been reevaluated. Patients are the third largest payer behind Medicare and Medicaid.[383] Think of all the processes and resources you have put in place to manage payer reimbursement. Patients are the new payer and they deserve equal time in the high-deductible health plan (HDHP) era. I tell folks, "It's no longer about estimation and transparency … it's about payment options." Patients can't afford it and they need a frictionless, tailored payment model. It's time for healthcare organizations to take the steps necessary to deploy these solutions.

And here's a news flash, gang: If you don't want to figure it out, Uncle Sam is going to create legislation that forces the industry to do it (see chapter 10). All you have to do is deliver payment options elegantly and watch the cash yield grow.

Strategy #2: Ensure Earned Revenue Gets Paid

After you've delivered care, it's important to maximize your reimbursements and reduce your bad debt. That sounds obvious, I know, but there are several areas in which many hospitals and health systems fall short. They're leaving money on the table—and often, they don't even realize it, because they haven't leveraged modern technology tools to identify and collect all of the revenue they've earned.

Think of it like golf—you need to have the right equipment and maximize each stroke (or claim touch). Now, I don't play a lot of golf anymore but I used to play a lot and loved it. Stick with me here, as I heard this analogy used at a Becker's conference—comparing the game of golf with the cost to collect—and I think it illustrates the point beautifully. For those who have not played, here is a primer: Golf involves a little white ball, clubs and a golf course with many holes to aim at.

The game of golf is scored by how many times (strokes) it takes you to hit the ball until it ends up in any one of those little hole marked by a flag hundreds of yards away. The fewer strokes, the better your score. For each hole (typically golf courses have 18 holes), one can receive par (professional average result, or 0), a birdie (one stroke under par for that hole), an eagle (two strokes under par), a bogey (one stroke over par), a double bogey (two strokes over par) and so on.

Back to revenue cycle: industry benchmark (par) on the average $1 billion hospital is 3–4 percent cost to collect, or $30–$40 million in collection costs, all in. In terms of par in golf, the average result for a professional (or "good") revenue cycle is $35 million for cost to collect. Birdie might be $20 million. Bogey? Well, that may be $50 million.

Now think of each patient account as a golf ball: your cost to collect depends on where you aim, how you hit it and how far it goes. It takes practice to be a pro and get those birdies and eagles I talked about. Each "ball" (err, claim) in your revenue cycle has the potential to be a birdie or even an eagle. This would mean getting paid at the maximum amount, in the shortest amount of time, with the least amount of effort—just like golf. You have to have the right clubs and the right amount of practice to consistently shoot under par, protecting your earned revenue effectively. Let's hit some balls and look at some examples.

Discover All Applicable Insurance (Insurance Discovery)

The Problem: Sometimes patients don't know their own insurance coverage. This happens more often than you might think. And if the patient can't accurately tell the registrar what payer(s) is responsible for their care, the hospital won't be able to appropriately bill the right payers. It's important to identify all billable insurance coverage from third-party payers as early in the process as possible.

A significant number of self-pay patients may be covered by payers but the patient is either unaware of the potential coverage or has chosen not to disclose. Even patients who present as insured may have secondary insurance. When additional insurance is discovered, it creates an opportunity for the potential coordination of benefits and/or Medicaid secondary, maximizing reimbursements.

Clearly, with all those scenarios looming, there are a lot of metaphorical sand traps and water hazards to get you off course as you take aim at your golf ball.

The Solution: A data-driven insurance discovery solution can help providers identify missed opportunities for payment. A comprehensive solution will continuously look for coverage on all accounts—not just self-pay. It will also streamline complex cases by looking for potential coordination of benefit opportunities, identifying commercial policy ID numbers for patients believed to be uninsured, and monitoring Medicare and Medicaid for retroactive Supplemental Security Income (SSI) certification. In the field, insurance discovery has been shown to have the potential to convert anywhere from 1 to 5 percent of a hospital's uncompensated care to paid accounts.[384] Using the right club, swinging and aiming in the right places can uncover hundreds of thousands to millions of dollars in unrealized revenue.

Review Transfer Diagnosis-Related Groups

The Problem: Providers stand to lose tens of thousands of dollars per patient when Medicare Transfer Diagnosis Related group claims—transfer DRG claims—are incorrectly coded. Under Medicare's post-acute transfer rules, if the care a patient receives after discharge from a post-acute care provider doesn't match the discharge status assigned by the acute care provider, the acute care provider may be underpaid. While CMS audits for overpayments on transfer DRGs, CMS does *not* audit for underpayments (per 42 CFR Parts 401 and 405).[385] Transfer DRGs account for about 41.6 percent of all Medicare discharges, so transfer DRG underpayments can contribute significantly to revenue leakage.[386]

Ideally, hospitals would be checking discharge logs/claims enrollment files on the Medicare side. Did a claim ever come from the skilled nursing facility we sent the patient to? What happened there and what didn't? Hospitals aren't really set up to do that kind of tracking. Missed the hole and Medicare took your ball!

The Solution: Post-acute care transfer reviews, internal audits and the adjustment of discharge disposition codes are essential for stopping this source of revenue leakage. However, conducting these tasks manually is time-consuming and subject to errors that put Medicare regulatory compliance at risk. Once again, data-driven technology solutions can streamline and automate this task, resulting in increased accuracy in coding and recapturing revenue from Medicare Transfer DRG underpayments. This is like having a really nice putter and a pro's guiding hand on your shots, then sinking them 100 percent of the time. Providers can leverage technology to assist with:

- Reviewing hospital and Medicare data sources
- Identifying where qualifying post-acute care was *not* provided
- Validating with Medicare and the post-acute care provider that care was not delivered
- Correcting and appealing claims with Medicare

Recover Medicare Beneficiary Bad Debt

The Problem: Medicare bad debt (MBD) is another place where hospitals can experience significant revenue leakage. The average hospital payer mix means that Medicare typically pays 40.8 percent of hospital costs.[387] So it's important for hospitals and health systems to maximize all types of Medicare reimbursement, including MBD.

There are three main types of MBD:

1. *Patients who are dually eligible for Medicare and Medicaid (a.k.a. "crossovers")*. In these cases, Medicaid

211

will rarely cover the entire Medicare coinsurance or deductible, but rules vary state by state, and you must follow your state's specific rules on how Medicaid pays secondarily to Medicare. Nationwide, about 60 percent of MBD cases fall into this category.[388]

2. *Traditional bad debt.* This includes patients who don't have a secondary insurer and may have been sent to collections for unpaid deductible or coinsurance amounts.

3. *Indigent bad debt.* Patients who can't pay because they are indigent—either on financial assistance programs or bankrupt, or are deceased without an estate.[389]

CMS regulations vary depending upon the type of bad debt incurred. Many hospitals struggle to optimize MBD reimbursement because of the differences in billing processes across the three types of MBD. If a provider doesn't follow the CMS regulations to the letter with respect to billing processes, they'll void their eligibility to collect MBD reimbursements. Most hospitals lack the internal resources and technology infrastructure they need to keep up with complex and changing Medicare rules and state regulations. This is basically like using the wrong club and hitting the balls too many times, too far or too short. Some golfers (hospitals) just give up, as it's too exhausting to be accurate and consistent. They find MBD has a very high cost to collect and a low yield.

The Solution: Leveraging a third-party Medicare cost-reporting solution can help providers maximize their MBD reimbursements—which can be significant, since providers can be reimbursed for 65 percent of the eligible MBD they incur.[390] The best example I can offer here is a good caddy. They carry your bag of clubs (burden of MBD claims), suggest the approach at each hole, and are a trusted adviser as you navigate each shot (claim recovery).

Validate Disproportionate Share Hospital Reporting and Documentation

The Problem: Medicare Disproportionate Share Hospital (DSH) payments are an important source of revenue for hospitals serving low-income populations. But aggregating, integrating and documenting the patient data needed to qualify for these payments can be really challenging. These are divots or hazards in the fairway on the golf course. It's not your fault … it's the community. Nonetheless, you have to hit the ball and navigate through them. You may even need a "ruling" from the course marshal; perhaps the hazards allow for your ball to drop in a better line to the hole.

The Solution: A third-party technology solution can help providers identify DHS-eligible patients and patient days by:

- Scrubbing patient encounter data to improve match results with Medicaid eligibility data
- Identifying all mother and baby matches
- Removing paid Medicare claims by matching the Medicare Provider Statistical and Reimbursement (PS&R) report to the final Medicaid log
- Leveraging analytics to ensure all appropriate Medicare records are removed from the Medicaid fraction, including those that are eligible but not paid
- Delivering the results with complete documentation as required for Medicare submission[391]

213

Leverage Uncompensated Care Analytics

The Problem: As I pointed out in chapter 3, uncompensated care costs are rising. According to the American Hospital Association (AHA), uncompensated care costs totaled $38.4 billion in 2017 and I suspect that number will reach $45 billion before 2025.[392] CMS uses Worksheet S-10 (part of the hospital's cost report) to determine a provider's eligibility for reimbursement based on uncompensated care.

Nonprofit hospitals that don't accurately report their charity care and bad debt on the S-10 worksheet risk losing significant reimbursement. Further, if a provider's written charity care or financial assistance policies aren't consistent with CMS regulations, providers risk losing out on uncompensated care payments.

In addition, the Internal Revenue Service (IRS) has been busting hospitals for not following regulations like 501(r), which requires charity screening prior to sending patients to collections.[393] You can get in a lot of compliance trouble if you don't do this right. This is basically like not following the rules in golf. You can't improve your lie (i.e., where the ball landed). Depending on how you hit the ball (charity), you have to hit it again from where it fell. And you want to hit it well so it ends up in the charity hole, not the lake (bad debt).

The Solution: Uncompensated care is another area of revenue that benefits from leveraging data, technology and analytic tools. Uncompensated care analytics can generate the data points needed to accurately complete the Worksheet S-10; provide documentation to facilitate the audit process; analyze the impact the results will have on your organization's uncompensated care payments; and provide benchmarking against peer hospitals. I would argue the caddy or your partners and colleagues have a role here, as trusted advisers. Perhaps they will suggest a different approach, different club or look at the hole together with you.

Strategy #3: Optimize Payment Strategies

Optimizing your collection strategies is all about deploying your resources efficiently so you aren't spending your efforts chasing dollars you're unlikely to ever recover. In golf, there are different types of clubs including the putter, irons and woods. We have probably all used putters: even if you don't play golf, you have probably used a putter to play mini golf. You can hit the ball with putters but they're truly designed for precise, short shots. Woods, on the other hand, are designed for distance—long distance. Irons of various sizes are designed to reach a distance somewhere in between and they also lift the ball up at different angles. Like payment strategies, in golf everything depends on the objective (driving/getting to hole/putting) and what club you use. The distance may represent the term of the payment plan and the hole may be payment or charity. And bad debt, yep—that's "the lumberyard, Danny" (see *Caddyshack*[394]). Driving to the desired outcome requires the right tool in order to optimize cash flow—it's like hitting the ball with the right club. Knowing how well you can hit each ball (patient account)—and how to hit it, how far and where—will drive just the right distance (yield in payments) with the least number of strokes (touches by your staff).

Make a Presumptive Determination When Charity Care Applies

The Problem: Your financial counselors often do not have access to the information they need to make appropriate decisions about patient financial assistance. The patient may be unable, or unwilling, to share information that will help your counselors accurately determine whether or not the patient is eligible for financial assistance. This is akin to someone hiding your ball—at the bottom of a pond on the course.

The Solution: First, it is important to develop a comprehensive and consistent interview tool, including questions about household size and income.

Web-based solutions are available to support financial counselors with these determinations. Data-driven solutions rely not just on patient-supplied information, but also on credit data based on the patient's financial status. This provides your counselors with objective and reliable information. The advantage of using a web-based charity-screening tool is that it supports your financial counselors in the fair and consistent application of your organization's unique financial assistance policies. At the same time, this type of solution also provides the documentation your organization needs to be audit-ready for 501(r) compliance reporting. This is like a "best ball" scramble approach. Without having to go to the ball, you can pick it up and move it up the fairway to the best location. Or—like the charity classification— the ball (account) can be moved or presumptively classified as a "charity" shot, because the data showed the patient fell into that category. It's a streamlined process of segmenting the bad debt portfolio (balls) into the most appropriate accounts (fairway, hazards or holes).

Leverage Insurance Discovery

The Problem: I talked about the challenges with eligibility, and how this is not about new technology but about applying technology in a new way that is hardwired to your processes. The same goes for insurance discovery. Insurance discovery solutions have been around for some time and I'm amazed they're still not being leveraged by some hospitals. A prominent revenue cycle management Vice President was recently on a panel I moderated and said, "Insurance discovery is standard practice for revenue cycle—it's a must-have."

Basically, this is a safety net for coverage. Patient access will tell you they did everything right with what they have. But there are still misses—there are things out of their control. This includes miskeyed policy numbers, misspelled names, secondary coverage that was not disclosed and Medicaid coverage that was unknown. There are a host of RCM insurance verification "black holes"; payment is there … you just have to check for it.

The Solution: Leverage insurance discovery as early as you can in the patient account life cycle. It's worth every penny. I have also heard RCM leaders liken insurance discovery to "printing money." These are reimbursable dollars the insurance company is not going to proactively tell you about. They aren't going to pick up the phone and say, "Hey, you forgot to check with us but we have that member on file and will pay his claim." The onus is on you—the provider—to check.

But can you possibly check them all? Of course you *can*—with an insurance discovery tool. These tools effectively leverage industry-leading eligibility technology to find coverage. These solutions can drive millions (with an *M*) of dollars of recovered revenue to an average-sized hospital annually. They can typically find 1–5 percent of net patient revenue in discovered coverage. In today's environment there's no excuse not to use an insurance discovery solution.

The golf analogy here would be if you were trying to use a putter to drive and hit every shot on the course. Insurance discovery is the TaylorMade AeroBurner Oversized Head Driver, baby (for the uninitiated, that's a high-end golf club). It hits the ball long and true, right in the middle of the fairway, so it's easy to spot. Combine this with a robust self-pay stratification process (see below), and you have 100 percent insurance verification for your patient population.

Transition from Denials to Maximized Revenue

The Problem: Most of the providers I encounter indicate denials are their number one issue and they don't see it getting better any time soon. Why? Probably because they're playing a losing round of golf. It's like the hole locations on the green are moved while your ball is in midair. You need to move from denials management to denials prevention, while also ensuring your earned revenue is paid at the maximal amount.

The Solution: Data and analytics can be leveraged here to provide insights that change behavior for denials by delivering insights for action and yield. There are solutions in existence *today* that can provide information in real time as to whether an authorization is required or not, and record or substantiate the "proof" and trend payment over time to ensure you weren't underpaid. These solutions can also tell you whether the "stroke" is worth it. Is touching this particular claim going to result in incremental revenue? Is this a real denial with dollars attached to it? How many other claims have this type of denial? Can I win this appeal? Did the payer pay this claim at the right amount?

All of these questions can be answered with advanced analytics for denials prevention and underpayments. This is like getting to the "19th hole"—the golf course bar and one of my favorite places. Instead of going through all the work and effort, you took just the right number of strokes and scored par (or maybe even birdie). You only touched the claims you needed to and you held the payers accountable to their payments.

Segment Accounts to Enable Collections Prioritization

The Problem: As I pointed out in my first book, over the past decade, the percentage of provider revenue that has shifted to patients has increased from less than 10 percent to more than 30 percent.[395] This means collection strategies have to change, because patients don't behave like commercial payers. A McKinsey & Company survey indicated, "Costs are likely to be significantly higher when collecting from individual patients on a per-transaction basis than when collecting from payers—on average, healthcare consumers pay more than twice as slowly as commercial payers."[396]

In the old days, you might have picked up the phone and worked your way through overdue patient accounts in an A-to-Z format. You had no way of prioritizing accounts, because you didn't have a lot of insight into which overdue accounts might give you the greatest yield.

It's not effective or efficient to approach collections manually anymore. If you do, you're going to leave cash on the table that you don't know about, or it's going to take you so long to recover it that you'll end up spending more money collecting it than what it's worth. This is like being in the "rough" in golf, or high grass. Land there and you can't see the fairway or even get your shot in without some help.

The Solution: Focusing staff efforts on accounts with the highest probability to pay will improve your collections yield. In order to do that, you need to have the right tools to stratify your bad debt portfolio according to each patient's unique financial position. Using a data-driven, technology-enabled collections strategy will help you keep more accounts in-house, resulting in lower collection vendor contingency fees.

Optimizing collections can reduce your bad debt and can also help with 501(c) reporting requirements. Optimizing collections works like a good "wedge" by lifting your ball up so you have the highest probability of getting back in the fairway and back on course. And as I mentioned above, the balls (patient accounts) are getting segmented into the correct hole with the least number of strokes (touches). Combining this approach with insurance discovery also offers 100 percent financial clearance for your patients. You'll drive the ball longer and more accurately and never have a bad shot again—with the right club and application.

The Bottom Line

The healthcare industry—including the revenue cycle—is data rich now, with increased complexity and volumes of data from disparate sources. This new revenue cycle environment demands transactional analysis and insights to help providers identify RCM problems and react to them quickly. That's what payers are doing now. And that's what patients want. Plus, that's what the government expects. They expect pro golfers.

The strategies and best practices I have outlined in this chapter can be summarized in a few key points:

1. Patients increasingly want and expect a personalized, customized experience. And that includes a personalized, customized *patient financial* experience.

2. The only way for hospitals and health systems to provide a customized experience is to appropriately leverage big data and analytics. Don't just capture data. Leverage that data into information, then insights, then action. Almost every other industry—including the clinical side of healthcare—is already leveraging big data and analytics to provide a more targeted consumer experience.

3. Because big data and analytics aren't necessarily core competencies of hospitals and health systems, they can benefit from partnering with organizations with expertise in these areas. In addition to expertise, partners with access to proprietary data can enhance the effectiveness of healthcare RCM solutions.

4. Leveraging big data and analytics can also have a big positive impact on revenue. Stopping revenue leakage in the 12 specific areas outlined in this chapter can significantly shift margins.

In other words, to get paid, you have to get rid of manual, antiquated workflows and leverage data technology to close the gaps in your RCM process, protect revenue from leakage and maximize revenue collection. Replace your golf clubs from 1985 (stop doing things manually) and leverage the savvy tools available now. Use your putter, drivers and woods (people, process and technology in combination) to improve your score, (i.e., your cost to collect). And get a good caddy—a partner who can help you deploy multiple solutions at once. I want you to do better than par. You're a pro. Your revenue cycle should reflect that. Go get those birdies and eagles. I know you can.

In the next few chapters, I'll talk about what the future looks like for healthcare, including short-term payment strategies, the legislative outlook, and some predictions and wishful thinking about how processes could be improved.

SECTION FOUR

A PROMISING FUTURE?

CHAPTER 9

RESCUE ME—NEAR-TERM STRATEGIES

In the short term, each group of stakeholders—patients, independent physicians, providers, payers and employers—is using different strategies to either maximize reimbursement (physicians, providers) or manage costs (employers, patients, payers). Until the healthcare industry payment model evolves, we will remain in an "everyone for themselves" payment system, where each stakeholder leverages the strategies at their disposal, regardless of the impacts on other stakeholders or the overall system.

Eventually, each stakeholder is going to have to disrupt their own area in a way that aligns their goals with those of the other stakeholders. At this point, however, I see little collaboration or alignment to the healthcare system. Patient, physician, payer and employer, for the most part, all seem to be doing their own thing. For meaningful change, we must have aligned incentives, and these stakeholders are going to have to stop thinking about themselves and start thinking holistically about costs and outcomes. In the meantime, here are a few of the strategies in play right now.

Patient Strategies

Patients have a significant role to play in managing their healthcare costs, but do they have all of the information they need to make the right decisions? A 2019 *New England Journal of Medicine* (NEJM) survey of healthcare executives, clinical leaders and clinicians found respondents believe patients generally lack the information they need to affect the cost of their care decisions (figure 9.1).

Figure 9.1 Patients Lack Information to Affect the Cost of Their Care Decisions

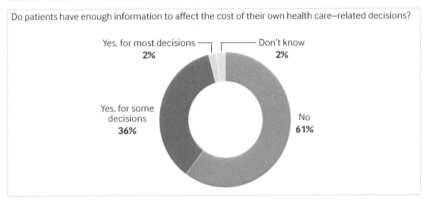

Do patients have enough information to affect the cost of their own health care–related decisions?

Yes, for most decisions — 2%

Don't know 2%

Yes, for some decisions 36%

No 61%

Source: Leemore Dafny, PhD and Chris DeRienzo, MD, MPP. "New Marketplace Survey: Patients Lack Information to Reduce the Cost of Care." Insights Report. NEJM Catalyst. March 7, 2019. Accessed October 26, 2019. https://catalyst.nejm.org/patients-lack-cost-of-care/

Throughout this book I've written in detail about ways providers can offer patients with the cost information they need to make more informed choices about care. For the first time in my career of 25 years, I'm starting to see the industry move, ever so slowly.

But this is only half the battle. Remember the saying about leading a horse to water but not being able to make it drink? You also can't make a horse do the backstroke.

Consumers have to own their empowerment, as they own any other experience in which they search for a service, evaluate it and purchase it. Providers can supply information about costs, but patients need to be engaged and informed enough to *care* about costs in the first place. They need to want to take a drink, regardless of how or where they are led. However, patients aren't currently engaged in the cost of healthcare, for many reasons.

I've thought hard about why patients aren't more engaged in understanding their personal healthcare costs. One reason is patients have been insulated from the true cost of care by third-party payers for so long and only recently have begun to feel the pain, in terms of things like high-deductible health plans (HDHP) and higher co-insurance. For the most part, third-party insurance from a large group employer insulates the patient from the true cost. They see the big number at the top (billed charges), then one that's smaller (contracted discount), then a significantly smaller one at the bottom (patient out-of-pocket), which really is all the patient cares about. And, in most cases that number is a fraction of the overall cost.

However, ask a patient who does not have insurance (self-pay) or one who has an HDHP—I'd wager they would tell you a different story about healthcare cost. I believe that same patient would wish they had taken the time to research options in advance before it was too late. Healthcare costs remain an afterthought for most patients—it's sticker shock. I'm going to make this crystal clear if I have not already: Healthcare has one of the most expensive price tags out there. It is right up there with automobiles, two-week vacations and designer jewelry, gang. My point remains, expensive healthcare is not new, and it is here to stay. Patients need a (big) wake-up call. Understanding coverage and exposure to out-of-pocket cost is integral to financial stability in today's healthcare environment.

Another reason patients are less engaged with healthcare costs is they're understandably more concerned with the life effect itself—the illness, disease or injury—than the cost. The healthcare need is likely not planned either. We experience something that doesn't quite feel right, so we ask a physician or phone a friend, and then we go see a healthcare professional.

We *might* ask about cost, but usually not. As we get more information about what's causing the illness, we may research costs a little more, but usually not—we just go as needed to fix a problem. When the bill comes, oh boy, do we research the cost, scrambling to look at our insurance plan or trying to remember the conversations that did or didn't happen with the provider: "They never told me ... or maybe they did and I forgot. I meant to go check. Oh well, it's too expensive, anyway. How can they live with themselves charging this much?! It doesn't cost *that* much. I'm not paying." But you went and now you have to pay.

Liken this to the restaurant example I used earlier—one of those restaurants where the menu is in a different language with no (zero, zilch, *nada*) numbers associated with each offering: The waiter (physician) suggested (ordered) it all. You thought about the cost, but—hey—they're the experts! You meant to check the prices, but you ate anyway. Then the bill comes and no matter how long you look at it, the numbers are the same. I know, you can't compare a lobster to a laminectomy. You *chose* to go eat and enjoyed it. Indeed, eating is way more fun than an unexpected event and being flat on your back in the emergency department (ED) in pain. My point is, we are distracted. We do not pause. We do not ask. We just go.

A third reason is the majority of us interact with the healthcare system pretty infrequently—most of us are doing well if we get in to see our physician once a year for an annual check-up. So, with something we do infrequently, we get lazy, err ... disengaged. We put our insurance card or checkup in the back of our minds and save it for later. Out-of-pocket costs for most common prescription drugs are very low. This is partly because they are mass-produced (large supply, low demand, low cost), and also because they are used often and, as such, we are price-sensitive to them. Prescription benefits, especially in the generic market, are purposely priced low (sometimes below cost), as prescriptions are the most frequently used piece of healthcare and the most consumer-facing, thus patients are highly engaged there. If our copays start going up, or our drugs are not covered or become expensive—suddenly, we care. We pay attention. We ask. We are *engaged*.

Patients simply need to be more engaged in their healthcare. They need to take responsibility for every aspect of healthcare, beginning with making healthy lifestyle choices and continuing on through asking questions about the financial impact of their choices before, during and after receiving healthcare services.

Below are examples of the strategies patients are—and aren't—using to control their cost of care.

Making Healthy Lifestyle Choices

As I discussed in chapter 2, chronic diseases have a big impact on U.S. healthcare costs. Americans with one or more chronic conditions account for 90 percent of all healthcare spending.[397] Many of these chronic conditions (including heart disease, cancer, chronic lung disease, diabetes and chronic kidney disease) are linked to lifestyle choices. Consumers who make good lifestyle choices—like not smoking, making healthy food choices, getting regular exercise and limiting alcohol use—can lower their chances of developing chronic disease and burdening the healthcare system.

Easier said than done, I know. I saw my physician recently for my annual visit, and he said, "You've got a fatty liver." I asked him, "What's that from?" and he said, "Well, most American males your age have a fatty liver." (I'm not sure whether that made me feel better or worse.) He also said my condition could be the result of a few different factors, including genetics and lifestyle. When I told him I don't have a family history of the disease, he said, "Well, then it's probably the result of your diet of steaks and bourbon." And I said, "Yep, it probably is." I eat a lot less steak and drink a lot fewer Manhattans now. I'm not happy about it, but I needed to make the choice for my health, my family and ultimately, my healthcare costs.

I share this because I'm not trying to be hypocritical here—this is a message we can all benefit from: Just put down the cheeseburger and go for a walk instead. Salads over fries. Hikes over TV. The dog loves to go for a walk. Trust me—making healthy lifestyle choices can be a very effective patient strategy for controlling costs.

Skipping or Deferring Healthcare

This isn't a strategy I recommend, and sometimes it's not a preferred choice, but it *is* a strategy that's trending upward for many patients, unfortunately. A 2018 survey found 40 percent of Americans have skipped a recommended medical test or treatment in the last 12 months due to cost.[398] In addition, 32 percent reported they were unable to fill a prescription, or took less of it, due to the cost.

The survey's most startling finding may be this—more Americans are afraid of paying for care than are afraid of getting seriously ill (figure 9.2). This is the wrong direction, gang. Costs have become a genuine fear in healthcare, and patients are scared as hell. Many are just skipping care, because they haven't been educated about available payment and charity options. If you ask a hospital, they'll tell you they "treat all regardless of their ability to pay." But are they also saying, "We reach out to all of our patients to ensure they don't have concerns about cost and get the care they need"? There's a large gap there and it matters.

Figure 9.2 More Americans Are Afraid of Paying for Care Than of Getting a Serious Illness

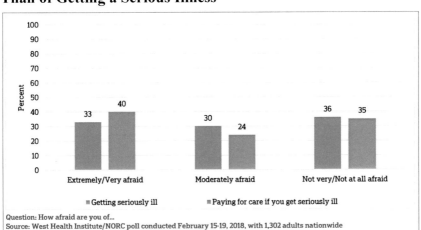

Question: How afraid are you of...
Source: West Health Institute/NORC poll conducted February 15-19, 2018, with 1,302 adults nationwide

Source: "Americans' Views of Healthcare Costs, Coverage and Policy." Issue Brief. West Health Institute/NORC Survey on Healthcare Costs, Coverage and Policy. NORC at the University of Chicago. March 2018. Accessed October 26, 2019. http://www.norc.org/PDFs/WHI%20Healthcare%20Costs%20Coverage%20and%20Policy/WHI%20Healthcare%20Costs%20Coverage%20and%20Policy%20Issue%20Brief.pdf

Skipping care is not a strategy I, or anyone else, recommend. As I mentioned previously, skipping care at the front end can ultimately lead to higher costs for everyone at the back end, when a healthcare condition becomes more acute. Patients end up paying more and so does the system. I call these "train wreck situations." A patient has diabetes but is scared of potential costs for the physician or their medications, so they don't engage. Things get really bad: Obesity, hypertension and A1Cs go through the roof, insulin shock, and then they hit the ED. Costs are 10 times more. Boom—bankruptcy. Nevertheless, as patients are faced with escalating costs, skipping care is a strategy they're using to lower the impact on their wallets. It costs them, the providers, the payer and the system in the long run. *Each diagnosed diabetic patient costs over $13,000 to treat, at a minimum.*[399] Overall, diabetes cost the United States over $400 billion (with a very large "B") in 2017, which equals an economic burden of $1,240 for every American (whether they have diabetes or not).[400]

Shop for Insurance Plans

Patients can—and do—shop for insurance plans. For a large part of the country, this is done "for you" by your employer or Uncle Sam. They give you a few plans to pick from (or there may only be one—for Medicaid, for example). I would argue patients' engagement in shopping for their insurance plans is still pretty limited at this point and could definitely be expanded. Most patients limit their plan "shopping" to once a year, when their employer's health insurance enrollment period opens up or, if they aren't eligible for insurance through their employer, they shop when the health exchange market opens up each year.

I've definitely shopped for health insurance as my life has changed. For example, when my wife and I decided to start a family, we bumped our plan up to a higher tier, because we knew we would hit the deductible between delivery costs, the inpatient stay and everything else that goes along with a new addition to the family. Perhaps because I work in the industry, it was easy for me to recognize when I needed to change my coverage and how to change it to my best advantage. It turns out not everyone understands insurance well enough to make good coverage choices.

Shopping for health insurance can be complicated. One survey found only 40 percent of Americans felt "very confident" they could choose the right health insurance plan.[401] Digging a little deeper, the same survey set out to determine whether Americans understand common health insurance terms.

The survey asked how confident respondents were in their understanding of certain health insurance terminology—and then tested those same people to see what their actual comprehension was. It turns out people generally overestimate their understanding of common insurance terms (figure 9.3).

Figure 9.3 Copay, Coinsurance, Co-what?

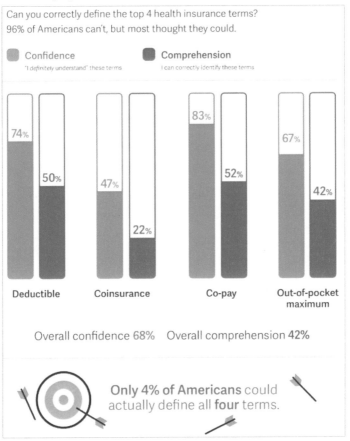

Can you correctly define the top 4 health insurance terms? 96% of Americans can't, but most thought they could.

Confidence — "I definitely understand" these terms

Comprehension — I can correctly identify these terms

Deductible — 74% / 50%
Coinsurance — 47% / 22%
Co-pay — 83% / 52%
Out-of-pocket maximum — 67% / 42%

Overall confidence 68%   Overall comprehension 42%

Only 4% of Americans could actually define all **four** terms.

Source: "4 basic health insurance terms 96% of Americans don't understand." PolicyGenius. January 24, 2018. Accessed October 27, 2019. https://www.policygenius.com/health-insurance/health-insurance-literacy-survey/

The survey results indicated only 4 percent of Americans could actually define all four terms correctly. And the younger the respondent the worse their comprehension: On average, only 36 percent of Millennials could correctly identify any of the four terms, compared to 47 percent of Baby Boomers.[402]

What's concerning is consumers are purchasing these insurance plans based on the copay—which they may or may not understand—and don't look beyond that detail. They're investing thousands of dollars in coverage and putting thousands more of their income at risk depending on how well they chose. Anything else a consumer spends thousands of dollars on is researched *exhaustively*—cars, TVs, plane rides, etc. Arguably, our industry has some work to do in educating the healthcare consumer better about their costs and coverage (see my first book), but again, wake-up call time, people! Opacity in pricing is no longer considered acceptable by today's healthcare consumer.

I would also argue patients are generally uninformed. We must overeducate to reach a disengaged population. We walked through some of these strategies in the earlier chapters: Empower the consumer to make an informed choice—inpatient ($$$$), ED ($$$), urgent care ($$) and clinic ($)—about the type of facility they visit. Set up a triage phone line for them to call 24/7. Hold town hall benefit forums in the library, with the employers, hospitals and citizens of the community. It's as simple as starting there. At the very least, patients should understand the ED is very expensive. But do they know about their other options or—more importantly—how to navigate them?

Providers can do right by their patients by *publishing* their "true" prices—the out-of-pocket cost to the patient—instead of requiring the patient to make a telephone call. Nobody calls on the phone anymore to get a price. We use our fingers and thumbs on our phones! Ideally, providers would structure their transparency strategy in a way that affords the patient the ability to get an estimate of their costs with little to no interaction with the provider. Have a chatbot at the ready or a phone line for patients, and don't assume they won't understand or it'll be too complicated. It needs to be done and patients are ready.

The same holds true when consumers shop for health insurance. The brokers and human resource representatives can brush up their game as well. Imagine, if you will, a conversation like this: "Mr. Wiik, it's time to sign up for your insurance. How's your health? Do you use your plan benefits to the level you feel you should? Do you know what these terms mean? Any life events coming up we can run through a calculator to help you understand your total annual costs?"

This happens with *everything* else you shop for that's a high dollar value, like the salesperson who runs up to you in the parking lot at the car dealership or at the electronics store and says, "Is this the right car (or TV) for you? What do you like? What's your price range?" This isn't hard; we're just not aligned for engagement on *both* sides. Providers must invest the same amount of time explaining costs to a patient as they do in bringing a patient out of anesthesia.

While the idea of smarter consumer shopping options for health insurance has merit, it's very apparent consumers need more education. If consumers don't understand basic health insurance terminology, like deductible, copay, coinsurance and out-of-pocket maximum, they can't make informed choices about their coverage. Consumers are suffering from "benefits illiteracy." It's clear this is an area where other stakeholders aren't yet meeting the needs of the patient as payer.

Selecting Healthcare Providers

Another strategy for patients to limit their exposure to higher healthcare costs is to shop for healthcare providers. This is an area where if the right information were available from providers and payers, patients could actually be in the cockpit and really drive change. It would transform the market if payers and providers had to compete to attract consumers based on cost and quality—"we have the highest outcomes, we have the happiest physicians, we have the lowest cost, and we have the happiest patients"—competing on the priorities that make up the Quadruple Aim (enhancing patient experience, improving population health, reducing costs and improving the work life of those who deliver care).[403]

There is not a lot of shopping going on right now. As I mentioned in chapter 1, even HDHPs don't drive a difference in shopping behavior right now: only 4 percent of patients with HDHPs compared costs across healthcare professionals during their last use of medical care, compared to 3 percent of enrollees without HDHPs who compared costs.[404] You just don't see patients asking questions like: "How much is this going to cost?" "Where should I go?" "Is that a good place to have this done?" "Why do I even need this done?" "Is there something cheaper that can be done?" "I already had one of those. Do I really need another one?"

These are the types of questions consumers will ask a plumber, a car mechanic or a house painter. But they typically don't ask these questions about their healthcare. I don't necessarily want to compare healthcare to a plumbing or car repair job, but just as consumers do when they're purchasing any other good or service, they tend to go through a checklist of questions—this just doesn't happen in healthcare yet. The industry is going to have to bridge that gap and advocate for the patient. Bring that horse to water and dump the trough of water on its head.

Now, some horses are thirsty. As noted in chapter 7, this is an area where the younger demographic is going to drive change in the industry. More and more patients are demanding all the information upfront. Baby Boomers aren't asking these questions but Gen Zers *are* asking these questions.[405] Providers who can't answer payment estimation questions are going to experience the younger generations leaving them for providers who are able to meet the patient as payer.

Clearly consumers need to engage more in the financial aspects of their healthcare, but they also need support and information from other stakeholders in the healthcare system if they're going to be able to engage in an effective and meaningful way with the cost of their care.

Physician Strategies

The current dysfunctional state of healthcare is impacting the way physicians do business. Physicians are seeing decreased reimbursement, sicker patients (because of the higher incidence of chronic disease), higher administrative costs and higher labor costs. It's become increasingly difficult to operate as a solo practitioner or small group practice. Solo practitioners and small group practices are putting the "for sale" sign on the lawn and joining larger organizations in order to survive.

Affiliations

Physician practice arrangements have changed dramatically over the past 36 years. Consider these statistics from the American Medical Association (AMA):

- In 1983, three out of four physicians (76 percent) owned their practices. As of 2018, less than half (45.9 percent) had an ownership stake in their practices.

- In 1983, 8 out of 10 physicians (79.6 percent) worked in practices with 10 or fewer physicians. As of 2018, that percentage dropped to just under 6 out of 10 physicians (56.5 percent).

- In 1983, more than 40 percent of physicians worked in solo practices. As of 2018, the percentage of physicians in solo practice dropped to 14.8 percent.
- In 2018, for the first time since the AMA has been tracking physician practice statistics, the percentage of physicians who are employees (47.4 percent) surpassed the percentage of physicians who are owners (45.9 percent).[406]

Physicians are finding strength in numbers, either by affiliating with each other or becoming employees of the health system. I think this is a trend that will continue, because there are benefits to affiliation. Physicians who are employees are incentivized to engage in behavior that aligns with hospital outcomes, including efficient reimbursement processes. As physicians become employees, you start seeing metrics like length of stay go down, because the physician is incentivized to do their dictation at 8:00 a.m. instead of 11:00 a.m. A lot of treatment and payment processes hinge on what the dictation says is next for the patient, so expediting dictation can have a significant impact.

Hospitals whose physicians are employees can also put other accountability measures in place to increase process efficiencies and decrease costs: Your dictations post-discharge will be completed within 24 hours. You will round on patients before noon. You will audit your orders for patient safety to ensure no more than two CTs are ordered on the same patient in one day. You will make sure you are looking at high-cost utilizations and try more conservative approaches first.

Obviously, physicians aren't happy when hospital cost-consciousness impacts clinical practice, but there has to be a balance, and I think that balance reaches an accord when the physician is employed by the hospital. When physicians are employees, it's easier to align physician practices with hospital health goals and payer strategies, which is quite meaningful.

The majority of rules and regulations impacting claims and denials have to do with the performing provider, not the referring provider—things like authorizations, medical necessity, notifications and documentation. If those details aren't in order, the hospital doesn't get paid. The physicians are the inputs for that, but if they aren't employees, there's no way to hold them accountable.

Most physicians typically don't check authorization rules before they order procedures, even though those rules are published. They typically don't check how much something costs before they order it either. They assume compliance with these types of rules falls mainly to the hospital, or even to the patient.

Physicians—in an effort to make their tasks faster—will pre-authorize in advance … since they know over time, they will be asked for it and without preauthorization the process may stop. And most (if not all) have completely separated themselves from the cost discussion with their patients.

Consequently, the responsibility falls on the patient. I understand physicians are practicing medicine, but the financial component should be on the agenda for everyone involved—it's that critical downstream for every stakeholder. If physicians want to help control costs, they need to understand the rules and also help consumers understand those rules. It's easier to get physicians to play by the rules when they are employees and their compensation is tied to the hospital's performance. It helps ensure the physician and the hospital are on the same team, pulling with each other instead of against each other to optimize both clinical and financial outcomes.

239

This is *Utilization Review 101*, gang. We had it 10 years ago, but it drifted. We became myopic on inpatient and observation status as a case management team, perhaps because that's where we were losing the most money and it was the biggest fire to put out. We need to move the fire truck over to the rest of the care: outcomes and evidence-based protocols that drive the Quadruple Aim (cost, quality, outcome and experience) on every patient, every order, every time. Yes, it will take resources and tenacity. It will be hard. You won't like it. The physicians will love it! (Riiiiiight). But it will be worth it.

Engaging with the Patient in their Financial Experience

As physicians become more aligned with providers—whether they are employed by providers or are practice owners working collaboratively with providers—they're going to have to become more involved in the patient financial experience, whether they like it or not.

Physicians, like hospitals, have long dragged their feet when it comes to discussing the cost of care with patients. Like hospitals, physicians claim they can't possibly know what an individual patient's cost of care will be, due to variables like who the insurer is, what the plan is, what the deductible is, what the copay is and where the patient is going to get the recommended care. And they have to draw from their most valuable resource—time—which is growing scarcer.

But I say to physicians—just like I say to hospitals—it's possible to give estimates to patients. Physicians, like hospitals, have a general sense of what different types of treatments or prescriptions are going to cost. And there are plenty of technology tools available to help providers refine estimates more precisely.

These automated tools are available right now, but physicians are choosing not to use them. They just don't seem to be moving toward getting on board this train and it's going to be to their detriment someday.

Back in 2014, Dr. Peter Ubel wrote:

> Like it or not, physicians cannot expect to practice medicine without discussing the cost of care with their patients. This is going to be difficult for a while. But I expect these cost conversations will get easier over time, as physicians gain experience holding such conversations and as they, and their administrative staff, become more familiar with how much various healthcare services cost. Rather than resist this inevitable trend, physicians should embrace the opportunity to help their patients better understand the full ramifications of their healthcare alternatives.[407]

I agree with this assessment of the situation and I believe it's even more applicable now than it was when he wrote this six years ago. Again, this will be hard. You won't like it. You are going to have to invest the time. But it will be worth it. Your patients (and your hospital) will thank you for it. And you will get paid.

Payer Strategies
Rules and Regulations

Rules, rules and more rules. One way payers are controlling costs is by making complex rules for providers to get paid. One study published in *Health Affairs* developed a measure of billing complexity across insurers based on detailed remittance data.[408] The study found fee-for-service Medicaid is the most challenging type of insurer to bill, but with varying levels of complexity across all payers (figure 9.4).

Figure 9.4 Measures of Billing Complexity

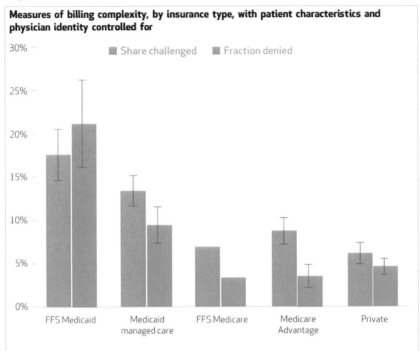

Measures of billing complexity, by insurance type, with patient characteristics and physician identity controlled for

■ Share challenged   ■ Fraction denied

FFS Medicaid — Medicaid managed care — FFS Medicare — Medicare Advantage — Private

SOURCE Authors' analysis of data for 2015 from the IQVIA Real-World Data Adjudicated Claims. **NOTES** The exhibit shows two billing complexity measures for each category of insurance in 2015, adjusted for differences across physicians and differences in patient complexity. Details on these adjustments are discussed on pages 2 and 3 of the appendix (see note 16 in text). The error bars denote 95% confidence intervals, which tested for differences relative to fee-for-service (FFS) Medicare.

Source: Jacqueline LaPointe. "Medical Billing Complexity Highest for Medicaid Fee-for-Service." RevCycleIntelligence. April 4, 2018. Accessed October 18, 2019. https://revcycleintelligence.com/news/medical-billing-complexity-highest-for-medicaid-fee-for-service; and Joshua D. Gottlieb, Adam Hale Shapiro and Abe Dunn. "The Complexity of Billing and Paying for Physician Care." Health Affairs. April 2018. Accessed October 18, 2019. https://doi.org/10.1377/hlthaff.2017.1325

I've already had plenty to say about rules in the preceding chapters of this book, so I won't go into more detail here, other than to say this: Payers need to stop with the excessive rules and denials and instead start focusing on making care better and more efficient. Work *collaboratively* with the provider. Develop shared goals. Reduce readmissions and ED utilization together. Reward physicians who pre-certify procedures appropriately, and sanction those who do not. Share risk and reward on performance in outcomes and cost.

Castell, Intermountain Healthcare's new, comprehensive health platform company, is doing just that.[409] In 2018, Intermountain introduced a value-based primary care model called Reimagined Primary Care.[410] After one year, the program produced strong results:

- A 60 percent reduction in Medicare Advantage admissions
- A 25 percent reduction in commercial insurance admissions
- A 20 percent decrease in per-member per-month costs
- Improved patient ratings
- Improved physician satisfaction

The Reimagine Primary Care program is now being rolled out to more providers via Castell. Check out Intermountain's website at: https://intermountainhealthcare.org/about/transforming-healthcare/innovation/castell/. Payers and providers are working together on shared outcomes. Look at that. Pass it on.

Narrowing Networks

Another way payers are trying to control costs is by narrowing their networks. They are realizing they can't contract with every single hospital in the country, or every doctor, or every clinic, or every freestanding ED. That would be apocalyptic, because no one could afford it. They have to limit choice to protect affordability.

In some ways, the move toward narrow networks is similar to the "old days" when Health Maintenance Organizations (HMO) were more popular. HMOs are health insurance plans that limit coverage to providers who work for, or directly contract with, the HMO.[411] They generally don't cover out-of-network care except in an emergency. The whole point of HMOs was to control costs by encouraging patients and providers to use healthcare services wisely, instead of offering unrestrained access to healthcare. HMOs peaked in popularity around 1996, when 31 percent of covered workers were enrolled in HMOs.[412] But consumers pushed back against the limited choices and burdensome restrictions that went along with HMOs.[413] Enrollment in HMOs declined to only 16 percent of covered workers by 2018.[414]

In the interest of cost savings, however, HMO-style narrow networks are making somewhat of a comeback. I think maybe HMOs rolled out too early, ahead of their time, but now they are relevant again. Today's narrow networks operate on the same principle: controlling costs by limiting choice. Today's consumer is more tolerant of narrow networks in the face of rising healthcare costs. They think, "Yes, choice is important, but it's not *that* important if it's going to cost me less."

Here's the deal: Payer tells provider, "Hey, you get more patients, more volume, and they can only come to you." The provider makes a concession on their rates and gives the payer a deep discount. The employer and employee (patient) get lower costs, with less choice.

Narrow networks are a legitimate way to control costs, as long as consumers are educated about it. It needs to be disclosed and transparent: "You bought a plan with a limited network. This one only has one place you can go. Do you like this place? Because you are going to have to use this doctor and these facilities under this plan as long as it exists."

It's a commitment, like getting married.

For the time being, narrow networks are making inroads only in very specific markets. Large employers are generally avoiding narrow network plans for logistical reasons. In a recent article on news website Axios, Drew Altman, Kaiser Family Foundation CEO, noted: "It's difficult for them [large employers] to satisfy a diverse workforce with a limited network of doctors and hospitals, especially in a tight labor market ... Where they are interested, they tend to promote what they regard as high performance networks that meet their guidelines for delivering high value care, not necessarily the lower cost networks more common in the non-group market."[415]

The 2019 Employer Health Benefits survey, conducted by the Kaiser Family Foundation, validates the reluctance of large employers to move to narrow network plans.[416] The survey found among employers who offer health benefits:

- Thirty-nine percent said they would *not* reduce network size for cost savings
- Eleven percent said they would need to realize cost savings of between 20 percent and 30 percent to shift to a narrower network
- Twenty-five percent said they would need to realize cost savings of *more than* 30 percent to shift to a narrower network[417]

When employers were asked what their biggest obstacles were to adopting narrow network plans:

- Twenty-eight percent cited employee considerations (disruption of provider relationships, employee backlash)
- Fourteen percent cited concerns about access or convenience for employees
- Twelve percent cited concerns about cost or quality of care

- Eleven percent said their employees are spread out over a large area
- Nine percent said they are in a rural area that lacks access to providers[418]

Narrow networks are more common in the individual and ACA marketplaces. People who have been uninsured, or who are responsible for their own coverage, are apparently "more willing to accept a tradeoff between provider choice and costs than workers in the group market."[419] This is another area where tradeoffs and compromises are going to have to come into play in order to reduce healthcare costs. One of our nation's largest employers, Walmart, is doing this today. (Take a look at the employer strategies section later in this chapter).

Steerage

Steerage is another strategy payers are using to control costs. An example of steerage is when an authorization is requested and the payer directs the patient to another facility, or when a patient actually calls the insurance company (like they are supposed to but never do) and asks where they should go.

In the first example, which I affectionately refer to as "hijacking," the payer intercepts the authorization request and redirects it. The referral then vanishes from the provider's view when, and if, the patient is informed. The patient subsequently chooses to go to the other, less expensive place for their care. In the other scenario, the patient actually calls the insurance company (which never happens) and questions, "Hey, my doctor ordered this. Where do you think I should go?" And the insurance company responds with information like, "Well, Mrs. Doe, you have four choices. You can go to the hospital, like your physician recommended and that will be $1,100 out-of-pocket. Or you can go to Specialty X-ray, which would be $930 out-of-pocket. Your third choice is to go to Discount Imaging for $450 out-of-pocket. Or you could go to our contracted imaging specialist for a $20 copay."

I didn't like it when I was on the receiving end of this at the provider level but I understood where the payer was coming from. I couldn't fault them—they were just trying to save the patient (and their employer buyer) some costs. It shows complete disregard for the patient-provider relationship (which appears to be less valuable these days anyway), but it was a good money play.

This "stealthy steerage" would often happen behind the scenes as well. When I worked at the hospital, we would call in an authorization for an MRI, for example, to the payer. I would not hear back from them, or the patient. The payer apparently made a call to the patient and said, "You have to go to XYZ Imaging Center," and that would take the referral away from the hospital.

I would get on the phone with the payer and say, "Hey, you can't really do that." Because that's how insurance contracts work: we give the payer a discount, and the payer sends patients to us for services. But payers would push back and say to me, "Well, we are trying to help our members save out-of-pocket expenses, and as a hospital, you are inefficient and expensive. Thus, we are within our rights to steer patients to a less expensive provider."

My next step would be to go back to the contract, but the payer would point out some provision, buried in the fine print, that read, "The carrier will act in the best interest of its members to provide care at the lowest cost, and the provider agrees to follow the carrier's recommended plan guidelines for referrals." In plain English, that meant the payer has the right to steer patients to the places they want.

I was less than pleased.

Patients can (and should) participate in the conversation—payers can incentivize patients to make lower-cost choices, but the patient can still make the decision. That's a role the payers can play—to help member patients pick the provider with the highest quality for the lowest cost. Steerage can even be built into the design of patient benefits. For example, UnitedHealthcare, Aetna and Medicare plans all feature lower copays for ambulatory surgery centers (ASC) than hospital outpatient departments (HOPD).[420]

This can work in a more transparent way. Providers need to keep their costs in check (really), and this should never happen. Consumers will decide where to go based on cost. There are lots of rules about the Emergency Medical Treatment and Active Labor Act of 1986 (EMTALA), indigent care, overhead and others I conveniently left out—I acknowledge that—while at the same time, providers need to be transparent as well.

Give the consumer the choice they deserve. If the industry keeps treating patients as patients and not consumers, they will lose them to someone who not only has their best clinical interests in mind, but also has their best financial interests in mind.

Provider (Hospital) Strategies

The old hospital strategy of "if you build it, they will come" is becoming less relevant. I just heard this at a HLTH conference in 2019. This saga is gone. For elective services, consumers want convenience and low cost. People go to the hospital when they are told to or when they want to, but they are no longer necessarily seeking or obtaining most of their elective services there.

According to the most recent data from the AHA, hospital inpatient admissions in community hospitals peaked around 2008 but have been declining since then—in spite of the aging American population (figure 9.5).

Figure 9.5 Inpatient Admissions in Community Hospitals, 1995–2016

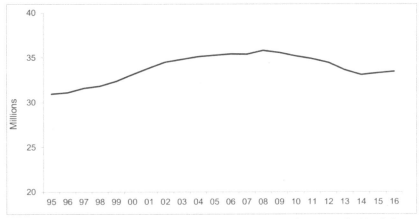

Source: Trendwatch Chartbook 2018. Chart 3.1: Inpatient Admissions in Community Hospitals, 1995–2016. Utilization and Volume. American Hospital Association. 2018. Accessed October 21, 2019. https://www.aha.org/system/files/2018-05/2018-chartbook-chart-3-1.pdf

Over a period of eight years—between 2008 and 2016—hospitals were losing more than 1 percent of inpatient volume each year.[421] That's a lot of income that is simply *gone*. And inpatient volume—supported by the right payer mix—is a hospital's bread and butter. It keeps the doors open. This isn't earth-shattering news. The transition from inpatient to ambulatory (outpatient) care has been happening for years.

My point is hospital care is migrating to freestanding centers based on a movement of *convenience* and *low cost*, not just payer reimbursement rules and care innovations. Patients are becoming very aware of cost, and are also tuned in to their family and friends telling them "how easy" it was to get in, and most importantly, these freestanding centers are affordable and make it easy for patients to pay.

Affiliations

Many services that used to be hospital inpatient services are being lost to outpatient, ambulatory facilities. At first, hospitals tried to address this dynamic by building their own outpatient centers with different fee schedules and different sets of rules to make it more convenient for patients. But this effort backfired due to Medicare's site-neutral payment rule.

Under Centers for Medicare & Medicaid Services' (CMS) previous payment system, hospital outpatient departments (HOPD) were paid more than office-based physician practices for the same services.[422] This meant ASCs could receive as little as 53 percent of the amount paid to HOPDs for the same service.[423] Not anymore. CMS has gradually been expanding the scope of site-neutral payments, meaning that regardless of where a patient accesses services—such as clinic services—the Medicare payment will be the same. And that payment will be at the lower rate: HOPDs will no longer receive the higher, differential payments. The AHA has argued against site-neutral payments on the grounds that hospitals are expected to provide 24/7 access for patients, serve as a safety-net provider and have resources in place to respond to disasters—none of which is required of office-based physician practices. According to AHA, higher fees for services provided by HOPDs help support the expenses associated with these additional expectations.[424]

CMS isn't buying that argument and has continued to expand site-neutral payment policies since the first such policies were initiated in 2017.[425] However, in September 2019, the U.S. District Court for the District of Columbia ruled for the AHA and against CMS's site-neutral payment policy in *American Hospital Association, et al.* v. *Azar*.[426] AHA responded to the decision with a statement noting, in part, "the [CMS] cuts directly undercut the clear intent of Congress to protect hospital outpatient departments because of the many real and crucial differences between them and other sites of care. Now that the court has ruled, it is up to the agency to put forth remedies for impacted hospitals and the patients they serve."[427]

As of this writing, the decision is still under appeal and CMS is progressing forward.[428] Until CMS changes things, hospitals are turning to affiliations as a strategy, rather than building their own outpatient facilities, to create intake paths for patients. If they don't pursue affiliations, they are going to get stuck, because they can't rely on patients just coming through the hospital doors anymore.

AHA statistics document this trend. Over the last 10 years, the number of hospitals that are part of health systems has slowly increased, while the number of independent hospitals (not in health systems) has steadily declined (figure 9.6).

Figure 9.6 Number of Hospitals in Health Systems, 2005–2016

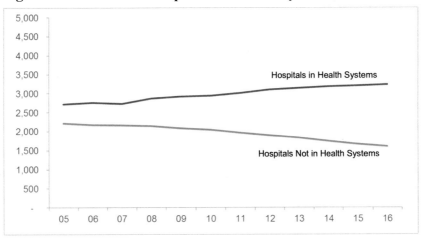

Source: Trendwatch Chartbook 2018. Chart 2.4: Number of Hospitals in Health Systems, 2005–2016. Organizational Trends. American Hospital Association. 2018. Accessed October 29, 2019. www.aha.org/system/files/2018-05/2018-chartbook-chart-2-4.pdf

Hospitals have to buddy up with physician practices and clinics of other hospitals, because if they do not, they are going to keep bleeding patient volume. At the same time, affiliations can be tricky. They can be tricky for providers because of regulatory and compliance issues. It can be tricky for patients, because they can get confused by the branding—who is working with whom. It can be complicated for the revenue cycle management (RCM) professional when they start sorting out network contracts, out-of-network contracts, and in-network rules and charges. It can create compliance issues.

For example, let's say "Smith Hospital" has a flower for their logo. The patient sees that logo and "Smith" on a building across town and they don't realize that's actually a separate physician's clinic that does "provider-based billing," so the price might be different there for some procedures or the ownership might be different. And then the patient comes to the hospital and finds out the price is different for the same procedure.

Technically, that shouldn't happen. The hospital should be watching for this but it happens with these affiliations, depending on the specifics of the arrangement and how the contractual reimbursement works. Patients receive what they believe is the same value for the same service but when they get billed its different based on sites of service, which in turn hits different benefits, with different reimbursements, which have different out-of-pocket impacts on the patient. The patient gets confused as to why that happens, and it becomes a service recovery issue for the RCM leader. Patients think the hospital is charging different prices for the same procedure and it gets really dicey.

So those are the complications that can arise with affiliations. But there are also positive aspects. Affiliations can help hospitals retain volume and treat as many patients as they can within their affiliation "net." Affiliations can give patients more options for care, so they don't have to rely as much on the ED. There is more availability for physician appointments, diagnostic testing, to fill your prescription, etc. For the self-pay patient, affiliations can increase the charity options available, which allows for a stratification of risk.

Ambulatory Strategy

Hospital ambulatory strategies are along the same lines. The question is: How are you going to treat outpatients differently? As I pointed out in chapter 7, hospitals are licensed as short-term acute care (STAC) facilities. There was a time when the CMS inpatient-only list actually helped prevent some of the bleed-off of patients to outpatient facilities. The CMS inpatient-only list specifies which procedures—typically complex or complicated surgical procedures requiring the services be provided safely in an inpatient setting—are not eligible for Medicare reimbursement if performed in an outpatient setting.[429]

The movement of procedures from an inpatient-only to an outpatient setting is accelerating the loss of inpatient volume being experienced by hospitals. As an example, total knee arthroplasty (TKA), a procedure that has been on the Medicare inpatient-only list seemingly forever, recently came off and can now be performed in an outpatient setting.[430]

Employer Strategies

I covered a lot of this in the prior chapters, and in my first book, so I will be brief. As noted, over 50 percent of U.S. citizens get their health insurance through their employer. Healthcare costs rank as one of the highest investments an employer has, second only to labor in most organizations.[431] As a major stakeholder, employers are taking back the reins. Haven, which I mentioned earlier, is building its integrated delivery model for hundreds of thousands of their employees—on their dime, to control outcome and cost. Walmart, one of the nation's largest employers, has started Walmart Health, a freestanding, full-service combination medical, dental and vision center.[432] Their own employees will be the guinea pigs, as well as consumers—so far, they only have one location, and it is in the state of Georgia, but I'm inclined to think Walmart Health will grow just as Walmart has.[433]

Employers have a lot of dollars sunk into healthcare costs for their employees. They would like to reinvest these dollars in an innovative way. I could write a whole book about that someday. My point is, you will see employers, as much as the patient, start to disrupt healthcare. Hospitals, payers and those who support them in the healthcare information technology (HIT) space will need to evolve as the largest purchasers innovate, create, deliver, fund, cover and pay for healthcare differently than our country has ever seen. Deloitte recently released a study for Healthcare 2040 and made this point:

> Along with companies that develop health products, other organizations will provide the structure that supports virtual communities. Consumer-centric health players will provide virtual, personalized wellness and care to consumers; leverage community to encourage behavior change; and drive consumer and caregiver education.[434]

There are many other innovative companies as well: Intel, CVS, Walgreens, Google, Boeing, Microsoft and many others are changing the way we receive healthcare.

We Are All in This Together

Each stakeholder holds a piece of the healthcare cost puzzle. As you can see by the strategies described above, right now each stakeholder is trying to leverage any means at their disposal to either optimize payment (physicians, providers) or manage cost (patients, employers, payers). Ultimately, lowering costs in the U.S. healthcare system will need to be a collaborative effort. A 2019 NEJM survey found healthcare executives, clinical leaders and clinicians believe responsibility for lowering healthcare costs is primarily in the hands of hospitals and health systems, followed by government, then clinicians, and finally, patients (figure 9.7). (Note: commercial payers weren't included as an option in this survey.) Employers will have to purchase healthcare differently than they do now by looking at direct-to-provider care, centers of excellence and other models. Employers that stick to traditional ways of purchasing healthcare plans won't benefit from cost controls generated by innovative care delivery models.

Figure 9.7 Responsibility for Lowering Cost of Care

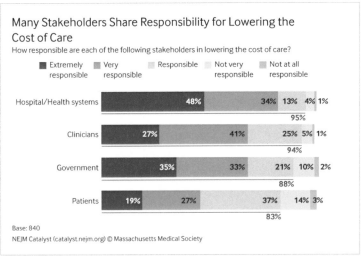

Source: Leemore Dafny and Chris DeRienzo. "New Marketplace Survey: Patients Lack Information to Reduce the Cost of Care." Insights Report. NEJM Catalyst. March 7, 2019. Accessed October 26, 2019. https://catalyst.nejm.org/patients-lack-cost-of-care/

At some point, all stakeholders are going to have to work together, and compromises are going to have to be made. There's no way to get around that reality. We can't provide universal access to care at the current cost of delivery because there's no way to fund it. We can't cap all payments at government rates because hospitals couldn't sustain their operations. We can't have affordable coverage for an unaffordable product. In other words, we need to find new solutions that lower costs without placing unsustainable burdens on any specific group of stakeholders.

The government is still trying to figure out what those solutions might look like. In the next chapter, I'll take a look at legislative solutions on the table at this time (with the caveat that legislative proposals seem to change hourly). Feel free to reach out to me for updates—I'm happy to chat about the latest developments.

CHAPTER 10

LEGISLATIVE OUTLOOK

First, a disclaimer: I once prepared a slide deck for a talk on the legislative outlook, particularly about the potential repeal of the ACA. President Trump had just been elected, and we had a Republican House and Senate. At that moment in time, it looked like the ACA repeal had significant momentum. I finished the slide deck and went on a weeklong rafting trip in the wilderness, well out of reach of emails, texts and the news. I got back Sunday night, feeling well prepared for my Tuesday speech. But when I checked in, I had literally dozens of text and voice messages that boiled down to, "You have to change your content. The ACA repeal didn't go through." I had one day to redo the entire deck.

I should have known ... nothing is *ever* guaranteed in Washington. You would think I would've learned my lesson. At that time, I swore to never write another legislative outlook or try to predict what our government was going to do to healthcare, because you could spin a roulette wheel and get closer. But I'm not one for learning fast lessons, so I'm going to go ahead and attempt a legislative outlook here, knowing the moment I write these words they may become obsolete. With that disclaimer in mind, here's what the legislative future looks like at this moment. Let's see how I do.

Affordable Care Act

On January 20, 2017—the day President Donald Trump was sworn in to office—he signed an executive order designed to begin the process of dismantling the ACA.[435] Prior to winning the election, he promised to "immediately repeal and replace Obamacare," but delivering on that promise has proven difficult.[436]

After five failed attempts to deliver a complete repeal and replace, the administration changed tactics and has been chipping away at different specific aspects of the ACA in an attempt to destabilize it.[437] As detailed in chapters 3 and 4, the current administration's changes include repeal of the ACA individual mandate penalty, cutting off funding for cost sharing reduction (CSR) and opening the market to "short-term health insurance plans" that don't have to comply with ACA minimum plan benefit requirements.[438] ACA opponents have continued to push legal challenges in the courts. In early 2018, "Texas and a group of Republican-led like-minded states challenged the constitutionality of the ACA."[439] This challenge has worked its way through the court process and the current ruling is the ACA is unconstitutional. At the time of this writing, a decision from the Fifth Circuit is still pending (figure 10.1).

Figure 10.1 Abbreviated Timeline of Texas, et al. v. U.S. (ACA Constitutionality Challenge)

ACTION	DATE
Complaint Filed by Texas, et. al.	February 26, 2018
District Court decision	December 14, 2018
Appeal to Fifth Circuit Court	January 2019
Fifth Circuit oral argument	July 9, 2019
Fifth Circuit decision	Expected fall 2019
Request cert. Supreme Court: possible that argument is in the 2019–2020 term, but the later the Fifth Circuit's decision, the less likely it makes this Supreme Court term	Expected fall-winter 2019

Source: "Texas, et. al., v. U.S. (ACA Constitutionality Challenge)." Groom Benefits Brief. Groom Law Group. September 26, 2019. Accessed October 29, 2019.
https://www.groom.com/resources/texas-et-al-v-u-s-aca-constitutionality-challenge/

What happens next is anyone's guess. The consequences of the Fifth Circuit's decision—and a possible, subsequent appeal of that decision to the Supreme Court—could range anywhere from validating the ACA to completely eliminating it. Sources close to me indicate the most recent ruling will get overturned by the Supreme Court. The stakes are high. Sabrina Corlette, director of the Center on Health Insurance Reforms at Georgetown University, said in an interview on National Public Radio (NPR) if the ACA is ruled unconstitutional:

> … the chaos that would ensue is almost impossible to wrap your brain around. The marketplaces would just simply disappear and millions of people would become uninsured overnight, probably leaving hospitals and doctors with millions and millions of dollars in unpaid medical bills. Medicaid expansion would disappear overnight … I don't see any sector of our healthcare economy being untouched or unaffected.[440]

A Kaiser Family Foundation (KFF) analysis of the impact of the possibility of *Texas* v. *U.S.* striking down the constitutionality of the ACA noted:

> More than eight years after enactment, ACA changes to the nation's health system have become embedded and affect nearly everyone in some way. A court decision that invalidated the ACA, therefore, would also affect nearly everyone in at least some way. It would be a complex undertaking to try to disentangle it at this point.[441]

KFF's point is well founded. As much as one may love or hate the ACA, it is a big part of our healthcare system today. It will take years to wind back if (big "if") the Texas ruling is upheld.

Medicaid Expansion

The fate of Medicaid expansion is closely tied to the fate of the ACA. ACA Medicaid expansion provisions led to a 26.1 percent increase in Medicaid enrollment over pre-ACA numbers.[442] The Kaiser Family Foundation reports Medicaid now "covers one in five Americans, accounts for one in six dollars spent on healthcare in the United States, and makes up more than half of all spending on long-term services and supports."[443]

A number of studies have concluded the Medicaid expansion has led to mostly positive outcomes. An August 2019 comprehensive literature review by the Kaiser Family Foundation concluded, "Research indicates the expansion is linked to gains in coverage; improvements in access, financial security and some measures of health status/outcomes; and economic benefits for states and providers."[444] Likewise, the Commonwealth Fund pointed out in a recent article "... a national study confirmed that during the two years when the federal government paid all of the costs for newly eligible enrollees, Medicaid expansion did not lead to any significant increases in state spending on Medicaid or to reductions in spending on other priorities such as education. But even at a lesser percent match, the fiscal case for expansion is compelling."[445]

As of September 2019, a total of 37 states and the District of Columbia have adopted Medicaid expansion (figure 10.2). States that have resisted the Medicaid expansion are clustered mainly in the southern and southeastern portions of the U.S.

Figure 10.2 Status of State Action on the Medicaid Expansion Decision

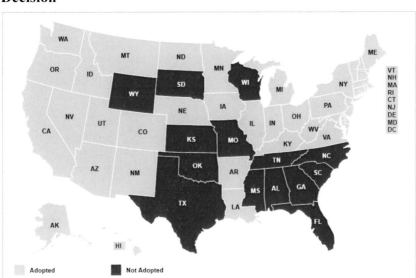

Source: Status of State Action on the Medicaid Expansion Decision. State Health Facts. Kaiser Family Foundation. September 20, 2019. Updated January 2, 2020 https://www.kff.org/health-reform/state-indicator/state-activity-around-expanding-medicaid-under-the-affordable-care-act/

A study by WalletHub found the average uninsured rate for states that didn't expand Medicaid (11.14 percent) is more than four percentage points *higher* than the average uninsured rate for states that expanded Medicaid (6.95 percent) (figure 10.3). This illustrates one of the significant benefits for providers:

> patients covered by the Medicaid expansion likely would have fallen into the uncompensated care bucket, prior to the expansion.

With the expansion, providers at least get paid Medicaid rates for services provided to these patients. Even though Medicaid payment rates are lower than provider's actual costs, at least Medicaid offers providers some compensation for care, rather than no compensation at all.

Figure 10.3 Average Uninsured Rate for States That Expanded Medicaid Versus States That Didn't Expand Medicaid (2018)

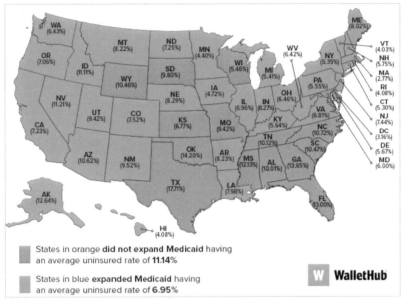

States in orange **did not expand Medicaid** having an average uninsured rate of **11.14%**

States in blue **expanded Medicaid** having an average uninsured rate of **6.95%**

Source: John S. Kiernan. "States with the Highest and Lowest Uninsured Rates." WalletHub. October 10, 2019. Accessed October 29, 2019. https://wallethub.com/edu/uninsured-rates-by-state/4800/#medicaid

In January 2018, the Trump administration introduced new guidelines for Medicaid expansion, allowing states to impose work requirements as a condition of eligibility for Medicaid.[446] As of October 2019, 18 states had submitted requests for work requirements, 6 have been approved, 9 are pending, and 3 have been set aside by the courts.[447] Only two of the approved work requirements were implemented (Arkansas and Indiana), but in March 2019, a court decision suspended Arkansas's work requirement implementation "until HHS [the U.S. Department of Health and Human Services] issues a new approval that passes legal muster or prevails on appeal."[448] After Arkansas initially implemented its work requirements, more than 18,000 people lost Medicaid coverage—not just because they weren't able to meet the work requirements, but also because many were unable to navigate the system to document whether they were meeting the requirements or eligible for an exemption.[449] As of this writing, Indiana had also backed away from implementing its Medicaid work requirements, following Arizona's lead.[450]

Based on the research I've done, the Medicaid expansion appears to have had a net positive effect for patients and for providers, with negligible fiscal impacts on the states. There have been lots of outcomes in the "pro" column, and very little in the "con" column. But just as with the ACA, the fate of the Medicaid expansion is now in the hands of the court system.

Health Benefit Exchanges

The ACA requires every state to offer a health insurance exchange where individual consumers and small businesses can shop for and purchase private health insurance coverage.[451] States have many options in offering these health benefit exchange (HBE) plans: they can operate their own exchanges (called state-based marketplace [SBM] or state-based exchanges [SBE]); offer a state-based marketplace using the federally facilitated marketplace IT platform (SBM-FP); offer a state-partnership marketplace (SPM), where HHS performs the majority of the marketplace functions; or rely on a Federally Facilitated Marketplace (FFM), where HHS is responsible for all marketplace functions (i.e., consumers enroll at Healthcare.gov).[452] As of this writing, there are 12 SBM/SBEs, 5 SBM-FPs, 6 SPMs and 28 FFMs. The 12 SBMs—though established per the ACA—don't rely on the federally funded technology platform to operate. The other three types of exchanges rely on healthcare.gov. Overturning the ACA could significantly disrupt the health benefit exchanges. Would the government stop supporting the federal technology platform

(Healthcare.gov) if the ACA were overturned? If so, 39 states that rely on Healthcare.gov could lose the technology they use to run their exchanges. Also, if the ACA were overturned, certain provisions could disappear, like the essential health benefit requirements for plans on the exchanges.[453] This could have a significant impact on the plans offered even on the HBEs.

Meanwhile, some Trump administration policies continue to impact health insurance exchange enrollment. For example, in 2017 the administration cut funding for outreach programs designed to help consumers navigate exchanges.[454] Dropping the CSR subsidies impacted plan affordability, hiking premiums and making them less appealing to consumers.[455] With respect to enrollment, the SBEs seem to be weathering the administration's storm better than federally-run exchanges. Over the past five years, enrollment in SBEs has remained relatively steady—around 3 million—while enrollment in Healthcare.gov-based exchanges has dropped to 8.4 million from 9.6 million in 2016 (figure 10.4).

Figure 10.4 Enrollment via Health Insurance Exchanges

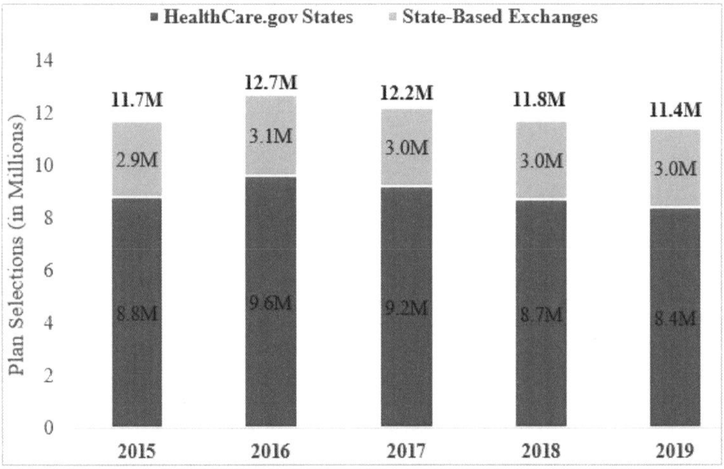

Source: "Health Insurance Exchanges 2019 Open Enrollment Report." Fact Sheet. CMS.gov. Centers for Medicare & Medicaid Services. Figure 1, Plan Selections during the 2015–2019 Open Enrollment Periods. March 25, 2019. Accessed October 29, 2019. https://www.cms.gov/newsroom/fact-sheets/health-insurance-exchanges-2019-open-enrollment-report

In addition to the policy changes impacting enrollment on the exchanges, insurers' experience of profits and losses have impacted insurer participation in the exchanges. The KFF reported that in 2014, there were an average of five insurers participating in each state's ACA marketplace.[456] In 2015, that number rose to an average of six insurers per state; in 2016, it dropped to 5.6; and in 2017, after insurance company losses, the average dropped to 4.3.[457] In 2018, it dropped even lower, to 3.5, and then in 2019, it rebounded to an average of only four participating insurers per state.[458]

Since that's an average it means the range was considerable. In 2019, 5 states (Alaska, Delaware, Mississippi, Nebraska and Wyoming) had only 1 company participating in the exchanges, while 3 states (California, New York and Wisconsin) had more than 10 companies participating.[459] In 2020, 67 percent of enrollees had a choice of three or more insurers (figure 10.5).

Figure 10.5 Participation on ACA Marketplaces, 2019–2020

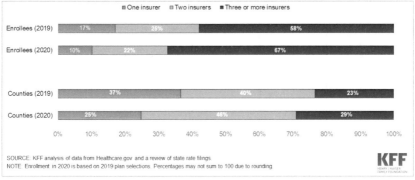

Source: Rachel Fehr, Rabah Kamal and Cynthia Cox. "Insurer Participation on ACA Marketplaces, 2014–2020." Kaiser Family Foundation. Figure 2, Insurer Participation on ACA Marketplaces, 2019–2020. November 21, 2019. Accessed November 29, 2019. https://www.kff.org/private-insurance/issue-brief/insurer-participation-on-aca-marketplaces-2014-2020/

The question remains: Are the health benefit exchanges going to survive or not? At the moment, the exchanges seem to be out of the intensive care unit and limping along, but will they still exist in 2025?

I tend to agree with the Robert Wood Johnson Foundation: "Stability has not been a major theme in the story of the Affordable Care Act marketplace, but since 2018, premium growth has slowed and issuer participation has increased. While enrollment has trended down somewhat in recent years, health plans seem newly interested in participating."[460] I think we will see them stabilize as we progress, as insurance carriers don't invest in programs that don't make money.

Value-Based Care

Value-based care is still in its infancy. As discussed in chapter 2, a study by the Health Care Payment Learning & Action Network (LAN) found as of 2017, a little more than one-third of total U.S. healthcare payments were tied to alternative payment models (APM) (i.e., value-based care plans).[461] Pure fee-for-service plans are slowly declining as a proportion of all healthcare business (see figure 6.4 in chapter 6), but the fee-for-service model is still deeply embedded in the industry.

Legislatively, I think that value-based care models are going to continue to grow. The government views value-based care as an effective cost containment measure, since they pay on *value* not *volume*. I expect the Centers for Medicare & Medicaid Services (CMS) will continue to support existing value-based care programs (the Hospital Value-Based Purchasing Program, the Hospital Readmission Reduction Program, the Hospital Acquired Conditions Reduction Program, etc.).[462] CMS will also continue its work to expand value-based care by introducing additional programs, such as the CMS Primary Cares Initiative, which is a set of value-based care payment models for primary care, introduced in April 2019.[463]

Transparency

Transparency continues to be a legislative hot topic, as alluded in earlier chapters. In August 2018, CMS published proposed rules clarifying the ACA's provisions around price transparency.[464]

And then on June 24, 2019, President Trump issued an executive order on Improving Price and Quality Transparency in American Healthcare to Put Patients First. [465]
These documents have not been well-received in the industry. The CMS final rule basically said that not only do providers have to display their chargemaster but they also have to display their negotiated rates.

Hospitals objected because they say, "If I display my negotiated rate, there will be a race to the top for all of my colleagues, which will make prices more expensive for patients, and that is the exact opposite of what we want to do." On the other hand, payers said, "There will be a race to the bottom for all of the insurance companies, because they'll all know what the lowest rate is in an area, causing massive disruption and rate setting in the market."

Two opposing views—but they're aligned in the fact they both oppose the price transparency rule as currently written. America's Health Insurance Plans (AHIP), the Association of American Medical Colleges (AAMC), the American Hospital Association (AHA), the Federation of American Hospitals (FAH) and the Healthcare Financial Management Association (HFMA) all published comments opposed to the rule.[466] Their disdain for the rule is shared by many providers.

A recent survey of 161 hospital health system executives found the industry is quite skeptical about the CMS price transparency rules:

- Two-thirds (66 percent) of respondents do not think the rules will ultimately go into effect
- Two-thirds (64 percent) of respondents do not think the rules will have a meaningful impact on consumers' ability to shop for care
- Forty-four percent are not taking any steps to prepare for the price transparency proposals
- Fifty-seven percent believe court challenges will likely change the transparency rules [467]

Well, at least the last point is correct. November 15, 2019, as this book was being finalized to go to press, CMS released the finalized rule addressing healthcare price transparency.[468] The final rule in the 2020 OPPS, which impacts providers, "requires hospitals to make their standard charges public, including the negotiated rates with payers."[469] The Transparency in Coverage Proposed Rule (CMS-9915-P) "would require most employer-based group health plans and health insurance issuers offering group and individual coverage to disclose price and cost-sharing information to participants, beneficiaries and enrollees up front."[470] The rule has an effective date of January 1, 2021.

Almost immediately, the AHA, AAMC, Children's Hospital Association and the FAH announced they planned to sue CMS over the final rule on price transparency.[471] As of this writing, the American Medical Association (AMA), FAH and several other organizations filed a lawsuit against the Department of Health and Human Services to challenge the final rule from CMS.[472] We can expect to see more debate—and litigation—about the issue of healthcare price transparency in 2020 and beyond.

The push for transparency is not going to go away, and I think by the time something gets implemented, it will be much more reasonable than originally proposed. My predictions are: the implementation period will be delayed, disclosure of procedure-specific contractual rates between payers and providers will not be required, and as further feedback from industry experts is considered, transparency will focus on prevailing or average rates rather than negotiated rates.

What's important is we need to remove opacity in patient cost. This was a step (perhaps a leap) in that direction, and we seem to have stepped back yet again. I urge the provider community to talk about what could actually work for the patient, versus what cannot, or the government will continue to find solutions for us.

Out-of-Network "Surprise Medical Bills"

"Surprise medical bills" are another topic that has received a lot of legislative attention recently. Surprise medical bills are the charges a patient incurs when they inadvertently receive care from an out-of-network provider. This can happen in emergency scenarios, when the patient isn't in a position to make choices about which emergency department (ED) to go to or which physician to use. But it can also happen in nonemergency situations, like when a patient receives planned care from an in-network provider but other treating providers (for example, the anesthesiologist, radiologist, etc.) are not from the same network.[473] The terms "balance billing" and "surprise billing" are sometimes used interchangeably, but they are not exact synonyms. The AMA differentiates the two terms as follows:

- *Balance billing* happens when a patient's health insurance company pays an out-of-network physician or other healthcare provider less than the amount the physician charges for care. Because the physician and the health plan have not agreed upon payment through a contract, the physician bills the patient for the remainder of the costs.

- *Surprise billing* refers to a type of balance billing where a patient receives care at an in-network facility, but the care is provided by an out-of-network physician or other healthcare provider without the patient knowing the provider is out-of-network. Surprise billing can also refer to emergency care provided by an out-of-network provider.[474]

Data on the incidence and impact of surprise bills is hard to come by, in part because the circumstances and billed amounts vary widely. Data from a Peterson-Kaiser study found on average, 18 percent of emergency visits result in at least one out-of-network charge and 16 percent of in-network patient admissions result in at least one out-of-network charge.[475] Rates vary considerably by state due to differences in state balance billing protections (figure 10.6).

Figure 10.6 States Vary in Their Approach to Surprise Bills

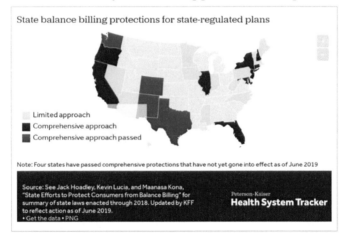

Source: Karen Pollitz, Matthew Rae, Gary Claxton, Cynthia Cox and Larry Levitt. "An examination of surprise medical bills and proposals to protect consumers from them." Peterson Center on Healthcare and Kaiser Family Foundation. Peterson-KFF Health System Tracker. October 16, 2019. Accessed October 29, 2019. https://www.healthsystemtracker.org/brief/an-examination-of-surprise-medical-bills-and-proposals-to-protect-consumers-from-them/

However, states' law protections are limited due to the Employee Retirement Income Security Act of 1974 (ERISA), a federal law that preempts state regulation of employer-provided health benefit plans.[476] That means states without legislation do not have protection from balance (or surprise) billing, so the federal government is leveling the playing field. In May 2019, President Trump called on Congress to develop bipartisan legislation to end surprise medical billing.[477] Subsequently, several bills (S 1895, HR 2328, HR 3502, HR 861, S 1266) were introduced with different approaches to managing surprise billing.[478]

At the time of this writing, federal legislation addressing surprise billing has unfortunately stalled. Several of the legislative proposals included reliance on a fixed payment standard to control surprise bills, an approach generally supported by employers and insurers.

To physicians and hospitals, however, a fixed payment standard reeks of government rate setting, to which they are adamantly opposed. A dark money group called Doctor Patient Unity spent almost $30 million on a campaign designed to undermine the leading congressional surprise billing legislation.[479] These ads interestingly ran precisely during Congress's recess.

Instead of using a government-set fixed standard or pay scale, these groups support the use of independent mediators to settle surprise billing payment disputes (a.k.a. arbitration).[480] Arbitration is an approach that has been enacted in Texas and New York.[481] Arbitration, however, has its own detractors. Opponents to arbitration say arbitration is not an effective way to control escalating out-of-network costs and will actually increase patient costs rather than resolve them.[482] They actually may also have the propensity to increase provider contracted rates.[483]

Even in the wake of the apparent stall of surprise billing legislation, the problem is not going away and will likely become worse. I expect we haven't yet heard the last of surprise billing legislation and anticipate several more bills will be introduced in 2020 and forward.

Medicare Advantage Plans

Medicare Advantage plans have been around in various forms since the late 1990s. President Bill Clinton signed Medicare+Choice into law in 1997; the name changed to Medicare Advantage in 2003.[484] Medicare Advantage plans include coverage of Part A (Hospital Insurance) and Part B (Medical Insurance) but are also sometimes bundled with Part D (Medicare Prescription Drug Plan) and/or other benefits that Original Medicare (A+B) doesn't cover.[485] These plans are managed in the private sector, often as an arm off the commercial insurance products.

The Medicare beneficiary "assigns" their benefits to the insurance carrier, and they operate the Medicare Advantage plans following Medicare, as well as their (often more stringent) rules. The upside is these plans often have a wider scope of benefits and are a relatively inexpensive way to bundle benefits. And they are growing like crazy. The downside is less choice for patients and more rules for providers.

Original Medicare offers unrestricted access to providers: Medicare Advantage plans can lower beneficiaries' out-of-pocket costs by leveraging managed care. In other words, Medicare Advantage plans (which are managed by private insurers) typically act more like a Health Maintenance Organization (HMO) and limit beneficiaries' choice of providers.[486] Medicare pays a fixed (capitated) amount to the insurers offering Medicare Advantage plans; because of that capitation, insurers are incentivized to manage patient care wisely. (The five types of Medicare

Advantage plans are: HMOs, Preferred Provider Organization (PPO) plans, Private Fee-for-Service (PFFS) Plans, Special Needs Plans (SNP) and Medical Savings Account (MSA) plans.[487]

Currently, about one-third (34 percent) of all Medicare beneficiaries are enrolled in Medicare Advantage plans, with the remaining two-thirds (66 percent) enrolled in Original Medicare. The majority (62 percent) of people enrolled in Medicare Advantage plans are enrolled in HMOs (figure 10.7)

Figure 10.7 Almost Two in Three People Enrolled in Medicare Advantage Plans Were in HMOs in 2019

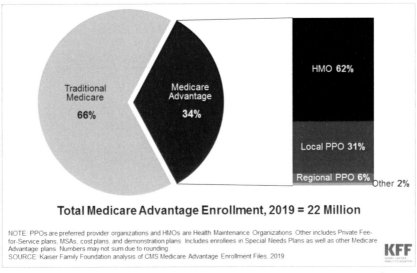

Source: "Medicare Advantage." Kaiser Family Foundation. Figure 3. June 6, 2019. Accessed October 29, 2019. https://www.kff.org/medicare/fact-sheet/medicare-advantage/

Initially, healthcare experts thought the ACA would impede growth of Medicare Advantage plans, due to federal payment cuts to the plans.[488] Instead, the opposite happened: more insurers are entering the Medicare Advantage market and enrollments are growing. Insurers made up for the federal budget cuts in two ways: (a) insurers gained revenue by identifying member conditions that entitled insurers to federal risk adjustment payments.[489] And (b) insurers qualified for federal bonus payments by scoring four or higher on the five-point Star Rating System.[490] It's become a very large growth model for the private insurance sector.

In 2019, CMS started allowing Medicare Advantage plans to cover supplemental, non-skilled home benefits.[491] This has allowed Medicare Advantage plans to move into areas related to social determinants of health, including "home-delivered meals following a hospital discharge, home safety interventions and nonskilled in-home caregiving."[492] The intention is to manage long-term costs by providing appropriate, lower-cost interventions up front. In this way, Medicare Advantage plans are leading the way in creating value-based care models.

This move is consistent with priorities expressed by Alex Azar, U.S. Secretary of Health and Human Services, in comments he made during a meeting in November 2018. Azar said:

> … we are eager to think about social determinants of health throughout the Medicare program, and one of the best ways we can do that is through the flexible, accountable, individual-driven system we already have: Medicare Advantage [MA]. Because MA plans hold the risk for their patients and they compete for their patients' business, they have an incentive to offer benefits that are both appealing to their members and that will bring down health costs—whether those benefits are traditionally thought of as health services or not. The key is just that we need to give them the flexibility to do this, which we generally haven't done. But starting next year, plans will now be allowed to pay for a wider array of health-related benefits, such as

transportation and home health visits. Starting in 2020, we are going to be expanding that range of benefits even more, to include home modifications, home-delivered meals, and more.[493]

Given Azar's perspective, it makes sense the Trump administration has encouraged the growth of Medicare Advantage plans through favorable policy changes:

In subtle and unsubtle ways, the Trump administration has seeded the ground for massive gains in Medicare Advantage enrollment. These include loosened restrictions on marketing Medicare Advantage plans, new consumer tools that accentuate the advantages of these plans, greater use of telehealth than permitted in original Medicare, the elimination of "meaningful difference" tests that limit the number of Medicare Advantage plans in a given market, and extra time for plan sponsors to secure a provider network.[494]

Considering these promising policy conditions, it's likely Medicare Advantage enrollment will continue to grow as a percentage of overall Medicare enrollment. The Congressional Budget Office has estimated 47 percent of Medicare beneficiaries will be enrolled in Medicare Advantage plans by 2029—which would mean a 13-percentage point increase over today's Medicare Advantage enrollment of 34 percent.[495]

Health Information Technology Outlook

As I pointed out in the introduction to this book, HIT is no longer optional. CMS's carrot/stick approach, with the EHR incentive program "worked": 96 percent of all nonfederal acute care hospitals have adopted certified health information technology systems.[496] The goals of the EHR Incentive Program/Meaningful Use have been updated and incorporated into CMS's Promoting Interoperability Program.[497] The Promoting Interoperability Program still requires eligible hospitals and critical access hospitals to use certified EHR technology (or prepare for a downward payment adjustment).[498]

The new program—as its name indicates—features an increased emphasis on interoperability: basically, data sharing between facilities for the good of the patient. Per the CMS website:

> Healthcare providers participating in the Promoting Interoperability Program must attest to certain statements to demonstrate that they have not knowingly and willfully taken action to limit or restrict the compatibility or interoperability of their CEHRT [certified electronic health record technology]. Collectively, these statements are referred to as the "prevention of information blocking attestation."[499]

This is interesting, because providers are probably the last ones who want to impede the achievement of interoperability. The biggest obstacles to interoperability are a lack of universally adopted data standardization and the reluctance of EHR vendors to "play nice" with other vendors. Of course, as EHR market consolidation continues, incompatibility between vendors may become less of a problem. According to the most recent U.S. Hospital EMR Market Share report by KLAS, the acute care market is dominated by a few key players: Epic (28 percent),

Cerner (26 percent), MEDITECH (16 percent), CPSI (9 percent), Allscripts (6 percent), MEDHOST (4 percent), athenahealth (2 percent).[500]

In addition to technical obstacles to interoperability, providers also deal with regulatory obstacles. The healthcare industry has always experienced tension between access to patient data and the protection of the privacy and security of that same patient data. I understand the Health Insurance Portability and Accountability Act of 1996 (HIPAA) requirements and regulations are in place to protect patient data, but at the same time, sometimes those protections seem to lock down data in a way that's incompatible with interoperability.

In February 2019, HHS and the Office of the National Coordinator for Health Information Technology (ONC) proposed new rules to promote the interoperability of electronic health information.[501] The proposed rules generated so much feedback from stakeholders that HHS extended the comment period.[502] By the time the comment period closed on June 3, 2019, the CMS proposed rule (CMS-9115-P) had received 1,761 comments and the ONC proposed rule had received 2,013 comments.[503] Many high-profile stakeholders, including the AHA, were against one or both of the proposed rules as written, feeling they were too burdensome.[504] At press time, neither rule has been published in final form.

Hospital Outlook

What does all of this mean for hospitals? Conditions are likely to remain volatile and uncertain for some time. Barring any dramatic changes in the industry, the patient will continue to assume increasing payment responsibility and payers will have more payment rules—with that increase, provider's cost to collect will continue to increase. The Medicare dollar doesn't stretch as far as it used to (cost-to-charge ratio), and as such, Medicare and Medicaid underpayments will continue to be problematic.

Providers will continue to be stuck in the middle, trying to achieve a sustainable operating margin in the face of these strong headwinds. As of August 2018, Moody's noted expense growth outpaced revenue growth for U.S. nonprofit and public hospitals for two consecutive years.[505] A year later, however, the nonprofit healthcare sector may have stabilized somewhat. A Fitch ratings report released in early September 2019 noted nonprofit health systems experienced an "improvement in financial medians for operating margins in 2019" breaking the previous two-year slump.[506] The report went on to say the nonprofit sector has displayed "considerable resiliency."[507]   .

Is this improvement or a flash in the pan? Does it signify a new direction for the industry? As the saying goes, "One data point doesn't make a trend." Hospitals and health systems are still navigating a rapidly changing market. They need to focus carefully on RCM in order to protect revenue and survive the challenges that still lie ahead. I know this: It will be a lot harder before it gets a lot easier. Our industry is receiving more legislation, more payer rules, more competition from non-traditional entrants and more demands from consumers. Notice I didn't say our industry is getting any more *money*. That means one thing—as the top line shrinks and the expense package grows, cost control will be mission critical. Automation and frictionless payment will represent the linchpins in the provider's revenue cycle strategy for the next decade.

What's next? In chapter 11 we'll explore some emerging trends that could make significant impacts on the industry in the future. These trends may seem far off, but they're closer than you think. We just need to have the desire to innovate and change.

CHAPTER 11

HEALTHCARE 2050: BEAM ME UP...

"Beam me up, Scotty." Most people recognize that phrase from the *Star Trek* series. While we don't have *Star Trek*–style transporters yet, the futuristic series did get a few things right about the future of medicine:

- Noninvasive scanning technologies
- Telemedicine (holographic physicians)
- Wireless telemetry
- Needle-free injectors (Dr. McCoy's "hypospray")
- Technology that helps people with visual impairments see

(Lieutenant Commander Geordi La Forge's visor)[508] The series even inspired a competition to develop a real-world *Star Trek* "tricorder"—a multifunctional, hand-held device that *Star Trek*'s clinicians used to scan medical patients for "immediate, comprehensive diagnoses of any condition or disease."[509] Qualcomm's Tricorder XPRIZE competition offered millions of dollars in prize money to teams that could develop a tricorder-inspired device that could (a) diagnose 13 medical conditions independent of a healthcare professional or facility; (b) be able to continuously monitor 5 vital signs; and (c) provide a positive consumer experience.[510] In 2017, the top prize was awarded to Final Frontier Medical Devices, a team led by brothers Dr. Basil

Harris (an emergency medicine physician) and George Harris (a network engineer).[511]

The winning design lives on today as DxtER™, produced by Basil Leaf Technologies. The current version of the device features an algorithm-based diagnostic engine that uses data from noninvasive sensors, plus a patient's personal and family medical history and a physical exam, to diagnose 34 different health conditions, including diabetes, atrial fibrillation, chronic obstructive pulmonary disease, urinary tract infection, sleep apnea, leukocytosis, pertussis, stroke, tuberculosis and pneumonia.[512] The creators have begun the process of going through clinical trials to get U.S. Food & Drug Administration (FDA) approval prior to bringing the solution to market.[513]

Harris, one of the founders of Basil Leaf Technologies, said, "An inevitable revolution in healthcare is coming. In this revolution, the consumers are the drivers and technology is the equalizer."[514] Tricorders aside, this consumer-driven revolution is shifting the dynamics of healthcare delivery. With the explosive growth of telemedicine and patient as payer, watch technologies start to take a front seat in healthcare delivery. The following are just a few of the ways the consumer revolution is changing healthcare.

Retail Healthcare

As I pointed out in chapter 7, the number of retail healthcare clinics in the U.S. is growing significantly. Between 2006 and 2017, the number of retail clinics grew from 351 to more than 2,800—an increase of nearly 700 percent over 10 years.[515] This makes sense in light of the fact today's consumers are interested in convenience. They want healthcare delivered where they are at—and "where they are at" is typically *not* in hospitals.

Retail medicine sees a "foot traffic" opportunity here.

Let's put this into perspective: according to the Centers for Disease Control and Prevention (CDC), the combined number of visits to physicians' offices, hospital outpatient departments and hospital emergency departments is about 1.25 billion per year—the equivalent of about 3.42 million per day.[516] Walgreens interacts with about 8 million customers each day.[517] CVS sees 4.5 million customers per day (yes, not per year, but per *day*).[518] Assuming these two are open 24/7, that is 333,333 customers an hour for Walgreens and 187,500 customers every hour for CVS. That's hundreds of thousands of visits an *hour*. They also represent the lion's share of retail clinic visits at 67.4 percent of all visits, with Walmart, Kroger and others not far behind.[519]

Consumers go to these stores primarily to fill their prescriptions and the stores know it. They're adding health clinics within them to capitalize on all that foot traffic—sometimes it's as simple as colocation—a clinic within a store. Consumers are showing up at these clinics, and that's disrupting traditional provider delivery models. Per a white paper on retail clinics by Civis Analytics, "Many patients (68 percent) who utilized these clinics made a purchase in the store during the same trip, and stated they had later made a subsequent visit to that store to purchase items (58 percent)."[520]

There are a lot of reasons patients choose retail clinics over traditional healthcare options. One reason is convenience.[521] Retail healthcare clinics are easy to access and they provide one-stop shopping. You can pick up a gallon of milk, pick up your prescriptions and get your cough checked out, all at the same time. You don't have to schedule your appointment weeks in advance— you can just walk in. And wait times are usually minimal. One survey found retail clinic visitors were either seen immediately (15.7 percent) or seen within 15 minutes (46.5 percent).[522] Only 5.7 percent of visitors reported waiting more than one hour.[523] Compare that to the traditional system: one survey found the average patient has to wait more than 29 days to see a family medicine practitioner.[524]

Retail clinics are also perceived as more affordable. A recent article in *Medical Economics* noted price can be a big differentiator for patients.[525] According to the article, "Urgent care centers are more cost effective than standalone ERs, which charge close to what hospital emergency departments do, but they charge more than physician practices do, on average. And, among physical sites, retail clinics charge the least for primary care."[526]

Data from the nonprofit research firm FAIR Health backs up this view. FAIR Health analyzes billions of privately insured healthcare claims annually for its FH Healthcare Indicators® and FH Medical Price Index® report.[527] As reported in *Medical Economics*, FAIR Health's 2019 analysis found these median prices for non-complex (CPT 99202) and more in-depth (CPT 99203) new patient visits:

> … median charges for a CPT 99202 visit ranged from $160 in an urgent center to $138 in an office to $104 in a retail clinic. Median allowed amounts for CPT 99202 were $93 for urgent care centers, $66 for offices, and $73 for retail clinics. CPT 99203 median charges were $213, $207 and $129, respectively. Urgent care centers were allowed $114, offices, $92, and retail clinics, $85, for CPT 99203. According to other reports, a telehealth visit may cost $50 to $80.[528]

While it's true that visiting your local CVS is a lot less expensive than driving to the nearest ED for a minor illness, it's also true that part of the perception of affordability is based on the price transparency offered by retail clinics. Price transparency is another reason why retail clinics are attracting consumers.[529]

Both CVS and Walgreens post detailed, fixed prices for their clinical services online[530]—no calling the provider in advance, trying to work out details like who your insurer is and what your copay is. Online price lists are simple, understandable and direct. Need to find out whether or not you have the flu? That'll cost you between $99 and $139, according to the CVS MinuteClinic website.[531] Need a vaccine for shingles? That'll run you $179.[532] Easy-to-understand online price lists help consumers make a quick decision about whether the cost of care with that provider is worth their time and money. The ability to make an informed decision is far more attractive than visiting a hospital where you are lucky to get an estimate before care is provided.

One final reason the retail clinic concept is taking off is consumers are generally pleased with their retail healthcare experiences. People love going to them. They seem to meet most needs consumers have for simple healthcare problems. They are convenient, efficient, affordable and effective. And to date, I've never heard a bad thing about any of these clinics. One survey of retail clinic patients asked, "Would you go back to a retail clinic in the future?" Eight out of 10 patients (81.7 percent) said yes.[533] The analysis concluded, "The reported convenience, lower price and overall satisfaction rates associated with retail clinic usage indicate retail clinics are doing a good job of creating happy customers who are likely to return."[534]

Interestingly, even though retail clinics may be diverting traffic from primary care physician offices and hospitals, they may not decrease overall healthcare spending. One study found only 3 percent of retail clinic visits replaced ED visits, and 39 percent replaced regular physician visits (figure 11.1).

However, 58 percent of visits were new visits—meaning the patient visited the clinic because it was there and easy to access, not because they had planned on going somewhere else and then changed direction.[535]

Figure 11.1 Increased Utilization in Healthcare Clinics Partially Offsets Savings

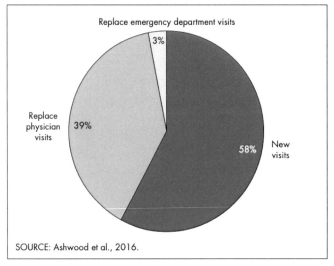

Replace emergency department visits

3%

Replace physician visits 39%

58% New visits

SOURCE: Ashwood et al., 2016.

Source: "The Evolving Role of Retail Clinics." Research Brief. RAND Corporation, RB-9491-2. 2016. Accessed November 4, 2019. https://www.rand.org/pubs/research_briefs/RB9491-2.html

What this means for healthcare spending is more than half of the retail clinic visits represented *new* healthcare utilization—that is, retail clinics actually increased healthcare utilization per person per year. From a preventive care perspective, this is good for healthcare—more patients interacting with the system early, before significant illnesses manifest. The benefits of reduced ED utilization have not yet come to fruition, but this is moving in the right direction: right care, right time and right cost.

What does the increasing popularity of retail healthcare clinics mean for hospitals? As we move forward, hospitals will lose patients to providers who can offer retail-style, positive patient experiences. Hospitals need to be prepared to offer retail-like experiences: frictionless experience in access, delivery and payment. Consumers are going where they find the least amount of friction, and retail clinics meet that expectation: they are convenient, easy to access and affordable.

Telehealth

Another example of healthcare delivery meeting the consumer where they are is telehealth. This is the future of healthcare. In this section, you will see how healthcare delivery is moving from brick and mortar to your living room.

Telehealth may seem pretty futuristic, but as researchers have pointed out, telehealth (defined broadly) has been around for a long time. One researcher pointed out that an article was published in *The Lancet* (a medical journal) in 1879 with the suggestion to "use the telephone to reduce unnecessary office visits."[536]

In 1925, *Science and Invention* magazine featured a cover showing a doctor diagnosing a patient via radio.[537] And in 1959, the Nebraska Psychiatric Institute used a closed-circuit television link with Norfolk State Hospital to conduct psychiatric consultations, therapy and medical student training.[538]Interest in telehealth continues to grow, although providers' interest in leveraging it may currently be ahead of consumers' interest in using it. A 2019 survey by American Well, an end-to-end telemedicine solution provider, found while 66 percent of consumers are willing to use telehealth, only 8 percent reported having actually tried it.[539] The survey also reported younger consumers, ages 18 to 34, are not only more willing to try telehealth (74 percent), but also more likely than other age groups to have actually had a video visit with a doctor (16 percent).[540] Nearly one-third of younger consumers (29 percent) indicated they would be willing to switch to a primary care physician (PCP) who offered video visits, while only 8 percent of seniors would be willing to switch PCPs in order to have access to video visits.[541]

Providers are interested in leveraging telehealth to expand access and reach patients. However, in a separate survey, providers identified concerns about reimbursement as a barrier to more widespread use of telehealth.[542] Barriers to telehealth reimbursement are changing—slowly. Nothing in healthcare is ever easy. If there is a way to overcomplicate something, we will. In January 2019, CMS's Medicare Learning Network published a 12-page booklet explaining the rules and HCPCS/CPT codes for billing Medicare Telehealth Services.[543] Overall telehealth reimbursement is quite complicated, because the Centers for Medicare & Medicaid Services (CMS)—as well as state regulations and requirements—vary in their definitions of reimbursable telehealth interactions.

CMS, and many states, differentiate reimbursable telehealth interactions from nonreimbursable telehealth interactions based on a number of conditions including:

- *Originating site*: the location of the patient (a.k.a. patient setting). (Under Medicare, the patient generally must live in a rural or underserved area and must receive services at a practitioner's office, hospital, rural health clinic or nursing home.)[544]
- *Distant site*: the location of the provider.

- *Distant site practitioner/provider type*: state laws dictate who can furnish and get payment for covered telehealth services.[545]

- *Type of service provided*: CMS, and states, often specify particular use cases for telehealth services, and won't reimburse for services provided outside of those defined use cases.[546]

- *Payer type*: states are more likely to regulate coverage and payment policies of private payers than their Medicaid programs.[547]

- *Type of technology/modality used*: some states consider audio-only interactions reimbursable; other states only reimburse real-time, interactive audio/video interactions (figure 11.2).

Figure 11.2 Different States Have Different Telehealth Restrictions Based on Modality

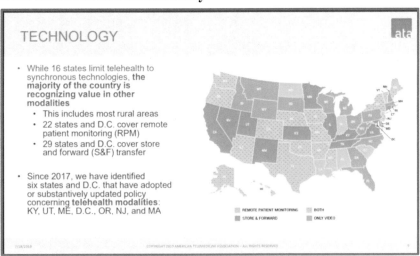

Source: "2019 State of the States Report: Coverage and Reimbursement." American Telemedicine Association. July 18, 2019. Accessed November 1, 2109.
https://www.americantelemed.org/initiatives/2019-state-of-the-states-report-coverage-and-reimbursement/

Telehealth reimbursement is so complicated the Center for Connected Health Policy (CCHP) publishes a semiannual compendium of state Medicaid telehealth laws and reimbursement policies. The most recent version of the CCHP compendium runs 440 pages (a 20-page increase from the spring 2019 edition).[548]

Telehealth services have the potential to increase access, curb costs and deliver the right level of care to patients. But for now, the growth of telehealth has stalled due to differing state policies on regulation and reimbursement. As CCHP states:

> Remarkably, no two states are alike in how telehealth is treated despite some similarities in the language used. For example, some states have incorporated telehealth-related policies into law, while other states address issues in their Medicaid program guidelines. In some cases, CCHP discovered policy inconsistencies within a single state. This variability creates a confusing environment for those who use (or intend to use) telehealth, especially health systems that provide healthcare services in several states.[549]

Mobile Technology

We've reached a point in time where there are now more mobile phones on the planet than people.[550] And smartphones certainly rule in the U.S. today. The Pew Research Center reports 96 percent of Americans now own a cellphone of some kind and 81 percent of Americans own smartphones.[551] Nearly 4 out of 10 Americans (37 percent) report they primarily use a smartphone to access the internet, rather than accessing the internet via broadband at home.[552] The younger respondents were more likely to use their smartphone for internet access: nearly two-thirds (58 percent) of adults ages 18 to 29 said they primarily access the internet using their smartphone (figure 11.3).

Figure 11.3 Americans of All Ages Are Increasingly Likely to Say They Mostly Go Online Using Their Smartphone

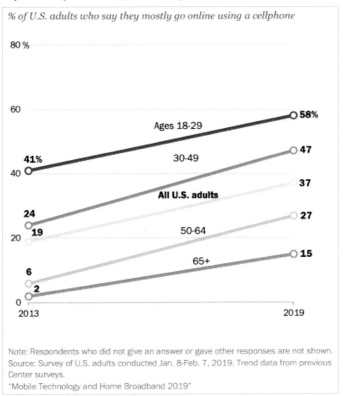

Source: Monica Anderson. "Mobile Technology and Home Broadband 2019." Pew Research Center, Internet & Technology. June 13, 2019. Accessed November 1, 2019. https://www.pewresearch.org/internet/2019/06/13/mobile-technology-and-home-broadband-2019/

Americans spend a lot of time on their smartphones: an average of 3.4 hours per day according to one study (that's more time than they spend watching TV).[553]

The same study found people spent the majority of that time (2 hours and 57 minutes) using apps on web browsers, while they spent about 26 minutes on a search engine.[554] The study found the most adopted retail mobile app is Walmart's, which resides on 58 million Americans' smartphones; in second place is Amazon's mobile app, downloaded on 54 million phones.[555]

Where does this leave healthcare? To reach consumers, healthcare has to be mobile. A separate study by American Well found 51 percent of consumers have used a mobile health app, with the level of engagement and type of app varying by the age of the consumer (figure 11.4).

Figure 11.4 Mobile Phone Health Apps Used

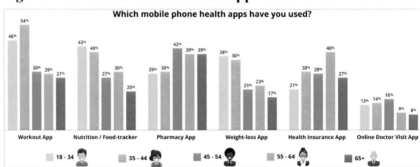

Source: "Telehealth Index: 2019 Consumer Survey." American Well. 2019. Accessed November 1, 2019. https://static.americanwell.com/app/uploads/2019/07/American-Well-Telehealth-Index-2019-Consumer-Survey-eBook2.pdf

The study noted all age groups are using pharmacy apps and health insurance apps to some degree and concluded,

"This shows these age groups are engaged with their health plan, and exposes a potential for health plans to integrate telehealth into these apps to drive telehealth awareness and usage."[556]

The same study found 65 percent of Americans have used a personal health monitoring device (a.k.a. "wearable"). Of those consumers who have used wearables, 60 percent have used a blood pressure monitor, 48 percent have used a step counter or pedometer, 32 percent have used a heart rate monitor, 24 percent have used a glucose monitor and 10 percent have used a Wi-Fi scale.[557]

These trends suggest providers who don't have consumer-friendly, retail-like, digital front doors are going to be left behind. It's not enough to have a website. You have to be mobile, pushing your services and relationship to the consumer.

And furthermore, you have to provide the mobile experience consumers are looking for. A study of why retail shoppers use e-commerce apps found 54 percent use them to compare products and prices.[558] The same percentage of respondents (54 percent) said they valued apps for helping them have purchasing flexibility.[559]

A separate study—again, focusing on retail shoppers using mobile apps—found 53 percent of respondents rated quality as the most important factor when making purchases, while 38 percent prioritized prices.[560]

Where does this leave healthcare when it comes to consumer expectations for a retail-quality mobile experience? I've already talked about issues with quality measures (too many different measures, not universally accepted, not consumer-friendly) and price transparency (we are not even close). I believe mobile is the path for both. But for right now, it's not easy for consumers to easily find and compare information about the quality and cost of various healthcare providers.

Even if they could find that information, most traditional providers (think: hospitals) don't provide any effective versions of the retail experience around financial engagement. Most don't even provide online estimates of the cost of care, and many typically don't provide billing or financing options online. A 2018 survey found nearly all hospitals, health systems and outpatient facilities are still billing patients using paper statements.[561] Yet more than half of the patients surveyed said they would prefer electronic medical billing and payment: patients would like to pay their financial responsibility to healthcare organizations "as they do for other bills."[562]

Someday—and hopefully sooner rather than later—providers are going to figure this out. They must implement a digital front door to let potential patients know about appointment availability, cost (including out-of-pocket) and quality ratings. This digital front door could provide wayfinding assistance and online, advance registration, so a patient's insurance eligibility and benefits could be verified prior to arrival. In addition, the app could screen the patient for financial needs, and immediately offer access to a payment plan, a charity assistance app or other appropriate financial assistance based on the patient's situation.

Finally, the app should offer mobile bill-pay (enabled with Venmo, ApplePay, Zelle, PayPal, patients' own bank accounts or others)—not just online bill-pay options—to meet the growing percentage of the population who access the internet primarily by using their smartphones. Mobile has got a lot of momentum going. A lot of healthcare organizations aren't prepared to take advantage of this momentum and they're going to be at risk of losing their patients.

Smart Care

This is where we start to get futuristic. Retail healthcare doesn't really have that *Star Trek* vibe; telehealth maybe has it somewhat. Mobile phones? Not really—unless we get to that tricorder. But advances in smart care—technology-enabled healthcare strategies and devices—is where healthcare meets the future. Here are a couple of examples of what I mean:

Smart Speakers

Voice technology is growing. And in combination with telehealth, watch out. We are going to see this technology start to grow rapidly, once consumers become familiar with it and trust the process. Decision trees will guide users through a process of elimination—meds will be delivered, appointments scheduled and ambulances dispatched.

In chapter 7 I wrote about Vanderbilt University Medical Center's (VUMC) flu tool, which uses a series of questions to help patients determine if they or a family member have the flu.[563] The tool can be used with Amazon's cloud-based voice service, Alexa. Patients simply say "Alexa, open Flu Tool" to access the application. It then uses a decision tree, based on a series of yes/no questions, to help patients analyze their symptoms and figure out what level of care they need.[564]

That's only the beginning of the possibilities for artificial intelligence-enabled (AI) smart speakers or other voice-enabled devices. For example, the Mayo Clinic has developed a Mayo Clinic First Aid skill for Alexa, which can be enabled at the Alexa Skills Store.[565] The First Aid skill offers self-care instructions for many "everyday mishaps" and "provides quick, hands-free answers from a trusted source."[566]

Examples of topics covered by the Mayo Clinic First Aid skill include:

- "How do I treat my baby's fever?"
- "Tell me about spider bites"
- "Help for a burn"
- "How to treat a cut"
- "Instructions for CPR"[567]

One study noted that as of January 2018, there were 47.3 million smart speakers installed in the U.S.; one year later, by January 2019, that number increased by 39.8 percent to 66.4 million installed smart speakers.[568] One in four U.S. adults now owns a smart speaker.[569] Amazon leads in market share (61.1 percent), followed by Google (23.9 percent).[570] The adoption of smart speakers is growing so quickly that smart speakers are expected to overtake tablets by 2021.[571] A separate study predicted more than 900,000 smart speakers will be used in healthcare facilities by 2021.[572]

I predict as smart speaker adoption becomes more common, patients will be able to interact with their smart speakers for healthcare purposes, just like they interact with everything else. And patients will pay for it. Maybe you will pay $10 a month for a "SMARTdoc" subscription. Think about who is creating that content and who is included in the directories for choices for care. Have you Googled your own facility? Will you show up in a list? How accessible are you online? Are your costs accessible? Are your costs competitive?

Elements of primary (and possibly urgent) care could fundamentally shift with the telehealth movement, as many interventions could be delivered in the home, through a speaker. We're not quite there yet, but consider this: smart speakers are less than five years old and we're already putting elements of healthcare though them, at a fraction of the cost, all automated, open 24/7.[573] The tech companies have their hands full with the Health Insurance Portability and Accountability Act of 1996 (HIPAA) and cybersecurity, but I'm confident they'll figure that piece out. Smart speakers will drive healthcare decisions—mark my words.

Providers, take notice.

Smart Pills

Just last year, the FDA approved a digital pill that helps track medication adherence.[574] Otsuka's Abilify MyCite System is an electronically enabled version of Abilify, which is used to treat schizophrenia and bipolar disorder. When a patient takes the pill, it records the information on a smartphone app. With the patient's permission, that information can also be forwarded to a healthcare provider or caregiver to provide medication adherence support.[575]

In a statement, Otsuka explained the system:

The Abilify MyCite System provides an opportunity for a connected care approach to treatment, and tracks if ABILIFY MYCITE (aripiprazole tablet with sensor) has been taken. The system comprises:

- An aripiprazole tablet embedded with an Ingestible Event Marker (IEM) sensor. This IEM sensor is the size of a grain of sand (1 mm) and is made up of ingredients found in food. The IEM sensor activates when in contact with stomach fluid and communicates to a wearable sensor, called the MYCITE Patch. The IEM sensor is then eliminated from the body.

- The MYCITE Patch detects and records the date and time of the ingestion of the tablet, as well as certain physiological data such as activity level, and communicates this and the tablet ingestion data to the MYCITE APP on a compatible mobile device.

- The MYCITE APP allows patients to review their objective medication ingestion and daily activity level, as well as enter their mood and rest if they wish to do so. They can also invite others to view their data.

- Web-based dashboards are provided to healthcare providers and caregivers. These dashboards give the healthcare provider the ability to display the individual's drug ingestion patterns over time. With patient consent, patient-selected caregivers can also access this information, as well as the individual's daily activity level, self-reported mood and rest.[576]

Kabir Nath, president and CEO of Otsuka North America Pharmaceutical Business, Otsuka America, Inc., said, "We are confident that being able to track drug ingestion in patients with serious mental illness will provide compelling insights for patients and their healthcare provider teams." This is too cool. Think of the applications here. Just from a patient safety standpoint this would revolutionize how drugs are administered outside the hospital. Patient self-medication dosage, timing and adherence could be remotely monitored.

In my first book, I noted medication adherence as a major cost driver for healthcare. This is a way to get that dialed in for patient and physician. Imagine your phone—or an implantable—"buzzing" when it's time to take the pill. Or alerts that go to the physician or family if the wrong pill (or no pill) is taken. Technology like this has significant potential to drive down pharmaceutical costs, and I can't wait until it comes to market.

Consumer-Direct Pricing

I've already addressed the barriers to transparent pricing in healthcare, and in the last chapter, I discussed how transparency legislation seems to have stalled in the legislature. Well, this is

America: if the government and providers can't figure out transparency and consumer-friendly pricing and payment models, the free market will.

In chapter 7, I mentioned MDsave (mdsave.com). MDsave was founded in 2011 and launched in 2013.[577] MDsave describes itself as "an online marketplace for healthcare."[578] MDsave cuts third-party payers out of the picture. It facilitates direct interaction between the patient and the provider. Consumers can search for the procedure they are interested in, from MDsave's list of more than 1,500 procedures.[579] For example, say you wanted to look up the cost of a tonsillectomy for a child under the age of 12. You type that into the MDsave website and up pops MDsave's average price for the procedure ($7,379 when I looked), the range of prices offered by providers in MDsave's network ($6,394–$9,383) and an estimated national average price ($14,619).[580]

You type in your zip code and MDsave presents you with a menu of providers in their network who are near you. Or, sometimes not so near you—at press time, MDsave claimed a network of 2,266 providers including 270 hospitals across the U.S.[581] (Tennessee-based MDsave's network of hospitals, clinics, labs and doctors does not yet extend across all 50 states. The network's providers are currently mostly found in Texas and the Southeastern U.S.).[582]

Once you find a provider and price you like, you pay upfront, using the shopping cart on the MDsave website. It's like eBay's "Buy It Now," but for healthcare. Patients can pay with a credit card, flexible spending account card or PayPal. If you need financing, you can apply for CareCredit (a health, wellness and personal care credit card) during the checkout process. (It doesn't get more frictionless than that!) MDsave doesn't accept insurance, but the website states some costs may be applicable to the patient's deductible, depending upon the procedure and insurer.[583]

The patient receives an email confirmation of the purchase, along with a voucher for the prepayment. The patient takes the voucher to the appointment. Vouchers expire one year from the date of purchase.

The quoted procedure prices are bundled, so they include the procedure and all related fees. Patients know exactly how much they will pay for a particular procedure, with no "surprise bills" afterward. MDsave founder Paul Ketchel said participating providers are willing to discount their fees for the increase in patient volume, as well as the elimination of the administrative work associated with billing insurance. Ketchel said: "Our healthcare providers are netting about 10–15 percent more per transaction with no claims to file. We're eliminating all these middlemen typically part of the transaction: claims processing companies, debt collectors, billing companies, the coding people [involved in] each claim."[584]

In addition to marketing their service to consumers and providers, MDsave also markets to employers, noting MDsave can help employees with high-deductible health plans (HDHP) lower their out-of-pocket costs, since many employees won't reach their annual deductible.[585]

MDsave is certainly offering an innovative model—one that is catching the attention of investors. MDsave's name is not well-known quite yet, but it will be. Savvy consumers will "buy now" when the options present themselves and will tell all their friends how much money they saved on their healthcare deal.

Another example of a company dealing directly with the consumer and eliminating middlemen is GoodRx. GoodRx began as a prescription savings website and mobile app in 2011. The GoodRx website and app (for iOS and Android) offer cost-comparison tools for prescriptions as well as medication discounts. Using the website or app is free for consumers: you just enter the name of the drug and the length of the prescription and dosage, and the app lets you know which pharmacies near you have it and what it will cost you at each one. The app also includes clinical information about the drug, including what conditions it's used to treat and possible side effects. The app provides the consumer with financial information as well, including whether or not it's typically covered by Medicare or insurance plans, the average retail price and links to free discount coupons that reduce patients' cost. Consumers don't have to print the coupons—they can simply pull them up on their smartphone and show the pharmacist.[586]

Consumers don't have to register or sign-up to use the GoodRx program. And it doesn't matter whether or not consumers have insurance coverage—according to the company, sometimes it is cheaper to pay cash directly at the GoodRx price than to run it through your insurance company.[587] (Note: Patients cannot combine insurance coverage and GoodRx discounts—they have to choose one or the other.)

This is frictionless, people—what I've been banging the drum about. The patient simply has to get online and search for their drug and they are *done*. They can proudly show their deal to the pharmacy, and again, tell all their friends how much money they saved on their drugs.

"That's awesome!" you might say. It gets better. GoodRx is now expanding into telemedicine. In September 2019, GoodRx bought telemedicine startup HeyDoctor.[588] GoodRx has rebranded it as GoodRx Care: by folding HeyDoctor's services into the company, they can now offer online physician visits for medical issues such as acne, birth control and HIV testing. Remember the speakers and voice technology I just mentioned? Here we go. The visits will cost $20 without insurance, and then the regular GoodRx app can direct the patient to the pharmacy with the best deal on any prescribed pharmaceutical treatment.[589]

With every innovation, there are also challenges. There have been some concerns about what exactly GoodRx's business model is. The company website states, "We do not collect your personal information. We make money from advertisements on our site and referral fees."[590] One critic points out that one of GoodRx's cofounders was a long-time Facebook employee.[591] Because of Facebook's business model—offering a free service but making money by collecting and selling personal data—this critic and others are skeptical of the GoodRx business model.[592]

GoodRx was recently valued at $2.8 billion—and this was in August 2018, before the HeyDoctor acquisition.[593] Similar to the MDsave model, GoodRx has no brick-and-mortar facilities for patients—just an easy-to-access, easy-to-use online platform with consumer-direct pricing. Insurers aren't part of either business model: both models work directly with consumers without the insurers as the middlemen. No friction, baby. Just a consumer, a service, a connection, transparent pricing and, most important, saved dollars.

The internet of things (IoT) also has a huge play here. This has already been leveraged with medical device technology (pumps, monitors, beds, etc.). Just imagine the possibilities with wearables: a buzzer goes off reminding you to take your pill, auto-orders the refill on the last one, and an Amazon PillPack drone drops it off at your front door tonight. That is medication adherence. *That* is the future.

Who Pays?

All this innovation is great, but who's going to pay for it? All of the approaches I've described in this chapter will require substantial investment in order to scale up enough to bend the curve on healthcare cost and efficiency. Retail clinics require investments in facilities and clinicians. Telehealth requires investment in telecommunications infrastructure, in the education of consumers and clinicians, and in the development of simplified regulations and payment models that encourage the practice of telehealth. Mobile technology requires investment in the user-friendly applications and back-end integrations and databases that will make mobile tech valid, accurate and consumer-friendly. Smart care technologies will require a whole lot of R&D before the government signs off on safety and quality, and consumers accept and adopt the technologies. Consumer-direct pricing requires investment in supporting partnerships, affiliations and technology platforms. And of course, there is the liability. The market will figure out these things just as it's figured out light bulbs, electricity and soon, self-driving cars. I just hope the rules don't take too long—potential improvements in the delivery and cost of care are anxiously waiting for these technology-enabled solutions.

Some good news: the government typically offers limited incentives for innovation—it may just take a while. As I discussed previously, government reimbursement for new ways of doing things (implantable cardiac pacemakers, telehealth) lags behind adoption by clinicians. In other words, the government typically requires a long period of unreimbursed demonstration before it supports payment models that reimburse for the innovation.

The one exception is the Center for Medicare & Medicaid Innovation (CMMI)—also known as the Innovation Center—

which supports the development and testing of innovative healthcare payment and service delivery models.[594] CMMI has initiated and investigated models such as Accountable Care Organizations (ACO), Medical Home Models and Bundled Payment Models (figure 11.5).

Figure 11.5 Center for Medicare & Medicaid Innovation Payment and Delivery System Reform Models (2018)

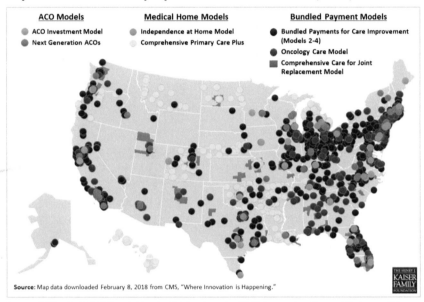

Source: Map data downloaded February 8, 2018 from CMS, "Where Innovation is Happening."

Source: "What is CMMI?' and 11 other FAQs about the CMS Innovation Center." February 27, 2018. Accessed December 1, 2019. https://www.kff.org/medicare/fact-sheet/what-is-cmmi-and-11-other-faqs-about-the-cms-innovation-center/

The problem is the scope of innovation funded by CMMI is limited, as are the funds available for investigating and supporting those innovations. The ACA funded CMMI with $10 billion from 2011 through 2019 and allocated $10 billion to CMMI for each subsequent decade.[595]

The Congressional Budget Office (CBO) estimated the CMMI initially increased government spending (associated with start-up costs for launching new payment models), but over time,

CMMI will save the government an estimated $34 billion between 2017 and 2026.[596] The jury is still out on whether these projections will be realized.

At any rate, we can't solely rely on the government to fund innovation in healthcare. Is that what we really want anyway? But if we don't rely on the government, who will "pay the monkey"? (See my first book if you can't remember this example.)

There is a cynical school of thought that suggests some healthcare stakeholders don't have real incentives to improve patient care. Some dark theories suggest providers want to keep raising prices in a fee-for-service model, insurers deny claims for the sake of it, and pharma has all sorts of drugs ready and waiting for the market at premium price. Just Google the phrase "Big Pharma wants people sick" and you will get nearly 2 million results.

According to this line of thinking, the sicker the population is, the more money Big Pharma makes, so why would they actually want to cure anyone? According to this view, the explosion of chronic disease in the U.S. has actually been a boon to Big Pharma's bottom line, because it means a growing population of life-long prescription drug customers.

Some people say the same thing about hospitals. Google the phrase "hospitals want you sick" and you get 170 million results. It's the same line of thinking as with Big Pharma: when hospitals are paid on a volume-based, fee-for-service model, more patients plus more services equals a better bottom line (which is the whole reason CMS is trying to redirect from fee-for-service to a value-based care model).

What about commercial payers? What are their incentives? One perspective is commercial payers want to support cost-effective healthcare to minimize claims costs. The counter-argument is commercial payers have many other levers they can pull to protect their profits: they can increase premiums, and they can increase rules and requirements, leading to an increase in denials. Even the medical loss ratio (MLR) standard imposed by the ACA has a kind of loophole for commercial insurers. The ACA MLR threshold for large group plans is they must spend 85 percent of premium dollars on healthcare and quality improvement.[597] So if the per person premium you are charging is $1,000 a month, you must spend $850 a month on healthcare, and you can keep $150 for administration, marketing and profit. Need more profit? Simply increase the premium amount; after all, 15 percent of a $1,500-a-month premium will net you $225 a month in profit—so what's to stop you?

I believe in my heart of hearts the hidden agendas I just described are not prevalent. My point is, we have created a system that perpetuates cost and profit over efficiency and cost control. The incentives are not aligned. We see very little collaboration between pharma, providers and payers. It's an all-out war. And on the battlefield, it's hard to innovate and focus on the long-term, like the Quadruple Aim (cost, quality, experience and outcome). That's why we've been stuck. So what are we going to do about getting technological advances out there that fundamentally change the cost and delivery of healthcare for the greater good?

There are only two stakeholders to "pay the monkey" for healthcare reinvention: employers and patients—the "purchasers" of healthcare. They're already paying the monkey—a lot! As I've discussed exhaustively in this book, patients are confused and strapped just trying to keep up with premiums and their increasing share of healthcare bills, not to mention the deductibles, copays and coinsurance.

Patients can vote with their feet to drive innovation (for example, by visiting retail clinics instead of their primary care physician's office, and by scheduling elective surgeries at ambulatory surgery centers [ASC] instead of the more expensive hospital outpatient departments [HOPD]), but they don't have the deep pockets to provide upfront funding for innovation. They also don't realize they really do have the most power as a consumer. Consumers will drive change in any market, it just takes time. Be that change.

That brings us to employers. Employers may be the only stakeholder in the current system where the incentives are truly aligned with providing the highest quality care at the lowest possible cost. Employers need and want healthy, productive workers. In this respect, employer and patient incentives are aligned: both the employer and the patient benefit when the patient is as healthy as possible.

At the same time, employers (and patients) want to minimize costs. The less employers have to spend on healthcare, the more they can spend on other important things like investing in business growth and recruiting and retaining good employees with competitive pay and benefits.

I am not a conspiracy theorist. I've worked in a health insurance company, and I have worked in a hospital. I never heard any of my colleagues say, or even imply, a sicker American population would be good for the bottom line. I do agree—and I argued this in my first book, as well as this one—incentives in the U.S. healthcare system are currently misaligned for most stakeholders. This misalignment is a big reason for the current dysfunction in the system.

Employers have been stuck ever since the Stabilization Act of 1942 was enacted to limit wage inflation during and after

WWII.[598] We're one of the few countries with healthcare benefits tied to compensation and employment. And because of this third-party arrangement, costs (and, I would argue some delivery) got all screwed up. Large employers are done paying the monkey. They want healthy employees and efficient healthcare that's accessible, frictionless and innovative. That's why employers are leading the way on innovations in healthcare delivery. From Haven—the Amazon/Berkshire Hathaway/JP Morgan collaboration—to Walmart's Centers of Excellence program and new ventures in care clinics with Walmart Health, employers are poised to be the most disruptive, innovative stakeholders in the system as we move toward "Healthcare 2050."

In what other areas could the U.S. healthcare system get innovative and align incentives? Chapter 12 includes my "wish list" for the industry going forward.

CHAPTER 12

WOULDN'T IT BE NICE?

As I mentioned in my first book, I like the Beach Boys. I concluded my first book with a chapter titled, "Wouldn't It Be Nice" after the Beach Boys song of the same name. [599] I wrote that chapter because I'm actively working in the healthcare finance business and constantly thinking about the challenges facing the healthcare industry, so the lyrics "Wouldn't it be nice ..." often play in my head. As in "Wouldn't it be nice if ... healthcare payments and coverage were fair?" and "Wouldn't it be nice if payers actually paid claims?"

Readers of my first book let me know "Wouldn't It Be Nice" was a favorite chapter so this is an encore version. In *Healthcare Revolution*, I focused on the idea the patient is the new payer. In this book, I've focused on the idea that in order for providers to survive this chaotic era of healthcare reform, they are going to have to innovate their revenue cycle management (RCM) strategies. The old ways of doing business no longer apply.

What I wrote three years ago is still true: providers have been slow to recognize this new reality and adapt quickly to it. For the well-being of both patients and providers, the industry must design and implement new revenue cycle management processes that engage patients in the financial aspects of their care.

Approaching the patient and payer payment challenges holistically is a win/win for all parties. A tailored patient financial experience can support patients in understanding their coverage and accessing funding to pay for their care. In addition, providers can increase revenue and decrease debt by engaging patients in financial discussions before treatment is delivered.

Holding payers accountable to payment also represents a critical RCM strategy. Securing earned revenue from patient and payer is table stakes in this chaotic era of healthcare reform.

Since the last book, a few of my "wouldn't be nice" ideas have actually gained some traction. Here's an update:

Employees Engaging in Healthcare Conversations with Their Employers

I recently had a phone call with a prominent news outlet reporter who was asking this exact question: "We see more employees looking at the deductible. Why is that important?"

You'll have to go look for the article for my answer, but my point is consumers (employees) are more engaged in their health benefits these days. They are looking to their employer to be innovative—*to disrupt*—healthcare delivery. We are seeing direct-to-provider contracting, patient care navigation portals and employer-sponsored shopping sites help the patient as payer engage with the system.

Engaging Millennials and Gen Z

I don't know with certainty we've made any headway with the insurance enrollment piece, but we are seeing engagement from a cost perspective. A 2019 consumer survey from TransUnion Healthcare showed Gen Z (85 percent) and Millennials (84 percent) research healthcare costs more often than Baby Boomers (65 percent).[600]

In addition, the ability to evaluate out-of-pocket cost information is impacting provider choices for 65 percent of Gen Zers and 60 percent of Millennials, compared to 34 percent of

Baby Boomers.[601] These younger generations will drive the change in this industry—just watch them.

Hospitals Collecting Upfront and Patient-Friendly Billing

Although adoption is lagging, I'm hearing these practices are starting to have more momentum now than in years past. Perhaps it is government-inflicted, but the conversation has changed from "this is too complex" to "how can we do it?" Many hospitals are looking to make patient experience a priority for their organizations in 2020 and subsequently experience less friction in billing and collections.

The Healthcare Financial Management Association (HFMA) is helping hospitals with their patient-friendly billing projects, and has an active attestation program where hospitals can self-assess and attest to their mission to meet the patient as payer.[602] Providers are beginning to engage the patient early and add cost to the conversation—ever so slowly.

We have made some progress, but alas, the beat goes on. We make progress on one issue and then three more manifest. Below are a few "wouldn't it be nice" ideas about how changing a few of the realities of the current healthcare system could make things better for patients and providers. Some of these are long-term challenges that won't be solved in the near future. Others are things you can do today. All of them are about frictionless payment from patient and payer, and I believe it's worth thinking about how much better the healthcare industry might function if what is now wishful thinking ("wouldn't it be nice") became reality.

If I could wave a magic wand and reorient the healthcare system to contain costs, become more patient-friendly, and empower patients to engage in more self-directed care, these are a few of the things I would change:

Wouldn't It Be Nice If ... the Government Stayed Out of It?

When the government tries to "fix" healthcare, do they actually make it better? Worse? Or have no impact at all? I think the jury is still out on that question. Sometimes, government solutions can have a positive effect.

I think if you ask providers, they would say certain provisions of the ACA—but not all—have had a positive effect. For example, I would argue the Medicaid expansion, the creation of health insurance exchanges and some of the access-related provisions of the ACA have benefitted providers.

But most of the solutions the government comes up with can tend to burden providers with useless regulations that don't improve patient care or improve payment. Sometimes it feels like hospitals are subject to more regulations than nuclear power plants. It's nuts!

Four government agencies are responsible for the majority of regulations impacting providers: The Centers for Medicare and Medicaid Services (CMS), the Office of Inspector General (OIG), the Office for Civil Rights (OCR) and the Office of the National Coordinator for Health Information Technology (ONC). Between them, these four agencies generate a *lot* of regulations.

In fact, a 2017 analysis by the American Hospital Association (AHA) found hospitals, health systems and post-acute care providers must comply with 629 discrete regulatory requirements across 9 domains.[603]

Just reading them at two documents per day would take you almost an entire year!

The nine domains include: quality reporting, new models of care/value-based payment models, meaningful use of electronic health records, hospital conditions of participation (CoP), program integrity, fraud and abuse, privacy and security, post-acute care, and billing and coverage verification requirements.[604]

I think we need some level of regulation in healthcare, but this amount of regulation is ridiculous. Because with all of these rules come administrative expenses. The AHA analysis estimated health systems, hospitals and post-acute care providers spend $39 billion (with a "B") each year on *nonclinical* regulatory requirements.[605] This means an average community hospital (161 beds) spends $7.6 million annually on administrative activities to support compliance—the equivalent of $1,200 each time a patient is admitted to a hospital[606]—$1,200, each time, for each patient, people. Tell me we aren't overregulated—I dare you.

Government regulation has gotten out of control. I understand regulations surrounding quality of care and patient safety have been put in place for good reasons. But there seems to be more and more regulation around getting paid. To give you one small example, the CMS Medicare Outpatient Observation Notification (MOON): At my hospital, I had a "utilization review" team with around 12 nurses, and honestly, I would probably have needed only one-third of that number if observation wasn't something I had to substantiate in the hospital. My poor team had to endlessly call the payers—every day—about most of the patients and argue why their patient was "sick enough" to meet inpatient criteria. When they approached the attending, the physician would snap, "I wouldn't have admitted them as an inpatient if they didn't need to be here!" It created an endless (and very expensive) game of ping-pong between staff, attending and the payer.

Overregulation means clinicians have less time to spend with patients. Overregulation creates barriers to access. And overregulation definitely contributes to higher healthcare costs. I think we need less regulation in hospitals specifically surrounding payment—and that's why it would be nice if the government stayed out of it.

Wouldn't It Be Nice If … Sick Care Became Healthcare?

In chapter 2, I wrote about how our current healthcare system is set up as a sick-care system, not a healthcare system. We treat patients in an episodic, siloed way. We don't treat the person holistically and longitudinally. For the most part, we treat only what is right in front of us at the moment, and then send the patient out the door. It's a variation on "treat 'em and street 'em," a phrase that's used in the industry to describe the ED practice of taking care of a patient and then quickly discharging them without much, if any, follow-up.

We know this doesn't work. It results in patients returning to the hospital over and over again, because we haven't addressed the root cause of the problem. As I described in chapter 2, stabilizing the blood sugar of a diabetic patient who presents with insulin shock is not going to address the long-term, chronic disease management needs of that patient. If you don't also address the social determinants of health (SDOH) needs of a patient, you can bet you will be seeing that patient again.

In this way, healthcare is like a horse with blinders on that just keeps running in circles around the track: "Oh, hello Mr. Smith, you are back again … and oops, you are back again … and oops, you are back again. Mr. Smith, that's your third lap." Maybe by the fourth lap hospitals will realize they have to do something fundamentally different.

I'm not suggesting hospitals become self-contained community wellness centers. What I'm suggesting is hospitals reach out to establish meaningful relationships with other providers in the community. You see examples of this in law enforcement.

There's a growing awareness of how mental health issues are intertwined with crime. As a result, are policeman becoming social workers? No. They are sticking to what they do best: law enforcement. But in some areas of the country, law enforcement is partnering with behavioral health service providers, so instead of taking a mentally ill person to jail, they can hand them off to a provider who specializes in mental health services.

The same concept can work in healthcare. Hospitals can keep focusing on what they do best (see my next point) but still address the patient holistically. By considering SDOH and chronic illness factors, and developing meaningful partnerships with other community organizations, hospitals can facilitate the development of a true healthcare system instead of a sick-care system.

From a reimbursement standpoint, it's going to be important to establish value-based care models that support the holistic care of the patient and still reimburse providers fairly. There are still some hospital proponents who say, "These outcome-based, bundled payments aren't set up fairly. They don't account for the variability that occurs in healthcare."

Well, let's figure that out. Let's figure it out and then maybe someday hospitals won't have to pay for Mr. Smith's second, third and fourth visits to the ED. They'll get paid the right amount the first time he visits to support a handoff to the providers who can address his long-term problems so he doesn't have to come back to the hospital again and again. Payment can address things like housing, transportation, nutrition and other SDOH elements to stop the madness. This kind of a system would make more sense than the system we have now.

Wouldn't It Be Nice If ... Hospitals Stuck to What They Do Well?

Hospitals are short-term acute care facilities (STAC). Since their inception, they were designed to treat short-term, acute medical conditions. The CMS Data Glossary defines an acute care hospital as "a hospital that provides inpatient medical care and other related services for surgery, acute medical conditions or injuries (usually for a short-term illness or condition)."[607]

Over time, hospitals have become a central hub for all kinds of healthcare—not just acute care. That has had both good and bad consequences. Now hospitals are like one-stop shopping centers: you can get your life saved *and* you can get your labs checked, get an ultrasound, buy your prescription and maybe even buy a wheelchair while you are there. Hospitals have become a potpourri, a hodge-podge of services with a lot of overhead and fixed costs. They've developed these large, broad footprints, which might be popular, but it doesn't do anything for cost or efficiency. Maybe consumers like it—because they like the convenience of one-stop shopping. Maybe physicians like it, because the facilities for all of the services they provide are centralized in one place. But someone has to "pay the monkey."

The "one-stop shopping" approach doesn't make sense for hospitals from an efficiency, outcomes or cost standpoint. The Triple Aim missed the bullseye. As Oliver Wyman Health reported last year:

> The community hospital model is increasingly challenged to deliver value and operate with sustainable economics. Despite years of effort to streamline processes and manage costs, the inherent complexity of offering a wide "whatever walks

through the door" set of services has left them
inefficient, expensive and ineffective. Delivering
low volumes of a wide variety of services limits the
ability to truly optimize on cost, quality or
outcomes. Hospitals thus represent the highest cost
factor in the current delivery system.[608]

In any industry, if you stray outside of your main niche,
you might not be as good at it as someone who focuses on just that
one area. If you overextend yourself, you risk becoming "a mile
wide and an inch deep." And I think this is where hospitals are
right now.

What if a grocery store decided to start selling lumber?
What if an airline started making cellphones?

Those choices wouldn't make any sense. But that's where
hospitals are now. They are investing time and staff and other
resources in areas that aren't related to their core mission—acute
care—and by doing so, they are creating a lot of waste and
inefficiency in the system.

In fact, all of this mergers and acquisitions (M&A) activity
I talked about earlier may be creating more inefficiencies in the
system. As referenced in chapter 7, M&A activity in the industry
has been associated with decreased competition and rising
healthcare costs—not exactly the direction we want to be heading.

In 2018, Pat Currie, president of hospital operations for
Baylor, Scott & White, wrote:

As the industry increasingly shifts toward
preventive care, the role of the hospital will see
significant changes ... Over the next decade, you

can expect to see fewer and smaller hospitals. Rather than large medical centers, hospitals will become more intensive care areas. The patients we treat in hospitals will be sicker and in need of more intensive care than they are today.[609]

I think more hospitals need to realize they aren't the center of the healthcare universe anymore—and that's OK. Hospitals can't compete on all aspects. They need to exit markets where they simply *cannot* succeed. Because when hospitals start providing services outside of their acute care scope, there's no reimbursement for it. Hospitals are bound to third-party reimbursement models so their scope of services can be limited, as well as their innovation. And hospitals rarely provide those services as well as specialized providers from a quality and cost standpoint.

I get it, gang—hospitals don't make money on ED and obstetrics (OB) and hospitals have (or had) to do the ambulatory services to subsidize the other services. It's a payment issue, not a care issue, and hospitals made up the difference by diversifying their portfolio—but times have changed.

We are now seeing Amazon (Haven), Walmart, CVS, Walgreens, Target and many other retailers provide their consumers with healthcare—and it is working. They are building on their consumer base and making it convenient to get primary care while you shop. It's more of an uphill battle for hospitals, as there are a lot of distractions and a lot of overhead. For hospitals to sustain their businesses into the next decade, they'll need to focus on what they do really, really well—acute care—and leave the rest to other types of providers.

Wouldn't It Be Nice If ... Providers Grew for the Patient, Not for the Money?

Look around your own community and you'll see hospitals still seem to be caught up in a building frenzy. They're adding wings. They're adding towers. They're building freestanding emergency departments. They're building new facilities in communities that already appear to have adequate facilities in place. All this infrastructure but what—truly—is the motivation? I understand there are some cases where there was an authentic need to expand and add services to best meet the needs of the patients in the community. But at the same time, in my observation, many cases involve market plays.

In some cases, hospitals are building out of a motivation to better serve their communities. They do it because they truly believe they are putting patients first: "This new wing will be updated and nice. Patients will like it; they won't have to wait as long, since we will have more beds, and we can get patients in and out more quickly." These hospitals have a mindset of "we will do what serves our community best, no matter the cost to the system." There is a cost to convenience.

In other cases, hospitals are building out to capture a larger market share. Their new freestanding ED serves as another "catcher's mitt" out in the community, to funnel patients into the system. In some cases, competing systems are even building new hospitals across the street from each other, or within just a short distance of each other, in order to capture market share. And then what happens? Both facilities end up operating at half capacity, adding inefficiency, waste and cost to the system as a whole.

Another interesting point is the decrease in occupancy rates at hospitals over time. Between 1980 and 2017, the average hospital occupancy rate dropped nearly 12 percentage points, from 77.7 percent to 65.9 percent.[610] It's been suggested the ideal hospital occupancy rate is between 85 and 90 percent.[611] A hospital occupancy rate higher than 90 percent suggests you might be a little closer to capacity than is comfortable in case of an unexpected surge in admissions. But a hospital rate below the ideal range suggests resources aren't being managed efficiently. Since the U.S. hospital occupancy rate is trending downward overtime, now hovering somewhere around 66 percent, what does that say about where we are headed in terms of creating an efficient healthcare system? Wrong direction again, gang.

If hospitals don't figure this out, legislators will—and, in some ways, already have. At the time I am writing this chapter, 35 states have some type of Certificate of Need (CON) laws or programs in place.[612] CON programs are designed to control healthcare facility costs and facilitate coordinated planning of new services and facility construction:

> The basic assumption underlying CON regulation is that excess capacity stemming from overbuilding of healthcare facilities results in healthcare price inflation. Price inflation can occur when a hospital cannot fill its beds and fixed costs must be met through higher charges for the beds that are used. Bigger institutions generally have bigger costs, so CON supporters say it makes sense to limit facilities to building only enough capacity to meet actual need or demand.[613]

From the point of view of accountability, I actually appreciate the government being involved when it comes to CONs or Certificates of Public Need (COPN), because I think if that happened more in our industry, we wouldn't have the overcapacity and high costs we now see from a plant and structure standpoint.

CONs and COPNs at least make healthcare systems take a step back and say, "Does this community need another MRI?" "Does the community need 50 beds added to this hospital?" "Is a third freestanding ED needed on that corner?" It's not American, and it is certainly not the capitalistic way to allow government to cap a hospital's growth. But right now, I'm not certain that some hospitals are growing for the right reasons.

It's not just hospitals at fault here. In our current dysfunctional system, each stakeholder—providers, physicians, the government and employers—aren't growing for the patient. They're growing away from each other to secure their own little piece of the pie, and that's not necessarily in the best interests of the patient or the healthcare system as a whole. Providers are contributing to the dysfunction by making decisions about plant and infrastructure that are based on short-term financial goals, but which have long-term cost consequences. Hospitals are replicating an inefficient footprint and delivery model. That has to change. Innovators in the industry (like Haven) recognize this and are exploring holistic coverage and delivery models for large populations, delivered in nontraditional ways. Sign me up.

Wouldn't It Be Nice If … Healthcare Coverage and Payment Were Fair and Equitable?

As I detailed in my first book, the U.S. has a unique healthcare system among developed countries, in which the key provider of health insurance is employers, rather than the government.[614] The employer-based insurance system has both pros and cons, depending on who is doing the arguing. Whether or not you believe this is the best system for the U.S., it's the system in place at the moment. The application of employer-sponsored insurance is applied universally in most cases and we are *all* paying for it.

Insurance is about calculating risk. If you build your house next to a river, in a flood plain, you are going to have to buy flood insurance. But if you build your house in an area without a risk of flooding, you won't have to buy flood insurance. In other words, the cost of your insurance premium is directly correlated with the risks you assume.

Health insurance premiums are also based on calculations of risk. In the U.S., that calculation is tied to a company's pool of employees. If a company's workers are engaged in a dangerous occupation—say, construction—your risk (and your premiums) are going to be higher than a company whose employees all have desk jobs.

If a company is large—say 3,000 employees—the risk is going to be lower because the claims risk is spread across a larger pool, and so premiums will be lower and benefits will be richer. If a company is small—a sole proprietorship, for example— premiums are going to be high because the risk pool is limited to a single person. In this sense—because premiums are directly correlated with risk—I think coverage is equitable in the current system. It may not be "fair" but it is equitable.

Life is about choices. Choices have consequences. These are facts. And in the U.S., your choices about your occupation and your employment are going to have consequences in terms of your health benefits. I have two school-aged children at home, and I have already talked to them about this idea. Because the same decisions we make about what we want to be when we grow up are the same types of decisions that will relate to the type of health insurance we will have when we grow up.

I have a friend who is really interested in a single-payer health insurance model. He is self-employed and works part-time. That may or may not have been a choice he made in his life based on where he grew up, who his parents are or, perhaps, his ethnicity. Regardless, health insurance for a single person based on a self-employed job will have a higher risk and ultimately higher out-of-pocket costs.

On the other hand, I work for a large company with a big risk pool. I have excellent insurance coverage with rich benefits. Why should I support a single-payer system, and the increase in taxes that would be associated, to cover my friend's health insurance? I am happy with my coverage, and it's the result of choices I made in my life, including the education I chose to pursue and the companies I have chosen to work for.

My friend and I each have health insurance coverage that aligns with the choices we made in our lives. To my mind, that seems equitable. It may sound selfish, but is it fair? I feel this is the crux of the universal healthcare coverage issue: Some need to pay for the needs of many. I'm not certain America will swallow that pill in 2020.

I realize some people—primarily those who do not have good coverage, including the underinsured and the uninsured—would like to see a single-payer system implemented in the U.S. The problem is a single-payer system couldn't work here without drastic changes to the healthcare delivery system.

If we airlifted the U.S. healthcare delivery system and dropped it in Europe, it would not work. The U.S. healthcare delivery system, as I've discussed throughout this book, is full of waste and fraud and it's over capacity. It's also part of the benefits package, and employment, the tax base and employer wages would all dramatically change. You couldn't just drop it into the European model—it would bankrupt the system. You would have to bring costs down first, by rationing healthcare or other means. The "Medicare for All" solution doesn't work either: It would mean bringing payments down to a level that would be unsustainable for providers, without commercial insurance to offset the costs.

For the U.S., it might be too late to try to implement something like a single-payer system. That ship has sailed. Many people are happy with the insurance coverage they have from their employers. They don't want to pitch in to pay for health insurance for people who made different life choices, or had unfortunate circumstances. And the government can't fill that gap, either. They can't afford it—it would be too expensive. As I pointed out earlier, the Democratic Party has released almost a dozen different proposals for government-sponsored health insurance in advance of the 2020 election. The ACA has its benefits and its faults, but when we try to shoehorn coverage across the nation, there are also costs and benefits. I'm fairly certain the U.S. tax base will not tender the change, no matter who gets voted in. The "benefits" have to change, not the "coverage" (access). As I have stated before, you cannot have affordable insurance for an unaffordable product. We cannot pay for waste—we simply can't cover everything and we may not be able to cover everyone. Sorry, but we're now on a path that frankly may be too difficult to reverse. Sure, there are ways we might modify the system—for example, by also tying premiums to specific lifestyle choices (like the tobacco surcharge that already exists in my plan, for example).

And we can make the consequences of choice more transparent so that people understand what their premiums and coverage are going to look like, based on the choices they make about their employment. Given that, we may not get to "fair," but we can certainly get to "equitable." We need to start looking at benefits, profits and costs as a system before we start talking about covering more people.

Wouldn't It Be Nice If … Healthcare Coverage and Payment Were Transparent? (Yeah, I Said the "T" -Word)

I talked about transparency—the T-word—in my first book. Since then, the transparency train has taken off, helped along by the finalized 2021 CMS rule defining what transparency looks like for providers (see chapter 2). Transparency is important, but it has to be defined correctly. When people hear the word "transparency" in healthcare, they immediately think of price. But my point is, the transparency we need in healthcare isn't only about price.

In the broadest sense, "transparency" means the buyer understands the goods they are purchasing; the person manufacturing the goods understands the costs associated with producing those goods; and third-party payers understand which goods have been effective and which haven't. This definition of transparency applies to any other industry you can think of.

The airlines are a great example of this. You know what kind of plane ticket you are going to buy. And the airlines know darn well what their costs are, from a fuel, staffing, safety and infrastructure standpoint. Now, airlines are not healthcare, but there is variability in airlines just as there is in healthcare. Car mechanics deal with variability, grocery stores deal with variability—but all of those industries have managed to figure out how to deal with that variability and still create a transparent process. The prices are posted, for the most part. Consumers have the information they need to make informed choices. Prices go up and down (quite frequently, I might add) based on what it costs, when it is provided and other factors. The consumer can choose when and where. Now, as I mentioned, a lot of healthcare is not a choice, it often can be an infliction. That said, when an event like this is presented, there's very little transparency from any party about when, where and what cost care should occur for the best clinical and financial outcome.

This information exists in healthcare, but it is not accessible to consumers. It is opaque and blocked. Payers certainly have a lot of that information; providers have some of that information; and patients and consumers have the least amount of information. This creates a lot of friction when consumers are trying to make healthcare choices: "Where should I go? "How much is this going to cost?" "Are you good at what you do?" "Who are some other people who are doing it?" "How can I compare that?" "What's my bill going to look like?" "How can I pay for it?" "How many times will I need to see the doctor?" "What is this course of treatment going to look like?"

The RCM leader can articulate a lot of those things to the patient. But the healthcare industry still has a defensive culture in that they don't want to put that type of information out there, upfront, because they will have to defend it later. That's why practices like providing patients with a guaranteed estimate upfront are so rare.

Hospitals also don't like showing their hand because that can put them at a disadvantage when they are negotiating contracts with payers. It undercuts their bargaining power. But I think there are ways around that. For example, what if the pricing of all hospitals for specific procedures was entered into a blind database? And then you could look up the hospital, and while it wouldn't tell you the exact price of the procedures, it could tell you what the hospital's rating was in terms of costs.

For example, it could tell you this provider is in the 95th percentile in terms of its prices (meaning, very high cost compared to peers) versus this provider in the 50th percentile (meaning costs are average for that procedure compared to peers). The first hospital would need to justify its ranking, and perhaps its costs as well. We have all shopped for other things—Whole Foods versus 7-Eleven, JetBlue versus United Airlines, Hyundai versus Porsche.

We have these choices (tiers), if you will, with accessibility for all, yet in healthcare it's flat and protected. A patient can walk into any ED, clinic or hospital, but the alternative price and quality aren't shared upfront—it's a blind transaction the majority of the time. The Emergency Medical Treatment and Active Labor Act of 1986 (EMTALA) certainly plays a role here, while at the same time, disclosure of these elements would help the patient make a better decision about the cost of their care.

Transparency for consumers—without undercutting provider negotiations with payers—is possible. This would help consumers identify where the best value is. And I would also argue if providers knew this information, about where they stood in terms of costs, it could drive change by helping hospitals understand where they are positioned in the market.

The bottom line is transparency is possible in healthcare. If you define it correctly—and don't just focus on the price listed on the chargemaster—you can provide transparency that helps consumers and also drives change in the industry. Consumers and payers want transparency and the government is now demanding it.

It's also starting to impact patients—we are making them choose between a financial and clinical priority with very little information. Transparent or not, the choice to go to the ED or forego care is a choice. The industry can't hide their heads in the sand on this issue—transparency is no longer optional.

Wouldn't It Be Nice If ... Providers Submitted Clean Claims?

Claim denials are a big problem, as I have discussed throughout this book. But one reason for high denial rates is providers. I'm going to pick on providers first (and then pick on payers in the next section). One of the reasons claims can get denied is providers make mistakes. They type in the wrong code. They misstate the diagnosis. They don't provide the right documentation. They submit claims twice. They *know* the rules, but submitted claims without *following* the rules.

For example, we had one recurring claims issue in our hospital that was just a matter of physician education. Prior to surgery, patients are routinely administered a partial thromboplastin time (PTT) test to catch any abnormalities in blood clotting. You've got to know this about a patient so they don't bleed out in surgery. But our physicians kept indicating "pre-op" as the reason for the test in the documentation. From their perspective, that *was* the reason, and when we asked the physicians, they would state "Yes, PTT is why." And we couldn't change it, because that's an order from the physician. But you couldn't code "pre-op," and even if you could code it, payers wouldn't pay for the test. The clinical reason for the test was to assess the clotting factor—and that's what had to be documented for Medicare to pay the claim. We cleaned up the process, but it took a massive educational effort to get the physicians to start indicating the PTT was for assessing the clotting factor, rather than mindlessly assigning it to "pre-op," which didn't meet the payers' documentation standards. This is just one example—don't get me started with "rule out," "motor vehicle accident," "status post-surgery," "follow-up," etc. None of these codes exist and yet they were on *a lot* of orders.

Providers need to literally clean up their act (claims), in order to reduce the time and expense associated with resubmitting claims. I worked for a time in an insurance company, and when I got a claim that was garbage, I denied and sent it back. Sometimes providers just become lazy about following the rules. Sometimes providers send in a partial claim they know will be denied, just to meet the initial timely filing deadline and give them more time to complete the claim when it comes back denied. They send it in knowing it's going to bounce, but figure they can put off finishing the documentation that way.

That's a waste of everybody's time—submitting a claim you know is going to be denied. Providers need to follow the rules given to them. Yes, they also need to advocate for the rules that make sense and fight tenaciously against unnecessary ones, but first, they need to follow the rules. Educate the coders, physicians and staff. Just like with any other business—if the form (claim) isn't right, no soup for you. It's worse than you think.

HFMA calculates the clean claim rate (CCR) by dividing the number of claims that pass all edits (i.e., require no manual edits), by the total number of claims accepted into the claims processing tool for billing prior to submission.[615] It's been estimated the average U.S. hospital has a CCR of between 75 and 85 percent.[616] Almost one in four claims spin because they are not clean. Hospitals and health systems could be doing a lot better. HFMA's Central Ohio group suggested healthcare organizations should aim to have a clean claims submission rate of around 97 percent.[617] At a minimum, putting best practices in place should bring your organization to a 90–95 percent CCR:

> Your claims management systems should thoroughly scrub claims before they leave your system, editing for coding and demographic errors. The cost for every re-touch of a claim is $1.40 and at that rate, hospitals spend tens of thousands of dollars in unnecessary claims handling. Once a claim is denied, there is only a 40 percent chance of that claim being paid, meaning 60 percent of denied claims will not be paid. Tweak your claims edits to check for demographic errors, insurance errors and coding errors. You will be able to achieve a 90–95 percent clean claim rate, meaning 90 percent or better of your claims are being paid on the first submission.[618]

This is not new—it just seems to be getting worse.

Wouldn't It Be Nice If … Payers Actually Paid the Claims?

Now I am going to pick on payers. Throughout this book I have talked about all of the different rules payers have put in place. Now, I am a pretty nice guy, but I can't tell you how many times I had conversations like this when I worked in a hospital:

> JONATHAN: Hi [insert name of payer], this is Jonathan over here at [insert name of hospital]. You have denied this claim with this particular diagnoses/CPT code every time I have submitted it. I've looked at your website. I've reviewed the contract. My coders have reviewed the claim. My

utilization review team has reviewed the claim. We've checked the patient's eligibility for benefits. We have given you the authorization code. We met criteria for payment. I want to follow your rules, but just tell me what they are. I can't figure out what is wrong.

PAYER: Just resubmit it. We will pay it.

JONATHAN: No, that's a waste of everybody's time. Why the #$@&%*! aren't these being paid the first time I send them to you? What is going on? This is costing me administrative time. And this is going to come up next year at renewal—all of these denials and nonpayments. I think you have too many #$*! rules, but I'm not in a position to get rid of them. I want to follow your rules. But you have to make your rules transparent so I can follow them.

Yes, conversations with payers about claims denials can drive you over the brink. Denials happen too many times because there are too many rules, and they are constantly changing, making it impossible for providers to keep up. I believe there is significant savings in reducing administrative expense here. Providers hire tons more staff (like 20 percent more) to meet payer rules, and payers, with their teams, have the same (or more) resources. It reminds me of the Revolutionary War—the "rebel" hospitals line up their patriots and fire their muskets, while the "redcoat" payers line up and fire a line of claim denials right back. It's wasteful and needs remedy.

There's not a lot of love for payers in the industry right now. I have tried to bridge this gap in my conversations (as I have worked both sides) and have been shut out. Payers and providers seem to have dug their heels in and neither will budge. I believe payers are best positioned to solve this. Payers have the resources, data, expertise and time to collaborate with providers on a holistic, clean claim, data-driven approach to improve outcomes and lower costs.

I think the providers might listen, too. It just has to be framed in a collaborative context, within the realm of a joint risk agreement, with both upside and downside risk. Pay for performance. Let's play it again and see if we can get anywhere.

Wouldn't It Be Nice If ... Computers Did What They Were Supposed to Do?

Once upon a time, we thought technology was going to solve all of our problems—especially digitizing health records and implementing electronic health records (EHR). Way back in 2004, in his State of the Union address, President George W. Bush said, "By computerizing health records, we can avoid dangerous medical mistakes, reduce costs and improve care."[619]

Unfortunately, it hasn't worked out quite the way he envisioned it. There's no doubt EHRs have offered some advantages. For example, one goal of EHRs was to reduce clinical errors related to the legibility of hand-written physician notes and orders. It's probably true that since the implementation of EHRs there are fewer medical errors related to illegible physician handwriting. But while EHRs have solved old problems they have also created new ones. This is especially true for RCM.

I worked in hospitals when billing claims was a manual, paper process, and I've worked with hospitals that use completely automated billing systems. I really do think the claims we submitted were cleaner when we were typing them versus submitting them electronically. Yes, the process was slower, but we used to be able to see the claims and evaluate them before sending them on. I am not advocating for a return to manual billing, but providers have to be aware of what can go wrong with automated billing processes when they don't work the way they are supposed to. I'll prove it to you: Go ask a CFO at a hospital what their return on investment (ROI) is on their EHR. They will *laugh*.

Case in point: Cerner, a well-known EHR vendor, recently settled a case related to significant, negative impacts on a hospital's billing processes and operating revenue after implementation of the EHR's medical billing component.[620] In 2019, Cerner settled with Glens Falls Hospital in New York after a post-conversion financial audit revealed "the billing system failed to send out about $38 million worth of bills in a timely manner or at all in 2017."[621] That $38 million represented 12 percent of the hospital's annual revenue from patient services.[622] In 2019, the hospital and Cerner agreed to a confidential settlement that included working together to resolve the billing issues.[623]

I'm not trying to pick on Cerner or EHRs—they have enhanced patient safety and created some efficiencies. Cerner is a large and trusted EHR vendor (and not the only vendor associated with negative impacts on operating revenue after implementation).[624] Other healthcare systems have reported losses associated with EHR installations or transitions.

In 2019, the Mayo Clinic reported $50 million in lost revenue, which was associated with their transition to Epic.[625] And that was over and above the $1 billion (with a "B") they invested to implement Epic in the first place.[626] There are lots of stories where the EHR is installed and claims get stuck and revenue gets lost. There are also stories where the EHR created better workflows. However, there are even more stories where some junk RCM software was installed and it did not drive the intended outcomes. CFOs are very weary of "BSOs" (bright shiny objects). CFOs are learning not to innovate just for the sake of innovation, and they've had too many experiences where the vendor has overpromised and the solution has underdelivered. For RCM professionals, the digitization and automation of billing processes haven't delivered like they were supposed to.

There are a lot of different reasons for this. One reason is there is a lot of "vaporware" in the market. Promises about RCM functionality are made—but not kept. Vendors promise solutions that will supposedly do everything for everyone, like those late-night infomercials on TV: "If you just buy this one solution, you will be able to replace three staff members, and you will never have to pick up the phone, or fax or copy a document again. You just push a button and it sends out a shiny, clean claim that will be paid immediately." The audience claps and cheers! But then you buy it and install it, and it turns out that instead of replacing staff, you actually had to hire more staff to manage it because it is not working as promised.

Another problem is the complexity created when you implement multiple one-off solutions simultaneously. The problem of lack of interoperability between different systems hasn't been solved on the clinical side, and it certainly hasn't been solved on the claims billing side, either.

At one time, the hospital I worked in was using 26 different systems to support revenue cycle. That was everything from the credit-card system, to the card-swiping devices, to the system that checked benefits eligibility, to the electronic funds transfer system (ACH), to the coding software, to the system that submitted claims to the carriers. My goal was to consolidate systems with more comprehensive solutions to try to eliminate complexity and inefficiencies.

Until technology starts delivering on its original promise, I have two suggestions for providers:

First, evaluate. Make sure what you are buying really does what it is supposed to do. Hold your vendors accountable to the solution they sold. It should do it faster, cheaper and with more cash—period.

Second, consolidate. Investing in dozens or hundreds of one-off solutions is going to decrease efficiency and increase costs, no matter how well those solutions do the one small task they are designed to do.

Providers should inventory and consolidate their software to focus on solutions that have demonstrated yield and ROI. I define yield as both quality and cost: Solutions driving good outcomes and cash or reducing expenses.

Wouldn't It Be Nice If ... Blockchain, Artificial Intelligence and Robotic Process Automation Really Worked for Payment?

Emerging technologies like blockchain, artificial intelligence (AI) and robotic process automation (RPA) are now getting the same kind of hype EHRs got when they were first introduced. "Will blockchain save the healthcare system?" was the title of a recent article in *Modern Healthcare*.[627]

The article points out while there is some promising experimentation going on, the technology is still immature and unproven in terms of what it can do for healthcare. Brian Kalis, managing director of digital health and innovation at Accenture, is quoted as saying, "It [blockchain] is not a cure-all for what ails the healthcare ecosystem."[628]

All the same, some big players are investing in blockchain to see what it can do. Six founding members—Aetna, Humana, MultiPlan, Optum, Quest Diagnostics and UnitedHealthcare—established the Synaptic Health Alliance in the spring of 2018. The goal of the alliance is "to explore how blockchain technology can help address some of the toughest problems in healthcare."[629] The group's pilot project is using blockchain to create a shared provider data exchange to ensure the most current information about healthcare providers is available in the provider directories maintained by health insurers (figure 12.1).

Figure 12.1 Creating a Blockchain to Maintain a Provider Directory

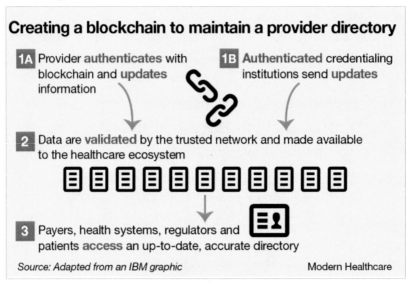

Source: Shelby Livingston. "Will blockchain save the healthcare system?" Modern Healthcare. February 9, 2019. Accessed October 17, 2019. https://www.modernhealthcare.com/article/20190209/TRANSFORMATION02/190209953/will-blockchain-save-the-healthcare-system

The initial results of Synaptic's pilot were promising. It showed "67–88 percent of the time the alliance could provide more information about a provider's status—whether active or inactive—compared with a member going it alone."[630] Since industry estimates show $2.1 billion is spent annually "chasing and maintaining provider data," the pilot project results could be good news.[631]

Blockchain has its caveats as well—scale and process time are challenging, as well as node connections. In plain English: It's slow, expensive and siloed. It'll get better, just like TVs, smartphones and laptops, but it may take a few years. Stay tuned for whether or not blockchain will fully deliver on its promises.

AI is another technology making inroads into healthcare. It's a broad term everyone talks about in healthcare, but no one seems to really understand. I hear revenue cycle leaders say, "We are using AI for that."

But when I get two or three questions deeper, those same people don't seem to have a good understanding of what they have or what they are actually doing. They've contracted with a vendor, and maybe they've automated a couple of tasks, but I have only seen pockets of any measurable ROI in terms of less labor, fewer touches, more yield or more efficiency. There aren't good baseline metrics and good outcome metrics that truly show the benefit of the automation.

We need a better definition of what AI means in the context of healthcare RCM and a better way to measure the impact before we can say AI is going to be the solution to many of healthcare's RCM issues. Don't get me wrong: I have seen it deployed elegantly in certain areas—eligibility, claims status and credit balances.

My point is it's a broad term with countless applications. Buyer beware—again, ensure the innovation is not just for the sake of innovation. It should have measurable impact in terms of yield and efficiency.

RPA is a technology physician's offices seem to be deploying effectively, but I haven't seen providers leveraging this technology to any great extent yet. An example of RPA payers have capitalized on is the technology involving automation in areas such as claims adjudication and provider directories. They have automated the tedious task of checking whether a claim was received, processed or paid by creating a "recording" macro of the activities. The login, the screen, the keystrokes, the results and the action are all automated. In the case of directories, they are taking in myriad detailed data sets from disparate sources and reconciling them. When a provider moves, changes networks or retires, the updated information is published to the claims clearinghouse. A McKinsey article stated, "Payers that have applied RPA in areas like claims adjudication and provider network lifecycle management have achieved significant improvements in productivity through a reduction in manual activities."[632]

You are also starting to see patient interactions with chatbots in the customer service space for common tasks like scheduling and billing. It's a robot, but it goes through a series of questions that are fairly easy to answer—like, "Do you need financial assistance to pay your bill?"—and can then help sort the patient into those buckets of charity care, bad debt risk, payment plans, full payment or collections. A lot of those solutions are doing a pretty good job. For some reason, physicians' offices are ahead of providers in leveraging these types of solutions. I think hospitals can probably learn from physicians' offices and other places to see how RPA is working from an access and payment standpoint.

All of these emerging technologies hold a lot of promise—wouldn't it be nice if these technologies panned out and delivered on the promise to enhance RCM and maximize revenue from patient and payer?

Wouldn't It Be Nice If … Data Was Actionable?

In the introduction to this book, I mentioned a quote by W. Edwards Deming that happens to be one of the mantras I live by. Deming said, "In God we trust, all others must bring data."[633] The flip side of that is the healthcare industry is overwhelmed with data right now.

Data—by itself—isn't very useful. If I have a solution that tells the provider a patient's credit score is 720, this piece of data alone isn't helpful. But if I have a solution to aggregate data and analytics in order to show the provider a person with a credit score of 720 typically pays all of their bills within 31 days, and they should be able to pay their hospital bill in full without financial assistance—*that* is actionable.

Or if I have a solution that tells the provider a patient's household income is less than 150 percent of the Federal Poverty Level which means they qualify for Medicaid in this specific state, and the same solution generates a pre-populated Medicaid application with the patient's information—that *is* actionable.

The key is—one number doesn't tell you anything, but if you put the numbers together in a meaningful way, they will tell you a story. Data must become information, which will lead to insight, which will lead to action.

Data and analytics are useless without action.

Herein lies the problem—the amount of data we are dealing with in healthcare today can be overwhelming, and we're still learning how to best leverage it effectively. As an industry, we have the bridle on the horse, we have the bit in the horse's mouth, but have we really figured out how to ride it yet? Do we have a data governance strategy? Are we just shipping meaningless reports back and forth between the provider and the payer without being able to analyze that data and collect actionable insights? How are patients benefitting from all of the data?

We're not yet at a point where all of the stakeholders are able to benefit from the data that's being generated. The Health Insurance Portability and Accountability Act of 1996 (HIPAA), cybersecurity and data permission squabbles have limited the stakeholder collaboration. To be frank, most providers and payers are hesitant to share their data with anyone, let alone each other. There are ways in which the data can be aggregated and de-identified and shared securely, which would have significant impacts on outcomes and costs. We are stuck in a "this is *my* data and I am *not* going to share!" mentality.

But I believe we'll be able to get there someday. The collaboration in one community alone would drive innovation in payment, outcomes and engagement beyond anyone's imagination—safely and securely.

∞

Over the course of this book I have touched on a number of ways hospitals and health systems can deliver a patient-friendly financial experience, maximizing revenue from patient and payer. Some providers are already experimenting with a variety of these approaches. Others are continuing to operate in the dark ages of revenue cycle management, with legacy processes still based on the assumption commercial and government payers are the way we will always get paid. It's important to think about where your organization falls on this continuum. Is your organization experimenting with new ways of effectively maximizing revenue, all while delivering a better patient financial experience? Or is your organization clinging to legacy solutions and processes, hoping this whole healthcare reform thing will "blow over"?

I have offered many suggestions throughout this book on strategies and best practices RCM professionals can begin to implement immediately to make a difference in their own sphere of influence and be prepared for the changes that lay head. Many of the tactical ideas I described in chapter 8, "Payment Strategies That Work," can be implemented directly by hospitals and healthcare systems.

Please feel free to reach out to me if you would like more information about how to implement some of those ideas within your own healthcare system. My philosophy is: If those of us who know better and in turn do something about the current state of affairs, the better our healthcare system will be—for the patient, the provider, the insurer and the employer. As you know by now, I'm a revenue cycle management guy and nothing gives me greater pleasure than working with hospitals and health systems to help their patients. I get goosebumps when I see them achieve long-term sustainability by adapting their revenue cycle management processes to create a positive patient experience and maximize revenue from both patient and payer.

Some organizations really excel at this change. Payer collaboration and patient financial experience is at the forefront for these change leaders, and their patient satisfaction surveys (Hospital Consumer Assessment of Healthcare Providers and Systems, or HCAHPS), financials, volumes and benchmark key performance indicators (KPI) prove it. I'm not going to name them but I bet you can. If not, send me a note and I'll fill you in on some of my favorites. Patient-friendly, payer-accountable, innovative revenue cycle management *is* achievable.

Each of us in the industry has a choice: We can lead, we can follow or we can get out of the way. That being said, I ask you to do me a favor: Take action. Don't be complacent; be *bold*. I dare you. Your patients, our industry and our future will ultimately thank you for your actions.

EPILOGUE

Kevin F. Brennan, CPA, FHFMA
Executive Vice President of Finance and Chief Financial Officer,
Geisinger Health System

As chair of the 40,000-member Healthcare Financial Management Association (HFMA) during 2018–2019, I had the opportunity to travel the country and hear many great speakers on topics important to those of us who care about the financial health of our industry. Jonathan Wiik was one such speaker with a powerful message on the effective use of data in meeting the challenges of delivering high-quality, cost-effective care to large populations. He has a deep understanding of the power of data while studying the link between the social determinants of health and the total cost of care in treating a population.

During my year as chair of the national board of HFMA, I carried a message of hope and promise embodied in my theme, "Imagine Tomorrow," while supporting the Institute for Healthcare Improvement (IHI) Triple Aim goals of consistently delivering high-quality care that improves the health of populations and is affordable to all.

It's this last goal, affordable cost of care, which plagues our industry and country. Where should healthcare financial professionals focus? This book, *Healthcare Evolution: Helping Providers Get Paid in an Era of Uncertainty,* advocates developing a better, more efficient revenue management system and offers countless observations on unleashing the power of data contained in our myriad systems operating within the complex healthcare environment.

As Chief Financial Officer (CFO) of large health systems for 35 years, including 23 at Geisinger Health, I developed a deep understanding of the lack of aligned incentives in our healthcare environment. At Geisinger, I gained valuable experience supporting innovations across an integrated delivery and financing system, keeping the patient/member at the center of everything. It was refreshing to focus on the health of a population while meeting the sick-care needs of thousands presenting to our emergency departments and specialists. It was hard work and fundamentally worked the best when the patient/member had a Geisinger doctor, used Geisinger hospitals and was insured by a Geisinger health plan.

Over the years there have been many trends swirling that increased the financial challenges managers were facing— economic trends highlighting our nation's rising cost of care and percentage of gross domestic product (GDP); societal trends demonstrating patients becoming more like activist consumers; technological trends and innovations bringing the industry new tools—and all while the industry was experimenting with new payment and delivery models. The implications of these trends on healthcare finance were, and are, profound, and the challenge to a CFO and a revenue management leader was to imagine what a future revenue management system could look like.

Geisinger participated in HFMA national efforts to design future systems through the Patient Friendly Billing Taskforce, the Price Transparency Task Force and the establishment of standardized metrics used to implement recognition for revenue management excellence. Geisinger changed everything. What followed was an unprecedented decade of HFMA recognition for revenue cycle excellence with consecutive MAP (Measure. Apply. Perform.) awards. A willingness to change and "Imagine Tomorrow" with a focus on opportunities identified with new tools and smart use of data was at the center of our performance improvement.

In the face of so many challenges in our delivery and financing systems, I'm glad Jonathan has turned his focus in this book to practical improvements in our revenue management systems with effective use of data. It's a worthy undertaking full of thought-provoking ideas while challenging us to reject the status quo.

ACKNOWLEDGMENTS

This book would not have been possible without God and His plan. Thank you, God, for all the gifts you have provided me and my family.

To my wife, Chelsea—my best friend and biggest fan (and most trusted critic)—the words are special because of you.

To my two boys—Kaden and Zane, who always wonder what their dad is up to when he's not on the river—this book will be meaningful when you get jobs and have to pay for healthcare, boys. I hope things change a little by then.

To my father, Hans, who talked me into a career in this crazy industry—thank you, Dad, for challenging me to do my best in all things.

I would also like to acknowledge all of the incredible support received from family, friends and colleagues throughout my career. Thanks for all the conversations, criticism and encouragement. Whether they occurred in the hospital hallways, at industry conferences, in the office, at a bar, on the ski lift, at the campfire or in rubber rafts—the dialogues were invaluable, and are most certainly, in this book. This book challenged how I think about U.S. healthcare, and I truly hope it will challenge all of you as well.

Finally, a special *thank you* to everyone at TransUnion Healthcare who touched this book in any way, especially John Yount and Manya Niman, who were with me every step of the journey.

Enjoy.

GLOSSARY

Abuse: Abuse is defined as excessive or improper use of a thing, or to use something in a manner contrary to the natural or legal rules for its use. Abuse can occur in financial or nonfinancial settings.[i]

Accountable Care Organization (ACO): An ACO is a voluntary network of healthcare providers (physician groups, hospitals and other health providers) who work together to provide high-quality, coordinated care to Medicare patients; participating providers share in the cost savings achieved for the Medicare program.[ii]

Ambulatory surgery center (ASC): An ASC is a specialized surgery center that provides surgical care for ambulatory patients.

America's Health Insurance Plans (AHIP): AHIP is a trade association and political advocacy group formed in 2003 by the merger of two other trade associations: The Health Insurance Association of America (HIAA) the American Association of Health Plans (AAHP). For more information, visit ahip.org.

American Hospital Association (AHA): The AHA is a national organization founded in 1898 that represents and serves hospitals and healthcare networks. Membership now includes nearly 5,000 hospitals, healthcare systems, networks, other care providers and 43,000 individual members.[iii] For more information, visit aha.org.

American Medical Association (AMA): The AMA is a national, professional association of physicians established in 1847. For more information, visit ama-assn.org.

Alternative payment model (APM): APMs are part of the Quality Payment Program (QPP), which the Centers for Medicare & Medicaid Services (CMS) launched in 2017. APMs use incentive payments to reward high-quality and cost-efficient care. For more information, visit https://qpp.cms.gov/apms/overview.

Artificial intelligence (AI): AI is technology used to replicate "intellectual processes characteristic of humans, such as the ability to reason, discover meaning, generalize or learn from past experience" to achieve goals without being explicitly programmed for specific action.[iv]

Balance after insurance (BAI): BAI refers to the patient responsibility portion of hospital charges after insurance has been applied.

Blockchain: Blockchain uses encryption and validation to record digital transactions, creating an immutable, digital public ledger.[v]

Centers for Medicare & Medicaid Services (CMS): CMS is one of 11 agencies operating in the U.S. Department of Health and Human Services (HHS). CMS provides oversight for Medicare, the federal share of Medicaid and the State Children's Health Insurance Program, the Health Insurance Marketplace, and related quality-assurance activities. For more information, visit cms.gov.

Centers of Excellence (COE): In healthcare, "Centers of Excellence" refer to "specialized programs within healthcare institutions which supply exceptionally high concentrations of expertise and related resources centered on particular medical areas and delivered in a comprehensive, interdisciplinary fashion."[vi]

Chargemaster or charge description master (CDM): The CDM is a hospital-specific pricing document that includes the itemized list price for each of the goods and services the hospital bills for, including the cost of the good or service, overhead costs and markups.

Children's Health Insurance Program (CHIP): Created as part of the Balanced Budget Act of 1997, CHIP is a federal-state partnership that provides health insurance coverage to low-income families who earn too much money to qualify for Medicaid.[vii]

Clean claim rate (CCR): The Healthcare Financial Management Association (HFMA) calculates the CCR by dividing the number of claims that pass all edits (i.e., require no manual edits), by the total number of claims accepted into the claims processing tool for billing prior to submission.[viii] A typical U.S. hospital has a CCR of between 75 and 85 percent.[ix]

Cost sharing reduction (CSR): The CSR is a feature of "silver"-level plans offered on the health insurance exchanges created by the Affordable Care Act (ACA). The CSR (essentially a subsidy) is a discount designed to lower a consumer's share of deductibles, copayments and coinsurance.[x] Eligibility for the cost-sharing subsidy is based on household income.

Current Procedural Terminology (CPT): CPT is a medical code set that is used to report medical, surgical and diagnostic procedures and services to entities such as physicians, health insurance companies and accreditation organizations.[xi] CPT codes are used in conjunction with International Classification of Diseases (ICD) diagnostic codes to document patients' diagnoses and treatments.

Diagnosis-Related Group (DRG): DRG is Centers for Medicare & Medicaid Services' (CMS) methodology for paying facilities for hospital inpatient services for Medicare patients. A DRG payment covers all charges associated with an inpatient stay from the time of admission to discharge. The DRG includes services performed by an outside provider.[xii]

Disproportionate share hospital (DSH) payments: Medicaid disproportionate share hospital (DSH) payments are statutorily required payments intended to offset hospitals' uncompensated care costs to improve access for Medicaid and uninsured patients as well as the financial stability of safety-net hospitals.[xiii]

Electronic health record (EHR): An EHR is a digital version of a patient's paper chart. EHRs are real-time, patient-centered records that make information available instantly and securely to authorized users. While an EHR does contain the medical and treatment histories of patients (a.k.a. an electronic medical record, or EMR), an EHR system is built to go beyond standard clinical data collected in a provider's office and can be inclusive of a broader view of a patient's care.[xiv]

Emergency Medical Treatment and Active Labor Act of 1986 (EMTALA): EMTALA is a federal law that ensures public access to emergency services regardless of an individual's ability to pay. EMTALA applies to all Medicare-participating hospitals that offer emergency services.[xv]

Employee Retirement Income Security Act of 1974 (ERISA): ERISA is a federal law that "sets minimum standards for most voluntarily established pension and health plans in private industry to provide protection for individuals in these plans."[xvi]

Federal Poverty Level (FPL): The FPL is a measure of income, issued annually by the U.S. Department of Health & Human Services (HHS), which is used to determine eligibility for programs and benefits such as subsidies for health insurance purchased on the federal health insurance marketplace, Medicaid and the Children's Health Insurance Program (CHIP).[xvii] For further information about the current FPL, visit https://aspe.hhs.gov/poverty-guidelines.

Fee for service (FFS): In the FFS reimbursement model, healthcare providers, including physicians and hospitals, are paid for each service performed.

Fraud: Fraud is defined as the wrongful or criminal deception intended to result in financial or personal gain. Fraud includes false representation of fact, by making false statements or concealing information.[xviii]

Fraud, waste and abuse (FWA): These three variables contribute significantly to excessive healthcare costs. Although each has a separate definition, together the three variables are often referred to as FWA.[xix]

Haven: Haven is the name of a joint healthcare venture established by Amazon, Berkshire Hathaway and JPMorgan Chase. The partnership was established in 2018.[xx]

Health & Human Services (HHS): HHS is the federal department charged with enhancing and protecting the health and well-being of all Americans.[xxi]

Health Benefit Exchange (HBE): Established by the Affordable Care Act (ACA), health benefit exchanges (also called health insurance marketplaces) are available in every state to help individuals, families and small businesses shop for and enroll in health insurance.

Health Care Payment Learning and Action Network (LAN): The LAN, established in 2015, is a group of public and private healthcare leaders dedicated to providing thought leadership, strategic direction and ongoing support to accelerate the U.S. healthcare system's adoption of alternative payment models (APM). For more information, visit hcp-lan.org.

Healthcare Financial Management Association (HFMA): HFMA is a not-for-profit membership organization for healthcare finance executives and leaders. HFMA helps its members achieve optimal performance by providing the practical tools and solutions, education, industry analyses and strategic guidance needed to address the many challenges that exist within the U.S. healthcare system. For more information, visit hfma.org.

Health Insurance Portability and Accountability Act of 1996 (HIPAA): HIPAA is a federal law that protects health insurance coverage continuity; establishes standards and rules to protect the privacy and security of individuals' health information; and outlines methods for transactions between covered entities for documentation, billing and reimbursement.

Health maintenance organization (HMO): An HMO is a type of health insurance plan whose member physicians closely manage enrollees' medical coverage, including limiting referrals to specialists outside the HMO network. HMOs reimburse providers using a capitated payment system.

Health savings account (HSA): An HSA is a tax-exempt account that eligible individuals (individuals with qualifying insurance plans) can set up to pay and/or reimburse qualified medical expenses.[xxii]

High-deductible health plan (HDHP): An HDHP is a health insurance plan with a higher deductible than a traditional health insurance plan. HDHPs typically have lower premiums, but members may pay more in out-of-pocket costs as they meet the deductible. For 2020, the Internal Revenue Service (IRS) defines a high-deductible health plan as any plan with a deductible of at least $1,400 for an individual or $2,800 for a family. An HDHP's total yearly out-of-pocket expenses (including deductibles, copayments and coinsurance) can't be more than $6,900 for an individual or $13,800 for a family (this limit doesn't apply to out-of-network services).[xxiii]

Hospital Consumer Assessment of Healthcare Providers and Systems (HCAHPS): HCAHPS is a national, standardized

survey designed to collect and measure patient satisfaction. All
hospitals subject to the Centers for Medicare & Medicaid
Services (CMS) Inpatient Prospective Payment System (IPPS)
must collect and report HCAHPS data annually. HCAHPS
results are available to the public on the Hospital Compare
website, medicare.gov/hospitalcompare.

Hospital outpatient department (HOPD): Hospital outpatient
departments are hospital-owned facilities for outpatient
procedures and services.

Hospital Readmissions Reduction Program (HRRP): HRRP is a
value-based care program launched by the Centers for Medicare
& Medicaid Services (CMS) in 2012. HRRP requires CMS to
reduce payments to hospitals with excessive readmissions,
defined as readmissions within 30 days of discharge.[xxiv]

Insurance discovery: Insurance discovery is a technology that combines
data mining with proprietary algorithms to identify insurance
coverage that a patient may not be aware of or has not
disclosed.[xxv]

International Classification of Diseases (ICD): The ICD is an
international diagnostic classification standard that defines
diseases, disorders, injuries and other health conditions using
standardized codes. The World Health Organization (WHO)
owns and publishes the ICD-10 classification, which is the
primary diagnostic coding structure for the U.S.[xxvi] Per a final
rule from the U.S. Department of Health & Human Services,
ICD-10 became the exclusive system used for medical coding.

Kaiser Family Foundation (KFF): KFF is a non-profit organization
focused on providing independent information on national health
issues. The KFF conducts policy analysis, polling and survey
research and journalism, focusing on how healthcare policy
affects people.[xxvii]

Long-term care hospital (LTCH): An LTCH is a hospital licensed to
provide medical and rehabilitative support for patients who
require greater than average (typically 25 days or more) acute
care support.[xxviii]

Meaningful use (MU): The American Recovery and Reinvestment Act
of 2009 (ARRA) authorized the Centers for Medicare &

Medicaid Services (CMS) to create an incentive program to encourage healthcare providers to adopt and use electronic health record (EHR) technology to improve the quality, safety and efficiency of healthcare delivery.[xxix]

Medicare Access and CHIP Reauthorization Act of 2015 (MACRA): MACRA is a pay-for-performance program that is focused on quality, value and accountability. The MACRA framework rewards healthcare providers for giving better care instead of more service. MACRA combines parts of the Physician Quality Reporting System (PQRS), Value-based Payment Modifier (VBM) and the Medicare Electronic Health Record (EHR) incentive program into one single program called the Merit-Based Incentive Payment System (MIPS).[xxx]

Medical loss ratio (MLR): MLR refers to the proportion of medical insurance premium revenues spent on clinical services and quality improvement, as opposed to other costs, such as administrative overhead and marketing. The Affordable Care Act (ACA) requires health insurance companies to issue rebates to consumers if their MLR percentage does not meet minimum standards.

Medical necessity: Medical necessity defines insurance payment standards for services or products provided by a physician to a patient. Medical care that does not meet this standard is denied by the insurance carrier.[xxxi]

Medicare Advantage Plans (MA): Medicare Advantage Plans, sometimes called "Part C" or "MA Plans," are an "all-in-one" alternative to Original Medicare. They are offered by private companies approved by Medicare.[xxxii] MA Plans typically "bundle" Medicare Part A (Hospital Insurance), Medicare Part B (Medical Insurance) and Medicare Part D (Medicare prescription drug benefits).[xxxiii]

Medicare bad debt (MBD): MBD is bad debt resulting from Medicare deductible and coinsurance amounts that are uncollectible from Medicare beneficiaries and are considered in the program's calculation of reimbursement to the provider if they meet the criteria specified in 42 CFR 413.89 and PRM-I, §§ 306-324.[xxxiv]

Merit-Based Incentive Payment System (MIPS): MIPS is a performance-based payment adjustment model for clinicians. For more information, visit qpp.cms.gov/mips/overview.

Minimum essential coverage (MEC): MEC is health insurance coverage that meets Affordable Care Act (ACA) minimum coverage requirements. To qualify, a plan must cover specified "essential health benefits," including specified preventive care for adults, women and children.[xxxv]

National Center for Health Statistics (NCHS): NCHS, part of the Centers for Disease Control and Prevention (CDC), is the principal health statistics agency in the United States. For more information, visit cdc.gov/nchs.

Outpatient Prospective Payment System (OPPS): OPPS is the system through which Medicare decides how much money a hospital or community mental health center will be reimbursed for outpatient care to patients with Medicare.[xxxvi]

Patient experience: Patient experience is the summation of all interactions that patients encounter within the healthcare systems, including access, care, follow-up visits, billing, etc., through any and all means of communication (including face-to-face, digital, telephone and direct mail).

Patient financial experience (PFE): PFE includes all of a patient's experiences related to their costs and coverage for medical services. A positive patient financial experience encompasses elements of transparent, tailored and useful interactions where the provider and patient have a clear understanding of the mutually agreed upon funding mechanisms for the patient's care.

Patient Protection and Affordable Care Act of 2010 (PPACA): Commonly referred to as the ACA or "Obamacare," the act was signed into law on March 23, 2010. The law expanded requirements for health insurance coverage; established subsidies to reduce the cost of health insurance premiums for low-income families; and expanded the Medicaid program. For more information, visit healthcare.gov/glossary/patient-protection-and-affordable-care-act.

Programs to Evaluate Payment Patterns Electronic Report (PEPPER): PEPPER is an electronic Medicare report that supplies provider-specific data and statistics for Medicare beneficiary discharges and services to help identify care delivery and payment outliers based on peer comparisons.[xxxvii]

Population health management (PHM): PHM is an interdisciplinary, customizable, care oversight approach that uses nontraditional partnerships among different sectors of the community to achieve positive health outcomes for the overall health and wellness of defined populations.[xxxviii]

Propensity to pay: Two of the factors that impact whether or not patients pay their medical bills include their ability to pay and their propensity—or likelihood—of paying. Automated solutions can help providers determine a patient's propensity to pay by using proprietary algorithms and data sources.

Protected health information (PHI): Protected health information includes all individually identifiable health information that is created, received, stored or transmitted by entities covered by the Health Insurance Portability and Accountability Act of 1996 (HIPAA) and their business associates.[xxxix]

Provider manual: A compilation of health plan policies, procedures, standards and definitions outlining the contractual requirements for coverage and payment of eligible plan benefits obtained by plan members at contracted provider facilities or parties.

Provider Reimbursement Manual (PRM, Medicare): Published by the Centers for Medicare & Medicaid Services (CMS), this manual provides the day-to-day operating instructions, policies and procedures used to administer CMS programs. The manual is available online at cms.gov/Regulations-and-Guidance/Guidance/Manuals/Paper-Based-Manuals.html.

Revenue cycle management (RCM): RCM is the administration of financial transactions that result from the medical encounters between a patient and a provider, facility and/or supplier. These transactions include billing, collections, payer contracting, provider enrollment, coding, data analytics, management and compliance.[xl]

Robotic process automation (RPA): Robotic process automation is the term used for software tools that partially or fully automate human activities that are manual, rule-based and repetitive.[xli]

Social determinants of health (SDOH): Social determinants of health are the conditions in which people are born, grow, live, work and age that shape health. [xlii]

Short-term acute care hospital (STACH): A STACH is a medical facility licensed to provide short-term (typically less than 25 days), acute care for patients. The vast majority of hospitals in the United States are licensed as STACHs.

Uncompensated care: Uncompensated care is the overall measure of hospital care provided for which no payment was received from the patient or insurer. It is the sum of a hospital's bad debt and the financial assistance it provides.

Value-based care: Value-based healthcare is a healthcare delivery model in which providers, including hospitals and physicians, are paid based on patient health outcomes. Under value-based care agreements, providers are rewarded for helping patients improve their health, reduce the effects and incidence of chronic disease, and live healthier lives in an evidence-based way.[xliii]

Waste: Waste is defined as the thoughtless or careless expenditure, mismanagement or abuse of resources to the detriment (or potential detriment) of the U.S. government. Waste also includes incurring unnecessary costs resulting from inefficient or ineffective practices, systems or control.[xliv]

ENDNOTES

1   Institute for Healthcare Improvement. IHI Triple Aim Initiative. (n.d.) Accessed May 24, 2019. http://www.ihi.org/Engage/Initiatives/TripleAim/Pages/default.aspx

2   American Hospital Association. Fast Facts on U.S. Hospitals. 2019. Accessed May 24, 2019. https://www.aha.org/statistics/fast-facts-us-hospitals

3   "Non-profit hospital margins just reached an all-time low. How should hospitals respond?" Sept. 14, 2018. Accessed May 24, 2019. https://www.advisory.com/daily-briefing/2018/09/14/moodys

4   Goldsmith, J., Stacey, R. and Hunter, A. "Stiffening headwinds challenge health systems to grow smarter." Sept. 2018 Accessed May 28, 2019. http://images.e-navigant.com/Web/NavigantConsultingInc/%7B7900bba7-87bd-4a9b-9cec-54cf0b6ea9d4%7D_HC_HealthSystemFinancialAnalysis_TL_0818_REV08.pdf

5   American Hospital Association. "Trendwatch Chartbook 2018: Trends affecting hospitals and health systems." 2018. Accessed May 28, 2019. https://www.aha.org/system/files/2018-07/2018-aha-chartbook.pdf

6   Bannow, T. "Ballooning costs, government mandates were hospitals' biggest challenges in 2018." Jan. 17, 2019. Accessed June 14, 2019. https://www.modernhealthcare.com/article/20190117/NEWS/190119923/ballooning-costs-government-mandates-were-hospitals-biggest-challenges-in-2018

7   Tseng P., Kaplan R.S., Richman B.D., Shah M.A. and Schulman K.A. "Administrative costs associated with physician billing and insurance-related activities at an academic health care system." JAMA. 2018;319(7):691–697. DOI:10.1001/jama.2017.19148. Accessed May 28, 2019. https://jamanetwork.com/journals/jama/article-abstract/2673148?redirect=true

8   The Office of the National Coordinator for Health Information Technology. Percent of Hospitals, By Type, that Possess Certified Health IT. Health IT Dashboard. 2015. Accessed June 13, 2019. https://dashboard.healthit.gov/quickstats/pages/certified-electronic-health-record-technology-in-hospitals.php

9   Henry J. Kaiser Family Foundation. The Uninsured and the ACA: A Primer. Table 1: Health Insurance Coverage of the Nonelderly. January 2019. Accessed May 31, 2019. http://files.kff.org/attachment/The-Uninsured-and-the-ACA-A-Primer-Supplemental-Tables

10 The Commonwealth Fund. "Uninsured rate rose from 2014 – 2018, with greatest growth among people in employer health plans." Feb. 7, 2019. Accessed June 26, 2019. https://www.commonwealthfund.org/press-release/2019/underinsured-rate-rose-2014-2018-greatest-growth-among-people-employer-health

11 Fontana, E. and Navarro, L. "At the margins: Our 2017 revenue cycle benchmarks are out. How do you stack up? Dec. 14, 2017. Accessed June 1, 2019. https://www.advisory.com/research/Revenue-Cycle-Advancement-Center/at-the-margins/2017/12/revenue-cycle-benchmarks

12 Peck, A. "Because of expanded numbers of patients with high-deductible health plans, patients are now responsible for 30% of hospital revenues." Sept. 22, 2017. Dark Daily. Accessed June 1, 2019. https://www.darkdaily.com/because-of-expanded-numbers-of-patients-with-high-deductible-health-plans-patients-are-now-responsible-for-30-of-hospital-revenues-920/

13 Peck, A. "Patients are now responsible for 30% of hospital revenues." Sept. 22, 2017.

14   Pellathy, T. and Singhal, S. Revisiting healthcare payments: An industry still in need of overhaul [PDF document]. McKinsey & Company. March 2010. Accessed June 2, 2019. http://healthcare.mckinsey.com/sites/default/files/776489_Revisiting_Healthcare_Payments_An_Industry_Still_in_Need_of_Overnaul.pdf

15   The W. Edwards Deming Institute. W. Edwards Deming Quotes. Accessed June 26, 2019. https://quotes.deming.org/authors/W._Edwards_Deming/quote/3734

16   Centers for Medicare & Medicaid Services (CMS). National Health Expenditures 2017 Highlights. 2018. Accessed June 11, 2019. https://www.cms.gov/Research-Statistics-Data-and-Systems/Statistics-Trends-and-Reports/NationalHealthExpendData/Downloads/highlights.pdf

17   Kamal, R., Cox, C., McDermott, D., Ramirez, R. and Sawyer, B. "U.S. health system is performing better, though still lagging behind other countries." *Peterson-Kaiser Health System Tracker.* March 29, 2019. Accessed June 11, 2019. https://www.healthsystemtracker.org/brief/u-s-health-system-is-performing-better-though-still-lagging-behind-other-countries/#item-start

18   Bruffey, W. "Cost of a car in the year you were born." Houston Chronicle. April 19, 2016. Accessed June 11, 2019. https://blog.chron.com/carsandtrucks/2016/04/cost-of-a-car-in-the-year-you-were-born/

19   Wiik, Jonathan. *Healthcare Revolution: The Patient Is the New Payer.* 2017.

20   Sawyer, B. and Cox, C. "How does health spending in the U.S. compare to other countries?" Kaiser Family Foundation. Dec. 7, 2018. Accessed June 11, 2019. https://www.healthsystemtracker.org/chart-collection/health-spending-u-s-compare-countries/#item-start

21   Centers for Medicare & Medicaid Services. NHE Fact Sheet. 2017. Accessed June 11, 2019. https://www.cms.gov/research-statistics-data-and-systems/statistics-trends-and-reports/nationalhealthexpenddata/nhe-fact-sheet.html

22   Centers for Medicare & Medicaid Services. NHE Fact Sheet. 2017.

23   Centers for Disease Control and Prevention. National Center for Health Statistics. Emergency Department Visits. 2016. Accessed June 13, 2019. https://www.cdc.gov/nchs/fastats/emergency-department.htm

24   Centers for Disease Control and Prevention. National Center for Health Statistics. Emergency Department Visits. 2016.

25   Centers for Disease Control and Prevention. National Center for Health Statistics. Emergency Department Visits. 2016.

26   Weinick R.M., Burns R.M., Mehrotra A. "Many emergency department visits could be managed at urgent care centers and retail clinics." Health Affairs. 2010;29(9):1630–1636. Accessed June 17, 2019. https://www.ncbi.nlm.nih.gov/pmc/articles/PMC3412873/

27   Castellucci, M. "Unnecessary ED visits from chronically ill patients cost $8.3 billion." Modern Healthcare.com. Feb. 7, 2019. Accessed June 13, 2019. https://www.modernhealthcare.com/article/20190207/TRANSFORMATION03/190209949/unnecessary-ed-visits-from-chronically-ill-patients-cost-8-3-billion

28   Castellucci, M. "Unnecessary ED visits." Modern Healthcare.com. Feb. 7, 2019.

29   Kate Perreault. "How freestanding emergency rooms impact your business' healthcare costs." *Phoenix Business Journal.* Aug. 1, 2018. Accessed June 17, 2019. https://www.bizjournals.com/phoenix/news/2018/08/01/how-freestanding-emergency-rooms-impact-your.html

30   Centers for Medicare & Medicaid Services. Emergency Medical Treatment & Labor Act. (n.d.). https://www.cms.gov/regulations-and-guidance/legislation/emtala/

31   The Henry J. Kaiser Family Foundation. Timeline: History of health reform in the U.S. [PDF document]. (n.d.) https://kaiserfamilyfoundation.files.wordpress.com/2011/03/5-02-13-history-of-health-reform.pdf

32   "Special note: What is the 250-yard rule and how does it affect these issues?" (n.d.) Emtala.com. http://www.emtala.com/250yard.htm

33   The Heritage Foundation. "The Crisis in America's Emergency Rooms and What Can Be Done." Dec. 28, 2007. Accessed June 17, 2019. https://www.heritage.org/health-care-reform/report/the-crisis-americas-emergency-rooms-and-what-can-be-done

34   Andre Maksimow and Dawn Samaris. "Optimizing a Health System's Post-Acute Care Network." HFMA. May 2018. Accessed June 17, 2019. https://www.kaufmanhall.com/sites/default/files/legacy_files/Optimizing-a-Health-Systems-Post-Acute-Care-Network.pdf

35   Insurance Information Institute. Facts + Statistics: Industry Overview. 2017. Accessed June 12, 2019. https://www.iii.org/fact-statistic/facts-statistics-industry-overview

36   Centers for Medicare & Medicaid Services. "CMS' Value-Based Programs." Last modified May 17, 2019. Accessed June 25, 2019. https://www.cms.gov/medicare/quality-initiatives-patient-assessment-instruments/value-based-programs/value-based-programs.html

37   Institute for Health Metrics and Evaluation (IHME). Healthcare Access and Quality Profiles. May 18, 2017. Accessed June 11, 2019. http://www.healthdata.org/results/country-profiles/haq

38   GBD 2016 Healthcare Access and Quality Collaborators. "Measuring performance on the Healthcare Access and Quality Index for 195 countries and territories and selected subnational locations: a systematic analysis from the Global Burden of Disease Study 2016." The Lancet. 2018. DOI: 10.1016/S0140-6736(18)30994-2. Accessed June 11, 2019. https://www.thelancet.com/journals/lancet/article/PIIS0140-6736(18)30994-2/fulltext#%20

39   Kamal, R. DB_Healthcare Quality and Access (HAQ) Index Rating, 2016 (charts). Peterson-Kaiser Health System Tracker. March 19, 2019. Accessed June 11, 2019. https://www.healthsystemtracker.org/chart/db_healthcare-quality-and-access-haq-index-rating-2016/#item-start

40   Anna D. Sinaiko, Ateev Mehrotra, and Neeraj Sood. "Cost-Sharing Obligations, High-Deductible Health Plan Growth, and Shopping for Health Care: Enrollees With Skin in the Game." JAMA Intern Med. 2016;176(3):395–397. Accessed April 24, 2019. DOI:10.1001/jamainternmed.2015.7554

41   James Frank Wharam, Fang Zhang, EM Eggleston, Christine Lu, Stephen Soumerai and Dennis Ross-Degnan. "Diabetes Outpatient Care and Acute Complications Before and After High-Deductible Insurance Enrollment: A Natural Experiment for Translation in Diabetes (NEXT-D) Study." JAMA Intern Med. 2017 Mar 1;177(3):358-368. DOI: 10.1001/jamainternmed.2016.8411.

42   James Frank Wharam, Fang Zhang, EM Eggleston, Christine Lu, Stephen Soumerai and Dennis Ross-Degnan. "Diabetes Outpatient Care and Acute Complications Before and After High-Deductible Insurance Enrollment: A Natural Experiment for Translation in Diabetes (NEXT-D) Study." JAMA Intern Med. 2017 Mar 1;177(3):358-368. DOI: 10.1001/jamainternmed.2016.8411.

43   American Hospital Association. "Fast Facts on U.S. Hospitals, 2019." Updated January 2019. Accessed June 24, 2019. https://www.aha.org/statistics/fast-facts-us-hospitals

44   American Hospital Association. "Fast Facts on U.S. Hospitals, 2019." 2019.

45   Kaiser Family Foundation. "Hospital Beds per 1,000 Population by Ownership Type." Accessed June 24, 2019. https://www.kff.org/other/state-indicator/beds-by-ownership/

46   John Elflein. "Hospital Occupancy rate in the U.S. from 1975 to 2017." Statistica. Last edited March 18, 2019. Accessed June 25, 2019. https://www.statista.com/statistics/185904/hospital-occupancy-rate-in-the-us-since-2001/

47   Dartmouth Atlas Project. "General FAQ." (n.d.) Accessed June 25, 2019. https://www.dartmouthatlas.org/faq/

48   Dartmouth Atlas Project. "General FAQ." (n.d.)

49   Dartmouth Atlas Project. "General FAQ." (n.d.)

50   Dartmouth Atlas Project. "General FAQ." (n.d.)

51   American Hospital Association. "Trendwatch Chartbook 2018: Trends Affecting Hospitals and Health Systems." Chart 2.5 Number of Medicare-certified Ambulatory Surgical Centers, 2010, 2011, 2015, 2016. Accessed June 26, 2019. https://www.aha.org/system/files/2018-07/2018-aha-chartbook.pdf

52   Cheryl Alkon. "What's behind the growth of urgent care clinics?" *Medical Economics*. August 29, 2018. Accessed June 25, 2019. https://www.medicaleconomics.com/business/whats-behind-growth-urgent-care-clinics

53   Michelle Andrews. "Congress Urged to Cut Medicare Payments To Many Stand-Alone ERs." *Kaiser Health News*. April 17, 2018. Accessed June 26, 2019. https://khn.org/news/congressional-advisers-urge-medicare-payments-to-many-stand-alone-ers-be-cut/

54   Michelle Andrews. "Congress Urged to Cut Medicare Payments." *Kaiser Health News*. April 17, 2018.

55   Michelle Andrews. "Congress Urged to Cut Medicare Payments." *Kaiser Health News*. April 17, 2018.

56   Medicare Program Advisory Commission (MedPAC). Report to the Congress: Medicare and the Health Care Delivery System. Chapter 8: Stand-alone emergency departments. June 2017. Accessed June 25, 2019. http://www.medpac.gov/docs/default-source/reports/jun17_ch8.pdf

57   Renee Y. Hsia, Jaime King and Brendan G. Carr. "Don't Hate the Player; Hate the Game." *Annals of Emergency Medicine*. Volume 70, Issue 6, 875 – 883. December 2017. Accessed June 26, 2019. DOI: https://doi.org/10.1016/j.annemergmed.2017.08.062

58   Medicare Program Advisory Commission (MedPAC). Report to the Congress: Medicare and the Health Care Delivery System. Chapter 8: Stand-alone emergency departments, Figure 8-3. June 2017. Accessed June 25, 2019. http://www.medpac.gov/docs/default-source/reports/jun17_ch8.pdf

59   Health Care Payment Learning & Action Network. Measuring Progress: Adoption of Alternative Payment Models in Commercial, Medicaid, Medicare Advantage, and Medicare Fee-for-Service Programs. October 22, 2018. Accessed June 28, 2019. https://hcp-lan.org/2018-apm-measurement/

60   Health Care Payment Learning & Action Network. Measuring Progress: Adoption of Alternative Payment Models in Commercial, Medicaid, Medicare Advantage, and Medicare Fee-for-Service Programs. October 22, 2018. Accessed June 28, 2019. https://hcp-lan.org/2018-apm-measurement/ and http://hcp-lan.org/workproducts/2018-APM-Progress-Press-Release.pdf

61   Health Care Payment Learning & Action Network. Measuring Progress. October 22, 2018.

62   MediGold. "Stars and HEDIS Overview." Updated October 2018. Accessed June 28, 2019. https://medigold.com/For-Providers/Tools-and-Resources/Stars-and-HEDIS/Stars-and-HEDIS-Overview

63   The Leapfrog Group website. Accessed June 28, 2019. https://www.leapfroggroup.org/

64   Lynn B. Rogut. "Searching for Quality Medical Care." *Health Affairs Blog*. February 9, 2018. Accessed July 2, 2019. https://www.healthaffairs.org/do/10.1377/hblog20180206.514753/full/

65   Robert Wood Johnson Foundation. "Right Place, Right Time: Improving Access to Health Care Information for Vulnerable Patients." January 2017. Accessed July 2, 2019. https://altarum.org/sites/default/files/uploaded-publication-files/RPRT%20Executive-Summary.pdf

66   Jayne O'Connell. "Low-rated US hospitals are deadlier due to mistakes, botched surgery, infections." *USA Today*. May 15, 2019. Updated May 16, 2019. Accessed July 2, 2019. https://www.usatoday.com/story/news/health/2019/05/15/patient-safety-d-and-f-hospitals-have-twice-death-risk-error/1183705001/

67   Nina Zhang. "Quality Metrics: The New Frontier for False Claims Litigation?" American Bar Association Health eSource. March 2019. Accessed July 2, 2019. https://www.americanbar.org/groups/health_law/publications/aba_health_esource/2018-2019/march/metrics/

68   Centers for Disease Control and Prevention. "Chronic Diseases in America." Last reviewed April 15, 2019. Accessed June 24, 2019. https://www.cdc.gov/chronicdisease/resources/infographic/chronic-diseases.htm

69   Centers for Disease Control and Prevention. "Chronic Diseases in America." 2019.

70   Christine Buttorff, Teague Ruder, Melissa Bauman. "Multiple Chronic Conditions in the
      United States." Rand Corporation. 2017. Accessed July 2019.
      https://www.rand.org/content/dam/rand/pubs/tools/TL200/TL221/RAND_TL221.pdf
71   C. Buttorff, T. Ruder and M. Bauman. "Multiple Chronic Conditions in the United States."
      Rand Corporation. 2017.
72   C. Buttorff, T. Ruder and M. Bauman. "Multiple Chronic Conditions in the United States."
      Rand Corporation. 2017.
73   Build Healthy Places Network blog. "The Pulse: Why Place Matters to Health." July 31,
      2015. Accessed June 25, 2019. https://www.buildhealthyplaces.org/whats-new/the-pulse-
      why-place-matters-to-health/
74   Fiscal Year (FY) 2019 Medicare Hospital Inpatient Prospective Payment System (IPPS)
      and Long-Term Acute Care Hospital (LTCH) Prospective Payment System Final Rule
      (CMS-1694-F), 83 Fed. Reg. 41144 *Federal Register: The Daily Journal of the United
      States*. Aug. 17, 2018. Accessed July 19, 2019. https://www.federalregister.gov/d/2018-
      16766. Also: 42 C.F.R. Parts 412, 413, 424, 495.
75   Fiscal Year (FY) 2019 Medicare Hospital Inpatient Prospective Payment System. 83 Fed.
      Reg. 41144. *Federal Register: The Daily Journal of the United States*. Aug. 17, 2018. See
      also: 42 C.F.R. Parts 412, 413, 424 and 495.
76   Advisory Board. "Hospitals question legality of CMS' price transparency proposal."
      Advisory Board. October 1, 2019. Accessed December 31, 2019.
      https://www.advisory.com/daily-briefing/2019/10/01/opps-comments
77   Fiscal Year (FY) 2019 Medicare Hospital Inpatient Prospective Payment System (IPPS)
      and Long-Term Acute Care Hospital (LTCH) Prospective Payment System Final Rule
      (CMS-1694-F), 83 Fed. Reg. 41144. *Federal Register: The Daily Journal of the United
      States*. Aug. 17, 2018. Accessed July 19, 2019. https://www.federalregister.gov/d/2018-
      16766. Also: 42 C.F.R. Parts 412, 413, 424, 495.
78   Medicare Program: Proposed Changes to Hospital Outpatient Prospective Payment and
      Ambulatory Surgical Center Payment Systems and Quality Reporting Programs; Price
      Transparency of Hospital Standard Charges; Proposed Revisions of Organ Procurement
      Organizations Conditions of Coverage; Proposed Prior Authorization Process and
      Requirements for Certain Covered Outpatient Department Services; Potential Changes to
      the Laboratory Date of Service Policy; Proposed Changes to Grandfathered Children's
      Hospitals-Within-Hospitals (CMS-1717-P), 84 Fed. Reg. 39398. Federal Register: The
      Daily Journal of the United States. Aug. 9, 2019. Accessed Aug. 10, 2019.
      https://www.federalregister.gov/documents/2019/08/09/2019-16107/medicare-program-
      proposed-changes-to-hospital-outpatient-prospective-payment-and-ambulatory-surgical.
      See also: 42 C.F.R. Parts 405, 410, 412, 416, 419 and 486, and 45 C.F.R. Part 180.
79   Medicare Program: Proposed Changes to Hospital Outpatient Prospective Payment. 84 Fed.
      Reg. 39398. *Federal Register: The Daily Journal of the United States.* Aug. 9, 2019. See
      also: 42 C.F.R. Parts 405, 410, 412, 416, 419 and 486, and 45 C.F.R. Part 180.
80   Emily M. Mitchell. Statistical Brief #521: Concentration of Health Expenditures and
      Selected Characteristics of High Spenders, U.S. Civilian Noninstitutionalized Population,
      2016. Figure 5. Agency for Healthcare Research and Quality (AHRQ). Medical
      Expenditure Panel Survey. February 2019. Accessed July 25, 2019.
      https://meps.ahrq.gov/data_files/publications/st521/stat521.shtml
81   Sarah Heath. "How Patient Experience in Billing Offices Impacts Patient Payments."
      Patient Engagement HIT. Oct. 15, 2018. https://patientengagementhit.com/news/how-
      patient-experience-in-billing-offices-impacts-patient-payments
82   Rachel Carollo. "Consumers Want Faster Delivery and They're Willing to Pay for It."
      Dropoff. March 20, 2018. Accessed July 2, 2019. https://www.dropoff.com/blog/retail-
      delivery-consumer-survey-shoptalk-2018
83   Rachel Carollo. "Consumers Want Faster Delivery." March 20, 2018.
84   Ayla Ellison. "13 hospital bankruptcies, state by state." *Becker's Hospital CFO Report.*
      June 17, 2019. Accessed Aug. 9, 2019. https://www.beckershospitalreview.com/finance/13-
      hospital-bankruptcies-state-by-state.html

85   National Health Expenditure Data, Historical. CMS.gov. Accessed Aug. 7, 2019.
      https://www.cms.gov/research-statistics-data-and-systems/statistics-trends-and-
      reports/nationalhealthexpenddata/nationalhealthaccountshistorical.html
86   National Health Expenditure Data, National Health Expenditure Projections 2018-2027,
      Forecast Summary. CMS.gov. Accessed July 23, 2019. https://www.cms.gov/Research-
      Statistics-Data-and-Systems/Statistics-Trends-and-
      Reports/NationalHealthExpendData/Downloads/ForecastSummary.pdf
87   Kimberly Amadeo. "US GDP Statistics and How to Use Them." *The Balance*. July 26,
      2019. Accessed August 8, 2019. https://www.thebalance.com/u-s-gdp-5-latest-statistics-
      and-how-to-use-them-3306041
88   Chris Girod, Sue Hart, Dave Liner, Tom Snook and Scott Weltz. Milliman Research
      Report: 2019 Milliman Medical Index. July 2019. Accessed July 26, 2019.
      http://assets.milliman.com/ektron/2019-milliman-medical-index.pdf
89   Helaine Olen. "Even the Insured Often Can't Afford Their Medical Bills." *The Atlantic*.
      June 18, 2017. Accessed Aug. 8, 2019.
      https://www.theatlantic.com/business/archive/2017/06/medical-bills/530679/
90   Board of Governors of the Federal Reserve System. "Report on the Economic Well-Being
      of U.S. Households in 2018." May 2019. Accessed July 23, 2019.
      https://www.federalreserve.gov/publications/files/2018-report-economic-well-being-us-
      households-201905.pdf
91   Board of Governors of the Federal Reserve System. "Report on the Economic Well-Being
      of U.S. Households in 2018." May 2019. Page 23. Accessed July 23, 2019.
      https://www.federalreserve.gov/publications/files/2018-report-economic-well-being-us-
      households-201905.pdf
92   Board of Governors of the Federal Reserve System. "Report on the Economic Well-Being
      of U.S. Households in 2018." May 2019. Page 23. Accessed July 23, 2019.
      https://www.federalreserve.gov/publications/files/2018-report-economic-well-being-us-
      households-201905.pdf
93   Board of Governors of the Federal Reserve System. "Report on the Economic Well-Being
      of U.S. Households in 2018." May 2019. Page 23. Accessed July 23, 2019.
      https://www.federalreserve.gov/publications/files/2018-report-economic-well-being-us-
      households-201905.pdf
94   Mike Ellrich and Lance Stevens. Americans Fear Personal and National Healthcare Cost
      Crisis. April 2, 2019. Accessed July 24, 2019.
      https://news.gallup.com/opinion/gallup/248108/americans-fear-personal-national-
      healthcare-cost-crisis.aspx
95   Ken Alltucker. Fear and health care: Gallup survey finds Americans skilled treatment,
      borrowed $88 billion to pay for costs. USA Today. April 2, 2019. Accessed August 10,
      2019. https://www.usatoday.com/story/news/health/2019/04/02/health-care-costs-gallup-
      survey-americans-borrowed-88-billion/3333864002/
96   Mike Ellrich and Lance Stevens. Americans Fear Personal and National Healthcare Cost
      Crisis. April 2, 2019. Accessed July 24, 2019.
      https://news.gallup.com/opinion/gallup/248108/americans-fear-personal-national-
      healthcare-cost-crisis.aspx
97   David U. Himmelstein, Robert M. Lawless, Deborah Thorne, Pamela Foohey and Steffie
      Woolhandler. "Medical Bankruptcy: Still Common Despite the Affordable Care Act."
      February 6, 2019. *American Journal of Public Health* 109, 431–433.
      https://doi.org/10.2105/AJPH.2018.304901
98   Kaiser Family Foundation. Health Insurance Coverage of the Total Population. 2017.
      Accessed July 24, 2019. https://www.kff.org/other/state-indicator/total-
      population/?currentTimeframe=0&sortModel=%7B%22colId%22:%22Location%22,%22s
      ort%22:%22asc%22%7D
99   Dan Witters. "U.S. Uninsured Rate Rises to Four-Year High." January 23, 2019. Accessed
      Aug. 9, 2019. https://news.gallup.com/poll/246134/uninsured-rate-rises-four-year-high.aspx

100   Dan Witters. "U.S. Uninsured Rate Rises to Four-Year High." January 23, 2019. Accessed Aug. 9, 2019. https://news.gallup.com/poll/246134/uninsured-rate-rises-four-year-high.aspx

101   Sara R. Collins, Herman K. Bhupal, Michelle M. Doty. "Health Insurance Coverage Eight Years After the ACA: Fewer Uninsured Americans and Shorter Coverage Gaps, but More Underinsured." The Commonwealth Fund, Survey Brief. February 2019. Accessed July 24, 2019. https://www.commonwealthfund.org/sites/default/files/2019-02/EMBARGOED_Collins_hlt_ins_coverage_8_years_after_ACA_2018_biennial_survey_sb_v4.pdf

102   Sara R. Collins, Herman K. Bhupal and Michelle M. Doty. "Health Insurance Coverage Eight Years After the ACA: Fewer Uninsured Americans and Shorter Coverage Gaps, but More Underinsured." The Commonwealth Fund, Survey Brief. February 2019. Accessed July 24, 2019. https://www.commonwealthfund.org/sites/default/files/2019-02/EMBARGOED_Collins_hlt_ins_coverage_8_years_after_ACA_2018_biennial_survey_sb_v4.pdf

103   David Blumenthal. "Americans can't afford to get sick — and limited plans could make things worse." The Hill. Nov. 1, 2018. Accessed July 24, 2019. https://thehill.com/opinion/healthcare/413960-americans-cant-afford-to-get-sick-and-limited-plans-could-make-things

104   Noam N. Levy. "Health insurance deductibles soar, leaving Americans with unaffordable bills." Los Angeles Times. May 2, 2019. Accessed July 25, 2019. https://www.latimes.com/politics/la-na-pol-health-insurance-medical-bills-20190502-story.html

105   "'We're Drowning': Financially Crippled Americans Are Reaching A Breaking Point As Health Insurance Drains Their Savings." Kaiser Health News. May 3, 2019. https://khn.org/morning-breakout/were-drowning-financially-crippled-americans-are-reaching-a-breaking-point-as-health-insurance-drains-their-savings/

106   Ken Alltucker. "Washington couple dies in a murder-suicide over angst about medical expenses." USA Today. August 10, 2019. Accessed August 11, 2019. https://www.usatoday.com/story/news/health/2019/08/10/medical-bills-factor-elderly-couples-murder-suicide-police-say/1978076001/

107   "Average Cost of Employee Health Care Makes Up 7.6 Percent of a Company's Annual Operating Budget." Aug. 30, 2016. The Society for Human Resource Management (SHRM). Accessed July 25, 2019. https://www.shrm.org/about-shrm/press-room/press-releases/pages/2016-health-care-benchmarking-report.aspx

108   Cohen, Robin A. and Zammitti, Emily P. "High-deductible health plan enrollment among adults aged 18–64 with employment-based insurance coverage." NCHS Data Brief, no 317. Hyattsville, MD: National Center for Health Statistics. 2018. Accessed July 25, 2019. https://www.cdc.gov/nchs/products/databriefs/db317.htm

109   John Tozzi and Zachary Tracer. "Sky-High Deductibles Broke the U.S. Health Insurance System." Bloomberg. June 26, 2018. Accessed August 9, 2019. https://www.bloomberg.com/news/features/2018-06-26/sky-high-deductibles-broke-the-u-s-health-insurance-system

110   Taylor Tepper. "The problem with health savings accounts." Bankrate.com. June 29, 2018. Accessed August 10, 2019. https://www.bankrate.com/banking/savings/problem-with-health-savings-accounts/

111   T. Tepper. "The problem with health savings accounts." June 29, 2018.

112   National Health Expenditures 2017 Highlights. CMS.gov. Accessed July 26, 2019. https://www.cms.gov/Research-Statistics-Data-and-Systems/Statistics-Trends-and-Reports/NationalHealthExpendData/downloads/highlights.pdf

113   J. Cubanski and T. Newman. The Facts on Medicare Spending and Financing. 2018.

114   J. Cubanski and T. Newman. The Facts on Medicare Spending and Financing. 2018.

115   J. Cubanski and T. Newman. The Facts on Medicare Spending and Financing. 2018.

116   J. Cubanski and T. Newman. The Facts on Medicare Spending and Financing. 2018.

117   J. Cubanski and T. Newman. The Facts on Medicare Spending and Financing. 2018.

118   Howard Gleckman. "Is President Trump Really Proposing to Cut Medicare by $845
        Billion?". *Forbes*. March 14, 2019Accessed July 26, 2019.
        https://www.forbes.com/sites/howardgleckman/2019/03/14/is-president-trump-really-
        proposing-to-cut-medicare-by-845-billion/#499b4f4b1d07
119   "Does the President's Budget Slash Medicare by $845 Billion?" March 12, 2019.
        Committee for a Responsible Federal Budget. Accessed July 26, 2019.
        https://www.crfb.org/blogs/does-presidents-budget-slash-medicare-845-billion
120   Tara Golshan. "Trump said he wouldn't cut Medicaid, Social Security, and Medicare. His
        2020 budget cuts all 3." Vox. March 12, 2019. Accessed July 27, 2019.
        https://www.vox.com/policy-and-politics/2019/3/12/18260271/trump-medicaid-social-
        security-medicare-budget-cuts
121   T. Golshan. "Trump said he wouldn't cut Medicaid." March 12, 2019.
122   T. Golshan. "Trump said he wouldn't cut Medicaid." March 12, 2019.
123   Andrew M. Harris and John Tozz. "Trump win on Health Plans Advances Effort to Undo
        Obamacare." Bloomberg. July 19, 2019. Accessed August 11, 2019.
        https://www.bloomberg.com/news/articles/2019-07-19/trump-s-short-term-health-insurance-rule-
        survives-lawsuit
124   Short Term Medical Plans brochure. UnitedHealthcare® Golden Rule Insurance Company.
        January 9, 2019. Accessed August 11, 2019.
        https://assets.documentcloud.org/documents/4448250/United-Golden-Rule-STLD-Plan-
        1.pdf
125   Sam Baker. "Workers' health care costs just keep rising." Oct. 4, 2018. *Axios*. Accessed
        July 26, 2019. https://www.axios.com/health-care-costs-premiums-deductibles-increasing-
        428c6244-6dc5-4f5a-94c3-8c6cb89500e9.html
126   Underpayment by Medicare and Medicaid Fact Sheet. January 2019. American Hospital
        Association (AHA). Accessed July 27, 2019. https://www.aha.org/system/files/2019-
        01/underpayment-by-medicare-medicaid-fact-sheet-jan-2019.pdf
127   Chapin White and Christopher Whaley. "Price Paid to Hospitals by Private Health Plans are
        High Relative to Medicare and Vary Widely." Rand Corporation. 2019. Accessed August
        11, 2019. https://doi.org/10.7249/RR3033
128   Underpayment by Medicare and Medicaid Fact Sheet. January 2019. American Hospital
        Association (AHA). Accessed July 27, 2019. https://www.aha.org/system/files/2019-
        01/underpayment-by-medicare-medicaid-fact-sheet-jan-2019.pdf
129   Underpayment by Medicare and Medicaid Fact Sheet. November 2008.
130   Change Healthcare Healthy Hospital Revenue Cycle Index: National medical claim denial
        trends and the impact on providers. June 26, 2017. Change Healthcare. Accessed July 27,
        2019. https://www.changehealthcare.com/blog/wp-content/uploads/Change-Healthcare-
        Healthy-Hospital-Denials-Index.pdf
131   The Advisory Board Company. "Elevating Revenue Cycle Performance." HFMA
        Presentation. January 2018. Accessed August 11, 2019.
        https://static1.squarespace.com/static/554b97b8e4b01f8ee692d265/t/5a5947538165f53cdc4475d9
        /1515800410085/9.+Optimizing+AR+-+Beadle+Ryby.pdf
132   Jonathan Wiik. *Healthcare Revolution: The Patient Is the New Payer*. 2017.
133   Christine Eibner and Sarah Nowak. "The Effect of Eliminating the Individual Mandate
        Penalty and the role of Behavioral Factors." The Commonwealth Fund. July 11, 2018.
        Accessed August 5, 2019. https://www.commonwealthfund.org/publications/fund-
        reports/2018/jul/eliminating-individual-mandate-penalty-behavioral-factors
134   Robin A.Cohen, Emily P. Terlizzi and Michael E. Martinez. Health insurance coverage:
        Early release of estimates from the National Health Interview Survey, 2018. National
        Center for Health Statistics. May 2019. Accessed September 1, 2019.
        https://www.cdc.gov/nchs/data/nhis/earlyrelease/insur201905.pdf
135   Dan Witters. "U.S. Uninsured Rate Rises to Four-Year High." Gallup. January 23, 2019.
        Accessed Aug. 9, 2019. https://news.gallup.com/poll/246134/uninsured-rate-rises-four-
        year-high.aspx

136   Rachel Garfield, Kendal Orgera and Anthony Damico. The Uninsured and the ACA: A Primer – Key Facts about Health Insurance and the Uninsured amidst Changes to the Affordable Care Act. Kaiser Family Foundation. January 25, 2019. Accessed August 5, 2019. https://www.kff.org/report-section/the-uninsured-and-the-aca-a-primer-key-facts-about-health-insurance-and-the-uninsured-amidst-changes-to-the-affordable-care-act-who-remains-uninsured-after-the-aca-and-why-do-they/

137   Key Facts about the Uninsured Population. Kaiser Family Foundation. December 7, 2018. Accessed July 25, 2019. https://www.kff.org/uninsured/fact-sheet/key-facts-about-the-uninsured-population/

138   Marshall Hargrave. Insurtech. Investopedia. May 2, 2019. Accessed August 15, 2019. https://www.investopedia.com/terms/i/insurtech.asp

139   Persons with overnight stays. National Center for Health Statistics. Centers for Disease Control and Prevention. 2017. Accessed August 15, 2019. https://www.cdc.gov/nchs/fastats/hospital.htm

140   Gary Claxton, Matthew Rae, Larry Levitt and Cynthia Cox. "The average price of laparoscopic appendectomy procedures has increased far faster than other prices in the economy." How have healthcare prices grown in the U.S. over time? Kaiser Family Foundation. May 8, 2018. Accessed August 8, 2019. https://www.healthsystemtracker.org/chart-collection/how-have-healthcare-prices-grown-in-the-u-s-over-time/#item-the-average-price-of-laparoscopic-appendectomy-procedures-has-increased-far-faster-than-other-prices-in-the-economy

141   Kaiser Family Foundation. Health Insurance Coverage of the Total Population. 2017. Accessed July 24, 2019. https://www.kff.org/other/state-indicator/total-population/?currentTimeframe=0&sortModel=%7B%22colId%22:%22Location%22,%22sort%22:%22asc%22%7D

142   100 Best Companies to Work For. Fortune. 2019. Accessed August 7, 2019. https://fortune.com/best-companies/2019/ultimate-software

143   Fortune 500. 2019. Filtered by Sector = Health Care; Profitable. Accessed August 16, 2019. https://fortune.com/fortune500/2019/search/?profitable=true&sector=Health%20Care

144   Rebecca Pifer. "UnitedHealth Q2 revenue growth fueled by Medicare, Optum." HealthcareDive. July 18, 2019. Accessed August 15, 2019. https://www.healthcaredive.com/news/unitedhealth-q2-revenue-growth-fueled-by-medicare-optum/558990/

145   Jack O'Brien. "UnitedHealth, CHS Among Healthcare Winners and Losers in Q2." HealthLeaders. August 8, 2019. Accessed August 16, 2019. https://www.healthleadersmedia.com/finance/unitedhealth-chs-among-healthcare-winners-and-losers-q2

146   Shelby Livingston. "UnitedHealth revenue cracks $200 billion mark." Modern Healthcare. January 16, 2018. Accessed September 1, 2019. https://www.modernhealthcare.com/article/20180116/NEWS/180119932/unitedhealth-revenue-cracks-200-billion-mark

147   Rachel Fehr, Cynthia Cox and Larry Levitt. Individual Insurance Market Performance in Mid-2018. Kaiser Family Foundation. October 5, 2018. Accessed August 8, 2019. https://www.kff.org/health-reform/issue-brief/individual-insurance-market-performance-in-mid-2018/

148   Epstein, L. A. (1964). "Income of the aged in 1962: First findings of the 1963 Survey of the Aged" [PDF document]. Reprinted in the *Social Security Bulletin, 51*(3). March 1964. Accessed August 8, 2019. https://www.ssa.gov/policy/docs/ssb/v51n3/v51n3p9.pdf

149   The Henry J. Kaiser Family Foundation. Medicare and Medicaid at 50 [Video file]. April 15, 2015. Accessed August 8, 2019. https://youtu.be/f9NUCvrrRz4

150   Total Number of Medicare Beneficiaries. Kaiser Family Foundation. 2018. Accessed August 9, 2019. https://www.kff.org/medicare/state-indicator/total-medicare-beneficiaries/?currentTimeframe=0&sortModel=%7B%22colId%22:%22Location%22,%22sort%22:%22asc%22%7D

151   Dan Diamond. "10,000 People Are Now Enrolling In Medicare - Every Day." Forbes. July
        13, 2015. Accessed September 1, 2019.
        https://www.forbes.com/sites/dandiamond/2015/07/13/aging-in-america-10000-people-
        enroll-in-medicare-every-day/#2d2101353657
152   An Overview of Medicare. Kaiser Family Foundation. February 13, 2019. Accessed August
        10. 209. https://www.kff.org/medicare/issue-brief/an-overview-of-medicare/
153   Erin Duffin. "Median age of the resident population of the United States from 1960 to
        2018." Statista. August 9, 2019. Accessed August 10, 2019.
        https://www.statista.com/statistics/241494/median-age-of-the-us-population/
154   An Overview of Medicare. Kaiser Family Foundation. February 13, 2019. Accessed August
        10. 209. https://www.kff.org/medicare/issue-brief/an-overview-of-medicare/
155   Medicaid enrollment changes following the ACA. Medicaid and CHIP Payment Access
        Commission (MACPAC). April 2019. Accessed August 10, 2019.
        https://www.macpac.gov/subtopic/medicaid-enrollment-changes-following-the-aca/
156   Medicaid enrollment changes following the ACA. April 2019.
157   The Affordable Care Act in 2019: Still alive. PwC (U.S.) Accessed August 12, 2019.
        https://www.pwc.com/us/en/industries/health-industries/top-health-industry-issues/aca-in-
        2019.html
158   Hits to ACA Pressure Not-for-Profit Hospital Revenues. August 14, 2019. Accessed August
        15, 2019. https://www.fitchratings.com/site/pr/10086143
159   Subsidized Coverage. Healthcare.gov. Accessed August 16, 2019.
        https://www.healthcare.gov/glossary/subsidized-coverage/
160   Cost Sharing Reduction (CSR). Healthcare.gov. Accessed August 16, 2019.
        https://www.healthcare.gov/glossary/cost-sharing-reduction/
161   Silver Health Plan. Healthcare.gov. Accessed August 16, 2019.
        https://www.healthcare.gov/glossary/silver-health-plan/
162   Kev Coleman. "Average Market Premiums Spike Across Obamacare Plans in 2018."
        HealthPocket. October 27, 2017. Accessed December 31, 2019.
        https://www.healthpocket.com/healthcare-research/infostat/2018-obamacare-premiums-
        deductibles#.XhUpedZKiL4 and "Average Market Premiums Decrease in 2019 For the
        First Time." HealthPocket. November 28, 2018. Accessed December 30, 2019.
        https://www.healthpocket.com/healthcare-research/infostat/2019-average-market-
        premiums-decrease#.XhUqxNZKiL4 and "Cost-Sharing for Plans Offered in the Federal
        Marketplace, 2014-2020." Kaiser Family Foundation. KFF.org. December 9, 2019.
        Accessed December 30, 2019. https://www.kff.org/slideshow/cost-sharing-for-plans-
        offered-in-the-federal-marketplace-2014-2020
163   Louise Norris. "The ACA's cost-sharing subsidies." Healthinsurance.org. June 21, 2019.
        Accessed August 16, 2019. https://www.healthinsurance.org/obamacare/the-acas-cost-
        sharing-subsidies/#funding
164   Louise Norris. "Silver Loading and Your Health Insurance Premiums." VeryWellHealth.
        August 17, 2019. Accessed September 1, 2019. https://www.verywellhealth.com/silver-
        loading-health-insurance-premiums-4174119
165   Louise Norris. "The ACA's cost-sharing subsidies." Healthinsurance.org. August 17, 2019.
        Accessed September 1, 2019. https://www.healthinsurance.org/obamacare/the-acas-cost-
        sharing-subsidies/#states
166   Jennifer Tolbert, Maria Diaz, Cornelia Hall, and Salem Mengistu. "State Actions to
        Improve the Affordability of Health Insurance in the Individual Market." Kaiser Family
        Foundation. July 17, 2019. Accessed September 1, 2019. https://www.kff.org/health-
        reform/issue-brief/state-actions-to-improve-the-affordability-of-health-insurance-in-the-
        individual-market/
167   Could Universal Health Care Work in the United States? Knowledge@Wharton podcast.
        February 22, 2019. Accessed August 13, 2019.
        https://knowledge.wharton.upenn.edu/article/could-universal-health-care-work-in-the-u-s/

168 Expanded & Improved Medicare For All Act, H.R. 676, 115th Cong. (2017-2018). History of legislation. Accessed August 14, 2019. https://www.congress.gov/bill/115th-congress/house-bill/676

169 "Medicare for All" Congress.gov. Accessed 081519. https://www.congress.gov/search?q=%7B%22congress%22%3A%22116%22%2C%22source%22%3A%22legislation%22%2C%22search%22%3A%22Medicare%20for%20All%22%7D&searchResultViewType=expanded

170 Compare Medicare-for-all and Public Plan Proposals. Kaiser Family Foundation. May 15, 2019. Accessed August 14, 2019. https://www.kff.org/interactive/compare-medicare-for-all-public-plan-proposals/

171 Sarah Kliff and Dylan Scott. "We read 9 Democratic plans for expanding health care. Here's how they work." Vox. June 21, 2019. Accessed August 14, 2019. https://www.vox.com/2018/12/13/18103087/medicare-for-all-explained-single-payer-health-care-sanders-jayapal

172 Erik Sherman. "U.S. Health Care Costs Skyrocketed to $3.65 Trillion in 2018." February 21, 2019. Accessed December 23, 2019. https://fortune.com/2019/02/21/us-health-care-costs-2/

173 Dylan Scott. "The revealing Medicare-for-all fact-check debate roiling the internet, explained." Vox. August 23, 2018. Accessed August 15, 2019. https://www.vox.com/policy-and-politics/2018/8/23/17769130/medicare-for-all-costs-bernie-sanders-mercatus-study

174 Health care reform for individuals. Mass.gov. 2019. Accessed August 12, 2019. https://www.mass.gov/info-details/health-care-reform-for-individuals#introduction-

175 Health care reform for individuals. Mass.gov. 2019.

176 Health care reform for individuals. Mass.gov. 2019.

177 Emily Delbridge. "These States Do Not Require Auto Insurance." The Balance. March 28, 2019. Accessed August 14, 2019. https://www.thebalance.com/states-with-no-car-insurance-requirements-4121731

178 Health Insurance Coverage of the Total Population. Kaiser Family Foundation. 2017. Accessed August 12, 2019. https://www.kff.org/other/state-indicator/total-population/?currentTimeframe=0&sortModel=%7B"colId":"Uninsured","sort":"asc"%7D

179 Health Care Access Rankings. US News & World Report. (n.d.) Accessed August 12, 2019. https://www.usnews.com/news/best-states/rankings/health-care/healthcare-access

180 Adam McCann. "2019's Best & Worst States for Health Care." WalletHub. 2019. Accessed August 12, 2019. https://wallethub.com/edu/states-with-best-health-care/23457/

181 2018 Annual Cost Trends Report. Massachusetts Health Policy Commission. February 2019. Accessed August 12, 2019. https://www.mass.gov/service-details/annual-cost-trends-report

182 QuickFacts: United States; Massachusetts. United States Census Bureau. Accessed September 1, 2019. https://www.census.gov/quickfacts/fact/table/US,MA/PST045218

183 Rural and urban health. Health Policy Institute. Georgetown University. (n.d.) Accessed September 8, 2019. https://hpi.georgetown.edu/rural/

184 Urban percentage of the population for states, historical. Iowa Community Indicators Program. Iowa State University. (n.d.) Accessed September 8, 2019. https://www.icip.iastate.edu/tables/population/urban-pct-states

185 U.S. States ranked by population, 2019. World Population. (n.d.) Accessed September 8, 2019. http://worldpopulationreview.com/states/

186 Urban percentage of the population for states, historical. Iowa Community Indicators Program. Iowa State University. (n.d.)

187 Teaching Hospitals Provide Significantly More Free Care to The Poor and Uninsured than Any Other Hospitals. The Commonwealth Fund. April 18, 2001. Accessed September 8, 2019. https://www.commonwealthfund.org/press-release/2001/teaching-hospitals-provide-significantly-more-free-care-poor-and-uninsured-any

188 2019 Reporting Cycle Teaching Hospital List. CMS.gov. October 2018. Accessed September 8, 2019. https://www.cms.gov/OpenPayments/Downloads/2019-Reporting-Cycle-Teaching-Hospital-List-pdf.pdf

189 Katie Jennings. "New Jersey will become second state to enact individual health insurance mandate." Politico. Accessed August 12, 2019. https://www.politico.com/states/new-jersey/story/2018/05/30/new-jersey-becomes-second-state-to-adopt-individual-health-insurance-mandate-442183

190 Morgan Haefner. "ACA's individual mandate is gone—Here are 4 places where insurance is still required." Becker's Payer Issues. January 4, 2019. Accessed August 12, 2019. https://www.beckershospitalreview.com/payer-issues/aca-s-individual-mandate-is-gone-here-are-4-states-where-insurance-is-still-required.html%20

191 Statistics (on Fraud). Blue Cross Blue Shield Blue Care Network of Michigan. (n.d.) Accessed August 18, 2019. https://www.bcbsm.com/health-care-fraud/fraud-statistics.html

192 Fraud. Office of Inspector General. U.S. Department of Health and Human Services. (n.d.). Accessed August 19, 2019. https://oig.hhs.gov/fraud/index.asp

193 Strike Force Operations. U.S. Department of Justice. December 6, 2018. Accessed August 19, 2019. https://www.justice.gov/criminal-fraud/strike-force-operations

194 Strike Force Operations. U.S. Department of Justice. December 6, 2018. Accessed August 19, 2019. https://www.justice.gov/criminal-fraud/strike-force-operations

195 "Nigerian Man Sentenced to Prison for Role in $8.3 Million Medicare Fraud Scheme and Related Money Laundering." Office of Public Affairs, U.S. Department of Justice. December 21, 2018. Accessed August 19, 2019. https://www.justice.gov/opa/pr/nigerian-man-sentenced-prison-role-83-million-medicare-fraud-scheme-and-related-money

196 "Justice Department Recovers Over $2.8 Billion from False Claims Act Cases in Fiscal Year 2018." Office of Public Affairs, U.S. Department of Justice. December 21, 2018. Accessed August 19, 2019. https://www.justice.gov/opa/pr/justice-department-recovers-over-28-billion-false-claims-act-cases-fiscal-year-2018

197 "Justice Department Recovers Over $2.8 Billion from False Claims." 2018.

198 "Justice Department Recovers Over $2.8 Billion from False Claims Act Cases in Fiscal Year 2018." Office of Public Affairs, U.S. Department of Justice. December 21, 2018. Accessed August 19, 2019. https://www.justice.gov/opa/pr/justice-department-recovers-over-28-billion-false-claims-act-cases-fiscal-year-2018

199 Alia Paavola. "AmerisourceBergen to pay $625M to settle civil fraud charges linked to repackaging scandal. Becker's Hospital Review." October 2, 2019. Accessed August 19, 2019. https://www.beckershospitalreview.com/legal-regulatory-issues/amerisourcebergen-to-pay-625m-to-settle-civil-fraud-charges-linked-to-repackaging-scandal.html

200 A.Paavola. "AmerisourceBergen to pay $625M."October 2, 2019.

201 Samuel Rubenfeld and Micah Maidenberg. "Former AmerisourceBergen Exec Blew Whistle That Led to Settlement." The Wall Street Journal. October 2, 2018. Accessed August 18, 2019. https://www.wsj.com/articles/former-amerisourcebergen-exec-blew-whistle-that-led-to-settlement-1538441841

202 "Nigerian Man Sentenced to Prison for Role in $8.3 Million Medicare Fraud Scheme and Related Money Laundering. Office of Public Affairs, U.S. Department of Justice. December 21, 2018. Accessed August 19, 2019. https://www.justice.gov/opa/pr/nigerian-man-sentenced-prison-role-83-million-medicare-fraud-scheme-and-related-money

203 Opioid Overdose. Centers for Disease Control and Prevention. May 20, 2019. Accessed August 20, 2019. https://www.cdc.gov/drugoverdose/index.html

204 2019 Appalachian Region Opioid Takedown. Office of the Inspector General. U.S. Department of Health and Human Services. (n.d.) Accessed August 19, 2019. https://oig.hhs.gov/newsroom/media-materials/2019/arpo/

205 2019 Appalachian Region Opioid Takedown. Department of Health and Human Services. (n.d.)

206 2019 Appalachian Region Opioid Takedown..S. Department of Health and Human Services. (n.d.)

207   Opioid Overdose Crisis. National Institute on Drug Abuse. National Institutes of Health. January 2019. Accessed August 18, 2019. https://www.drugabuse.gov/drugs-abuse/opioids/opioid-overdose-crisis

208   Florence C.S., Zhou C., Luo F. and Xu L. "The Economic Burden of Prescription Opioid Overdose, Abuse, and Dependence in the United States, 2013." Med Care. 2016;54(10):901–906. doi:10.1097/MLR.0000000000000625 Accessed August 19, 2019. https://www.ncbi.nlm.nih.gov/pubmed/27623005

209   Fifth Annual Study on Medical Identity Theft. Ponemon Institute, LLC. February 2015. Accessed August 20, 2019. http://www.medidfraud.org/wp-content/uploads/2015/02/2014_Medical_ID_Theft_Study1.pdf

210   Fifth Annual Study on Medical Identity Theft. Ponemon Institute, LLC. February 2015

211   "Medical Identity Theft. Money Scams & Fraud." AARP. February 15, 2019. Accessed August 18, 2019. https://www.aarp.org/money/scams-fraud/info-2019/medical-identity-theft.html

212   Fifth Annual Study on Medical Identity Theft. Ponemon Institute, LLC. February 2015.; and Michelle Andrews. The Rise of Medical Identity Theft. Consumer Reports. August 25, 2016. Accessed September 8, 2019. https://www.consumerreports.org/medical-identity-theft/medical-identity-theft/

213   Daniel P. O'Neill and David Scheinker. "Wasted Health Spending: Who's Picking Up The Tab?" Health Affairs Blog. May 31, 2018. DOI: 10.1377/hblog20180530.245587 Accessed August 26, 2019. https://www.healthaffairs.org/do/10.1377/hblog20180530.245587/full/

214   Tanya G.K. Bentley, Rach M. Effors, Kartika Palar and Emmett B. Keeler. "Waste in the U.S. Health Care System: A Conceptual Framework." The Milbank Quarterly. 2008 Dec.; 86(4): 629–659. doi: 10.1111/j.1468-0009.2008.00537.x Accessed August 28, 2019. https://www.ncbi.nlm.nih.gov/pmc/articles/PMC2690367/#

215   T. Bentley et al. "Waste in the U.S. Health Care System" The Milbank Quarterly. 2008.

216   Insurance Information Institute. Facts + Statistics: Industry Overview. 2017. Accessed June 12, 2019. https://www.iii.org/fact-statistic/facts-statistics-industry-overview

217   David U. Himmelstein, Miraya Jun, Reinhard Busse, Karine Chevreul, Alexander Geissler, Patrick Jeurissen, Sarah Thomson, Marie-Amelie Vinet, and Steffie Woolhandler. "A Comparison Of Hospital Administrative Costs In Eight Nations: US Costs Exceed All Others By Far." Health Affairs 2014 33:9, 1586-1594. Accessed August 28, 2019. https://www.healthaffairs.org/doi/full/10.1377/hlthaff.2013.1327

218   Daniel P. O'Neill and David Scheinker. "Wasted Health Spending: Who's Picking Up The Tab?" Health Affairs Blog. DOI: 10.1377/hblog20180530.245587. May 31, 2018. Accessed August 26, 2019. https://www.healthaffairs.org/do/10.1377/hblog20180530.245587/full/

219   Henry J. Aaron. "The Costs of Health Care Administration in the United States and Canada—Questionable Answers to a Questionable Question." N Engl J Med 2003; 349:801–803 DOI: 10.1056/NEJMe030091. August 21, 2003. Accessed August 27, 2019. https://www.nejm.org/doi/10.1056/NEJMe030091

220   Tanya G.K. Bentley, Rach M. Effors, Kartika Palar and Emmett B. Keeler. "Waste in the U.S. Health Care System: A Conceptual Framework." The Milbank Quarterly. 2008 Dec.; 86(4): 629–659. DOI: 10.1111/j.1468-0009.2008.00537.x Accessed August 28, 2019. https://www.ncbi.nlm.nih.gov/pmc/articles/PMC2690367/#

221   Susan Morse. "Claims processing is in dire need of improvement, but new approaches are helping." Healthcare Finance. May 28, 2017. Accessed August 28, 2019. https://www.healthcarefinancenews.com/news/claims-processing-dire-need-improvement-new-approaches-are-helping

222   Juliette Cubanski, Tricia Neuman, Shannon Griffin and Anthony Damico. "Medicare Spending at the End of Life: A Snapshot of Beneficiaries Who Died in 2014 and the Cost of Their Care." Kaiser Family Foundation. July 14, 2016. Accessed August 26, 2019. https://www.kff.org/medicare/issue-brief/medicare-spending-at-the-end-of-life/

223   J. Cubanski et al. "Medicare Spending at the End of Life." Kaiser Family Foundation. July 14, 2016.

224   J. Cubanski et al. "Medicare Spending at the End of Life." Kaiser Family Foundation. July 14, 2016.

225   Carmen DeNavas-Walt and Bernadette D. Proctor. Current Population Reports, P60 252, Income and Poverty in the United States: 2014. U.S. Census Bureau. U.S. Government Printing Office, Washington, DC, 2015. Accessed August 27, 2019. https://www.census.gov/content/dam/Census/library/publications/2015/demo/p60-252.pdf

226   "Medicare Advantage Provider to Pay $270 Million to Settle False Claims Act Liabilities." U.S. Department of Justice. October 1, 2018. Accessed August 20, 2019. https://www.justice.gov/opa/pr/medicare-advantage-provider-pay-270-million-settle-false-claims-act-liabilities

227   "Medicare Advantage Provider to Pay $270 Million." U.S. Department of Justice. October 1, 2018

228   "Medicare Advantage Provider to Pay $270 Million." U.S. Department of Justice. October 1, 2018

229   "Medicare Advantage Provider to Pay $270 Million." U.S. Department of Justice. October 1, 2018

230   Jonathan Montrose, Courtney McClure, Hannah Rector and Janis Coffin. "Medicare fraud and abuse." Medical Economics, Vol. 95, Issue 24. December 12, 2018. Accessed August 21, 2019. https://www.medicaleconomics.com/medical-billing-collections/medicare-fraud-and-abuse

231   Ingrid S. Martin. "Big Data: Medical Billing Fraud and Abuse Claims Increasingly Based on Data Analysis." Healthcare Business Today. February 27, 2018. Accessed August 21, 2019. https://www.healthcarebusinesstoday.com/medical-billing-fraud-abuse-claims/

232   Compliance Projects. CMS.gov. June 20, 2018. Accessed August 27, 2019. https://www.cms.gov/Research-Statistics-Data-and-Systems/Monitoring-Programs/Medicare-FFS-Compliance-Programs/Data-Analysis/index.html

233   Programs to Evaluate Payment Patterns Electronic Report (PEPPER). Compliance Projects. CMS.gov. June 20, 2018. Accessed August 27, 2019. https://www.cms.gov/Research-Statistics-Data-and-Systems/Monitoring-Programs/Medicare-FFS-Compliance-Programs/Data-Analysis/index.html

234   Good Use of PEPPER Data Makes a Difference in Quality. Relias Media. April 1, 2017. Accessed August 29, 2019. https://www.reliasmedia.com/articles/140333-good-use-of-pepper-data-makes-a-difference-in-quality

235   Welcome to PEPPER Resources. PEPPERresources.org. (n.d.) Accessed August 29, 2019. https://pepper.cbrpepper.org/

236   How insurance companies set health premiums. Healthcare.gov. (n.d.) Accessed September 4, 2019. https://www.healthcare.gov/how-plans-set-your-premiums/

237   How insurance companies set health premiums. Healthcare.gov. (n.d.)

238   James Lightwood and Stanton A. Glantz. "Smoking Behavior and Healthcare Expenditure in the United States, 1992–2009: Panel Data Estimates." PLOS Medicine. Vol. 13,5 e1002020. DOI:10.1371/journal.pmed.1002020 May 10, 2016. Accessed September 4, 2019. https://www.ncbi.nlm.nih.gov/pmc/articles/PMC4862673/#

239   Abigail S Friedman, William L. Schpero and Susan H. Busch. "Evidence Suggests That the ACA's Tobacco Surcharges Reduced Insurance Take-Up And Did Not Increase Smoking Cessation." Health Affairs (Project Hope). Vol. 35,7 (2016): 1176–83. DOI:10.1377/hlthaff.2015.1540. Accessed September 4, 2019. https://www.ncbi.nlm.nih.gov/pmc/articles/PMC5589079/

240   Phil Galewitz. "Feds Say Smokers Are Lying on Obamacare Enrollment Forms." MedCity News. May 4, 2016. Accessed September 4, 2019. https://medcitynews.com/2016/05/smokers-lying-obamacare/

241   Cigna Healthy Rewards Program. Cigna.com. (n.d.) Accessed September 4, 2019. https://www.cigna.com/individuals-families/member-resources/healthy-rewards

242   Get rewarded. Aetnamedicare.com. Accessed September 4, 2019. https://www.aetnamedicare.com/uawtrust/en/live-well/get-rewarded.html

243   Accenture Study Finds Growing Demand for Digital Health Services Revolutionizing Delivery Models: Patients, Doctors + Machines. Accenture. March 6, 2018. Accessed

September 17, 2019. https://newsroom.accenture.com/news/accenture-study-finds-growing-demand-for-digital-health-services-revolutionizing-delivery-models-patients-doctors-machines.htm

244   Aine Cryts. "The Future of Healthcare Wearables." Managed Healthcare Executive. Vol. 29, Issue 8. August 11, 2019. Accessed September 17, 2019. https://www.managedhealthcareexecutive.com/technology/future-healthcare-wearables

245   A. Cryts. "The Future of Healthcare Wearables." Managed Healthcare Executive. August 11, 2019.

246   A. Cryts. "The Future of Healthcare Wearables." Managed Healthcare Executive. August 11, 2019. Accessed September 17, 2019.

247   Stephen Miller. "Employers' Health Costs Could Rise 6% in 2020." SHRM. August 20, 2019. Accessed September 4, 2019. https://www.shrm.org/resourcesandtools/hr-topics/benefits/pages/2020-large-employer-health-costs-expected-to-rise.aspx

248   S. Miller. "Employers' Health Costs Could Rise 6% in 2020." SHRM. 2019.

249   Bureau of Labor Statistics, U.S. Department of Labor, Occupational Outlook Handbook, Actuaries. September 4, 2019. Accessed September 5, 2019. https://www.bls.gov/ooh/math/actuaries.htm

250   U.S. Department of Labor. Occupational Outlook Handbook, Actuaries. Bureau of Labor Statistics, U.S. Department of Labor. September 4, 2019. Accessed September 5, 2019. https://www.bls.gov/ooh/math/actuaries.htm

251   Kirchhoff, S. M. Medical loss ratio requirements under the Patient Protection and Affordable Care Act (ACA): Issues for Congress [PDF document]. August 26, 2014. Accessed September 5, 2019. https://fas.org/sgp/crs/misc/R42735.pdf

252   The Henry J. Kaiser Family Foundation. Explaining health care reform: Medical loss ratio (MLR). February 29, 2012. Accessed September 5, 2019. http://kff.org/health-reform/fact-sheet/explaining-health-care-reform-medical-loss-ratio-mlr/

253   The Henry J. Kaiser Family Foundation. Explaining health care reform. February 29, 2012.

254   Centers for Medicare & Medicaid Services (CMS). The Center for Consumer Information & Insurance Oversight, Medical loss ratio. n.d. Accessed September 5, 2019. https://www.cms.gov/CCIIO/Programs-and-Initiatives/Health-Insurance-Market-Reforms/Medical-Loss-Ratio.html

255   Kirchhoff, S. M. Medical loss ratio requirements under the Patient Protection and Affordable Care Act (ACA): Issues for Congress [PDF document]. August 26, 2014. Accessed September 5, 2019. https://fas.org/sgp/crs/misc/R42735.pdf

256   Rate Review & the 80/20 Rule. Health Insurance Rights and Protections. n.d. Accessed September 17, 2019. https://www.healthcare.gov/health-care-law-protections/rate-review/

257   Aquilina O. "A brief history of cardiac pacing." Images in Paediatric Cardiology. 2006;8(2):17–81. Accessed September 5, 2019. https://www.ncbi.nlm.nih.gov/pmc/articles/PMC3232561/#

258   Decision Memo for Cardia Pacemakers: Single-Chamber and Dual-Chamber Permanent Cardiac Pacemakers (CAG-00063R3). Decision Summary. CMS.gov. August 13, 2013. Accessed September 6, 2019. https://www.cms.gov/medicare-coverage-database/details/nca-decision-memo.aspx?NCAId=267

259   CMS' Program History. CMS.gov. August 5, 2019. Accessed September 17, 2019. https://www.cms.gov/About-CMS/Agency-information/History/

260   Fraud, Waste, and Abuse in the Medicare Pacemaker Industry. Special Committee on Aging, United States Senate. September 1982. Accessed September 17, 2019. https://www.aging.senate.gov/imo/media/doc/reports/rpt882.pdf

261   Decision Memo for Cardiac Pacemakers: Single-Chamber and Dual-Chamber Permanent Cardiac Pacemakers (CAG-00063R3). Decision Summary. CMS.gov. August 13, 2013. Accessed September 6, 2019. https://www.cms.gov/medicare-coverage-database/details/nca-decision-memo.aspx?NCAId=267

262   What are the value-based programs? Centers for Medicare & Medicaid Services (CMS.gov). July 16, 2019. Accessed September 6, 2019.

https://www.cms.gov/Medicare/Quality-Initiatives-Patient-Assessment-Instruments/Value-Based-Programs/Value-Based-Programs.html

263   Jeff Lagasse. "Healthcare payments tied to value-based care on the rise, now at 34 percent." Healthcare Finance. October 24, 2018. Accessed September 6, 2019. https://www.healthcarefinancenews.com/news/healthcare-payments-tied-value-based-care-rise-now-34-percent

264   Jacqueline LaPointe. "Implementation of Risk-Based Contracts in Healthcare Stalling." Revenue Cycle Intelligence. March 12, 2019. Accessed September 6, 2019. https://revcycleintelligence.com/news/implementation-of-risk-based-contracts-in-healthcare-stalling

265   Numerof & Associates and David Nash. The State of Population Health: Fourth Annual Numerof Survey Report. Numerof & Associates, Inc. March 2019. Accessed September 6, 2019. http://nai-consulting.com/numerof-state-of-population-health-survey/

266   Numerof & Associates and D. Nash. The State of Population Health. Numerof & Associates, Inc. March 2019.

267   Robert Pearl. "Healthcare's Dangerous Fee-For-Service Addiction." Forbes. September 25, 2017. Accessed December 23, 2019. https://www.forbes.com/sites/robertpearl/2017/09/25/fee-for-service-addiction/#60e0b379c8ad

268   Jenny Gold. "Accountable Care Organizations, Explained." Kaiser Health News. September 14, 2015. Accessed September 7, 2019. https://khn.org/news/aco-accountable-care-organization-faq/

269   Accountable Care Organization. Glossary. HealthCare.gov. (n.d.). Accessed September 4, 2019. https://www.healthcare.gov/glossary/accountable-care-organization/

270   Shared Savings Program Fast Facts. CMS.gov. July 1, 2019. Accessed September 7, 2019. https://www.cms.gov/Medicare/Medicare-Fee-for-Service-Payment/sharedsavingsprogram/Downloads/ssp-2019-fast-facts.pdf

271   Shared Savings Program Fast Facts. CMS.gov. July 1, 2019.

272   "What are the different types of Medicare ACO models?" Medicare Delivery System Reform: The Evidence Link. Kaiser Family Foundation. (n.d.) Accessed September 7, 2019. https://www.kff.org/faqs-medicare-accountable-care-organization-aco-models/

273   Shared Savings Program Fast Facts. Centers for Medicare & Medicaid Services. CMS.gov. July 1, 2019. Accessed September 7, 2019. https://www.cms.gov/Medicare/Medicare-Fee-for-Service-Payment/sharedsavingsprogram/Downloads/ssp-2019-fast-facts.pdf

274   "What's MACRA?" Centers for Medicare & Medicaid Services. CMS.gov. June 14, 2019. Accessed September 7, 2019. https://www.cms.gov/Medicare/Quality-Initiatives-Patient-Assessment-Instruments/Value-Based-Programs/MACRA-MIPS-and-APMs/MACRA-MIPS-and-APMs.html

275   "What's MACRA?" Centers for Medicare & Medicaid Services. CMS.gov. 2019.

276   MIPS Overview, 2019. Quality Payment Program. (n.d.) Accessed September 8, 2019. https://qpp.cms.gov/mips/overview

277   APM Scoring Standard, 2019. MIPS Alternative Payment Models (APMs). Quality Payment Program. (n.d.) Accessed September 8, 2019. https://qpp.cms.gov/apms/mips-apms

278   2018 Quality Performance Category Scoring for Alternative Payment Models (Table 3.1). Quality Payment Program. Centers for Medicare & Medicaid Services. CMS.gov Accessed September 8, 2019. https://qpp-cm-prod-content.s3.amazonaws.com

279   Quality Measures Requirements. Quality Payment Program. Centers for Medicare & Medicaid Services. CMS.gov 2019. Accessed September 8, 2019. https://qpp.cms.gov/mips/quality-measures?py=2019

280   Explore Measures & Activities, MIPS Overview. Quality Payment Program. Centers for Medicare & Medicaid Services. CMS.gov. 2019. Accessed September 8, 2019. https://qpp.cms.gov/mips/explore-measures/quality-measures?py=2019&specialtyMeasureSet=Family%20Medicine&measureType=Outcome

281   Explore Measures & Activities, MIPS Overview. Quality Payment Program. CMS.gov.
        2019. Accessed September 8, 2019. https://qpp.cms.gov/mips/explore-
        measures/improvement-activities?py=2019&measureWeighting=High
282   Explore Measures & Activities, MIPS Overview. Quality Payment Program. 2019.
283   Explore Measures & Activities, MIPS Overview. Quality Payment Program. 2019.
284   "What Is Pay for Performance in Healthcare?" NEJM Catalyst. March 1, 2018. Accessed
        September 8, 2019. https://catalyst.nejm.org/pay-for-performance-in-healthcare/
285   "What Is Pay for Performance in Healthcare?" NEJM Catalyst. March 1, 2018.
286   Value-Based Purchasing (VBP). Glossary. HealthCare.gov. (n.d.). Accessed 8, September
        2019. https://www.healthcare.gov/glossary/value-based-purchasing-vbp/
287   Non-federal Acute Care Hospital Electronic Health Record Adoption. The Office of the
        National Coordinator for Health Information Technology. Health IT Dashboard. 2017.
        Accessed September 18, 2019. https://dashboard.healthit.gov/quickstats/pages/FIG-
        Hospital-EHR-Adoption.php
288   Jared Sorensen. "Can We Make The Revenue Cycle More Like Retail?" 3M Health
        Information Systems. Presentation at 2018 HFMA Annual Conferences, June 24-27, Las
        Vegas, NV. June 2018.
289   TransUnion Healthcare. "News Reports about a Weakening Economy Impacting How
        Some Patients Seek Medical Treatment." September 17, 2019. Accessed September 30,
        2019. https://newsroom.transunion.com/news-reports-about-a-weakening-economy--impacting-
        how-some-patients-seek-medical-treatment/
290   TransUnion Healthcare. "News Reports about a Weakening Economy." September 2019.
291   Wayne Wood. 'Think it's flu? Now you can ask Alexa." My Southern Health. Vanderbilt
        University Medical Center. February 21, 2018. Accessed September 18, 2019.
        https://www.mysouthernhealth.com/alexa-flu-tool/
292   Wayne Wood. "Think it's flu? Now you can ask Alexa." My Southern Health. 2018.
293   Wayne Wood. "Think it's flu? Now you can ask Alexa." My Southern Health. 2018.
294   Casey Ross. "Amazon Alexa is now HIPAA-compliant. Tech giant says health data can
        now be accessed securely." STAT. April 4, 2019. Accessed September 18, 2019.
        https://www.statnews.com/2019/04/04/amazon-alexa-hipaa-compliant/
295   "NTT DATA Study Finds Nearly Two-Thirds of Consumers Expect Their Healthcare
        Digital Experience to Be More Like Retail." NTT Data. March 5, 2018. Accessed
        September 18, 2019. https://www.businesswire.com/news/home/20180305005288/en/NTT-
        DATA-Study-Finds-Two-Thirds-Consumers-Expect
296   "NTT DATA Study." NTT Data. March 5, 2018
297   TransUnion Healthcare. "News Reports about a Weakening Economy Impacting How
        Some Patients Seek Medical Treatment." September 17, 2019. Accessed September 30,
        2019. https://newsroom.transunion.com/news-reports-about-a-weakening-economy--impacting-
        how-some-patients-seek-medical-treatment/; and Engage Patients Early: Optimal Outcomes
        for Patients and Providers. TransUnion Healthcare. (n.d.) Accessed October 15, 2019.
        https://solutions.transunion.com/pfe-lookbook/
298   Tara Bannow. "Hospital megamergers continue to drive near-historic M&A activity."
        Modern Healthcare. July 22, 2019. Accessed September 19, 2019.
        https://www.modernhealthcare.com/mergers-acquisitions/hospital-megamergers-continue-drive-
        near-historic-ma-activity
299   Hospitals, beds and occupancy rates, by type of ownership and size of hospital: United
        States, selected years, 1975-2015. Table 89. National Center for Health Statistics (NCHS).
        Centers for Disease Control and Prevention. 2017. Accessed September 19, 2019.
        https://www.cdc.gov/nchs/data/hus/2017/089.pdf
300   Jack O'Brien. "Top 5 Healthcare Mergers of 2018." HealthLeadersMedia. December 26,
        2018. Accessed September 19, 2019. https://www.healthleadersmedia.com/finance/top-5-
        healthcare-mergers-2018; and Ayla Ellison. "Post-merger results: Advocate Aurora sees
        revenue, outpatient volume grow." Becker's Hospital CFO Report. April 1, 2019. Accessed
        September 19, 2019. https://www.beckershospitalreview.com/finance/post-merger-results-
        advocate-aurora-sees-revenue-outpatient-volume-grow.html

301   Advocate Aurora Health website (n.d.) Accessed September 19, 2019.
        https://www.advocateaurorahealth.org/; and Advocate Aurora Health to Become 10th
        Largest Health System in the U.S. Advocate Health Care. March 22, 2018. Accessed
        September 19, 2019. https://www.advocatehealth.com/news/advocate-aurora-health-to-
        become-10th-largest-health-system-in-the-u.s

302   Beth Jones Sanborn. "LifePoint Health, RCCH HealthCare Partners merger finalized."
        Healthcare Finance. November 19, 2018. Accessed September 19, 2019.
        https://www.healthcarefinancenews.com/news/lifepoint-health-rcch-healthcare-partners-
        merger-finalized

303   B. Jones Sanborn. "LifePoint Health, RCCH HealthCare Partners merger finalized."
        Healthcare Finance. November 19, 2018.

304   John Commins. "Dignity Health, CHI Finalize $29B CommonSpirit Health Megamerger."
        HealthLeadersMedia. February 1, 2019. Accessed September 19, 2019.
        https://www.healthleadersmedia.com/strategy/dignity-health-chi-finalize-29b-commonspirit-
        health-megamerger

305   Alex Kacik. "Beth Israel Deaconess and Lahey Health complete merger." Modern
        Healthcare. March 1, 2019. Accessed September 19, 2019.
        https://www.modernhealthcare.com/mergers-acquisitions/beth-israel-deaconess-and-lahey-
        health-complete-merger

306   "Beth Israel Lahey Health Begins Journey to Transform Health Care." Lahey.org. March 1,
        2019. Accessed September 19, 2019. https://www.lahey.org/lhmc/article/beth-israel-lahey-
        health-begins-journey-to-transform-health-care/

307   Hospital concentration. Healthy Market Index. Health Care Cost Institute (HCCI). (n.d.)
        Accessed October 1, 2019. https://www.healthcostinstitute.org/research/hmi/hmi-
        interactive#HMI-Concentration-Index

308   The Impact of Hospital Consolidation on Medical Costs. NCCI Insights. July 11, 2018.
        Accessed September 20, 2019.
        https://www.ncci.com/Articles/Pages/II_Insights_QEB_Impact-of-Hospital-Consolidation-
        on-Medical-Costs.aspx

309   Executive Order on Improving Price and Quality Transparency in American Healthcare to
        Put Patients First. President Donald J. Trump. June 24, 2019. Accessed September 20,
        2019. https://www.whitehouse.gov/presidential-actions/executive-order-improving-price-
        quality-transparency-american-healthcare-put-patients-first/

310   Executive Order on Improving Price and Quality Transparency. June 24, 2019.

311   Katie Keith. "Unpacking The Executive Order on Health Care Price Transparency and
        Quality." HealthAffairs. June 25, 2019. Accessed September 20, 2019.
        https://www.healthaffairs.org/do/10.1377/hblog20190625.974595/full/

312   California Department of Justice Conditionally Approves Affiliation of Dignity Health and
        Catholic Healthcare Initiatives with Strong Community and Patient Protections. State of
        California, Department of Justice, Attorney General. November 21, 2018. Accessed
        September 20, 2019. https://oag.ca.gov/news/press-releases/california-department-justice-
        conditionally-approves-affiliation%C2%A0of%C2%A0dignity

313   Alex Kacik. "Beth Israel Deaconess and Lahey Health complete merger." Modern
        Healthcare. March 1, 2019. Accessed September 20, 2019.
        https://www.modernhealthcare.com/mergers-acquisitions/beth-israel-deaconess-and-lahey-
        health-complete-merger

314   A. Kacik. "Beth Israel Deaconess and Lahey Health complete merger." March 1, 2019.

315   Anita Wadhwani. "Medical monopoly in rural Appalachia: 6 things to know about the
        Ballad Health merger." Nashville Tennessean. June 23, 2019. Accessed October 2, 2019.
        https://www.tennessean.com/story/entertainment/2019/06/23/ballad-health-merger-6-things-
        know/1506340001/

316   A. Wadhwani. "Medical monopoly in rural Appalachia." June 23, 2019.

317   Tara Bannow. "Ballad Health at odds with community over controversial changes."
        Modern Healthcare. September 18, 2019. Accessed October 1, 2019.
        https://www.modernhealthcare.com/providers/ballad-health-odds-community-over-controversial-
        changes

318   T. Bannow. "Ballad Health at odds." September 18, 2019.
319   Chad Mulvany. "Analysis: Yes Virginia (and Tennessee), controlling healthcare costs requires hard choices." Healthcare Financial Management Association (HFMA) blog. September 25, 2019. Accessed October 1, 2019. https://www.hfma.org/topics/operations-management/article/analysis-yes-virginia-and-tennessee-controlling-healthcare-costs-requires-hard-choices.html
320   Anita Wadhwani. "Medical monopoly in rural Appalachia: 6 things to know about the Ballad Health merger." Nashville Tennessean. June 23, 2019. Accessed October 2, 2019. https://www.tennessean.com/story/entertainment/2019/06/23/ballad-health-merger-6-things-know/1506340001/
321   "Certificate of Public Advantage (COPA)." COPA. Tennesse Department of Health. TN.gov. (n.d.) Accessed December 8, 2019. https://www.tn.gov/health/health-program-areas/health-planning/certificate-of-public-advantage.html
322   Anita Wadhwani. "Medical monopoly in rural Appalachia: 6 things to know about the Ballad Health merger." Nashville Tennessean. June 23, 2019.
323   Anna Wilde Mathews. "Cigna and Express Scripts Seal $54 Billion Merger." The Wall Street Journal. December 20, 2018. Accessed September 20, 2019. https://www.wsj.com/articles/cigna-and-express-scripts-seal-54-billion-merger-11545327979
324   A.W. Mathews. "Cigna and Express Scripts Seal $54 Billion Merger." 2018.
325   Berman, Ken. "Big Pharma, Big Dividends." Forbes. Forbes Magazine. January 18, 2018. Accessed December 6, 2019. https://www.forbes.com/sites/kenberman/2018/01/18/big-pharma-big-dividends/#6eb408d0a654
326   "Cigna Completes Combination with Express Scripts, Establishing a Blueprint to Transform the Health Care System." Cigna Press Release. December 20, 2018. Accessed September 20, 2019. https://www.cigna.com/about-us/newsroom/innovation/cigna-completes-combination-with-express-scripts
327   Anna Wilde Mathews. "Cigna and Express Scripts Seal $54 Billion Merger. The Wall Street Journal. December 20, 2018." Accessed September 21, 2019. https://www.wsj.com/articles/cigna-and-express-scripts-seal-54-billion-merger-11545327979
328   Anna Wilde Mathews and Aisha Al-Muslim. "CVS Completes $70 Billion Acquisition of Aetna. The Wall Street Journal." November 28, 2019. Accessed September 21, 2019. https://www.wsj.com/articles/cvs-completes-70-billion-acquisition-of-aetna-1543423322?mod=article_inline
329   "CVS Health Completes Acquisition of Aetna, Marking the Start of Transforming the Consumer Health Experience." CVS Health Press Release. November 28, 2019. Accessed September 21, 2019. https://cvshealth.com/newsroom/press-releases/cvs-health-completes-acquisition-of-aetna-marking-the-start-of-transforming-the-consumer-health-experience
330   "CVS Health Completes Acquisition of Aetna." November 28, 2019.
331   Bill Copeland. "Convergence is innovation for health care, but converge to what?" Perspectives. Deloitte. April 10, 2018. Accessed September 21, 2019. https://www2.deloitte.com/us/en/pages/life-sciences-and-health-care/articles/health-care-current-april10-2018.html
332   B. Copeland. "Convergence is innovation." April 10, 2018.
333   B. Copeland. "Convergence is innovation." April 10, 2018.
334   "Number of U.S. Retail Health Clinics will Surpass 2,800 by 2017." Accenture Forecasts. Accenture. November 12, 2015. Accessed September 21, 2019. https://newsroom.accenture.com/news/number-of-us-retail-health-clinics-will-surpass-2800-by-2017-accenture-forecasts.htm
335   Tara Bannow. "CVS to aggressively expand healthcare services in stores." Modern Healthcare. June 4, 2019. Accessed September 22, 2019. https://www.modernhealthcare.com/patient-care/cvs-aggressively-expand-healthcare-services-stores

336	T. Bannow. "CVS to aggressively expand healthcare." June 4, 2019.
337	T. Bannow. "CVS to aggressively expand healthcare." June 4, 2019.
338	The Evolving Role of Retail Clinics. Research Brief. Rand Corporation. 2016. Accessed October 2, 2019. https://www.rand.org/pubs/research_briefs/RB9491-2.html
339	2016 Health Care Cost and Utilization Report. Health Care Cost Institute (HCCI). June 19, 2018. Accessed September 22, 2019. https://www.healthcostinstitute.org/research/annual-reports/entry/2016-health-care-cost-and-utilization-report/
340	Amer Kaissi and Tom Charland. "Hospital-Owned Retail Clinics in the United States: Operations, Patients and Marketing." Journal of Primary Healthcare: Open Access. ISSN: 2167-1079. March 25, 2013. Accessed September 22, 2019. https://www.omicsonline.org/open-access/hospital-owned-retail-clinics-in-the-united-states-operations-patients-and-marketing-2167-1079.1000130.php?aid=12067
341	"Why Choose Us: Clinical affiliations enhance quality, access and continuity of care." CVS Pharmacy, MinuteClinic. (n.d.) Accessed September 22, 2019. https://www.cvs.com/minuteclinic/why-choose-us/quality-clinical-affiliations
342	Shelby Livingston. "Left out of the game: Health systems offer direct-to-employer contracting to eliminate insurers." Modern Healthcare. January 27, 2018. Accessed September 22, 2019. https://www.modernhealthcare.com/article/20180127/NEWS/180129919/left-out-of-the-game-health-systems-offer-direct-to-employer-contracting-to-eliminate-insurers
343	"2020 Large Employers' Health Care Strategy and Plan Design Survey, A National Business Group on Health Publication." Press Briefing. August 13, 2019. Accessed September 22, 2019. https://www.businessgrouphealth.org/pub/?id=6EC458A6-F948-D81C-644E-A6F919D3C412
344	"Henry Ford Health System Launches 'Direct to Employer' Healthcare Contract with General Motors." Henry Ford Health System Press Release. August 6, 2018. Accessed September 22, 2019. https://www.henryford.com/news/2018/08/direct-to-employer-announcement
345	"Henry Ford Health System Launches 'Direct to Employer' Healthcare Contract." August 6, 2018.
346	"Henry Ford Health System Launches 'Direct to Employer' Healthcare Contract." August 6, 2018.
347	Centers of Excellence: The best possible care for serious conditions. Walmart. (n.d.) Accessed September 22, 2019. https://one.walmart.com/content/usone/en_us/me/health/health-programs/centers-of-excellence.html
348	Centers of Excellence. Walmart. (n.d.) https://one.walmart.com/content/usone/en_us/me/health/health-programs/centers-of-excellence.html
349	"Walmart offers its workers free surgery (with a catch). Now it wants others to do the same." Advisory Board Briefing. March 19, 2019. Accessed October 2, 2019. https://www.advisory.com/daily-briefing/2019/03/19/walmart-coe
350	"Hospital networks: Perspective from four years of the individual market exchanges." McKinsey Center for U.S. Health System Reform. May 2017. Accessed October 15, 2019. https://healthcare.mckinsey.com/sites/default/files/2017%20Hospital%20networks%20-%20Perspectives%20from%20four%20years%20of%20the%20individual_%20exchanges%20vF.pdf
351	Steven Findlay. "In Search Of Insurance Savings, Consumers Can Get Unwittingly Wedged Into Narrow-Network Plans. Kaiser Health News. November 1, 2018. Accessed October 15, 2019. https://khn.org/news/in-search-of-insurance-savings-consumers-can-get-unwittingly-wedged-into-narrow-network-plans/#targetText=%E2%80%9CNarrow%20networks%20are%20a%20trade,be%20successful%20when%20done%20well.
352	S. Findlay. "In Search Of Insurance Savings." November 1, 2018.
353	S. Findlay. "In Search Of Insurance Savings." November 1, 2018.

354   Christina Farr. "Everything we know about Haven, the Amazon joint venture to revamp health care." CNBC. March 13, 2019. Accessed September 23, 2019. https://www.cnbc.com/2019/03/13/what-is-haven-amazon-jpmorgan-berkshire-revamp-health-care.html

355   "How is Haven going to improve healthcare?" Vison/FAQs. Havenhealthcare.com. (n.d.) Accessed September 23, 2019. https://havenhealthcare.com/vision

356   Mike Brown. "Should Amazon Get Into Virtual Currency? Banking? Insurance?" LendEDU Survey. February 27, 2018. Accessed September 23, 2019. https://lendedu.com/blog/amazon-virtual-currency-banking-insurance/

357   M. Brown. "Should Amazon Get Into Virtual Currency?" February 27, 2018.

358   "Big data," definition. From Lexico, powered by Oxford. (n.d.) Accessed October 2, 2019. https://www.lexico.com/en/definition/big_data

359   Victoria Greene. "Top 7 examples of big data retail personalization." Big Data Made Simple. October 11, 2018. Accessed October 2, 2019. https://bigdata-madesimple.com/7-examples-of-big-data-retail-personalization/

360   V. Greene. "Top 7 examples of big data retail personalization." October 11, 2018.

361   Devon McGinnis. "Please take my data: Why consumers want more personalized marketing." Salesforce blog. December 2, 2016. Accessed October 2, 2019. https://www.salesforce.com/blog/2016/12/consumers-want-more-personalized-marketing.html

362   Matthew Bayley, Sarah Calkins, Ed Levine and Monisha Machado-Pereira. "Hospital revenue cycle operations: Opportunities created by the ACA" [PDF document]. May 2013. Accessed October 3, 2019. http://healthcare.mckinsey.com/sites/default/files/793544_Hospital_Revenue_Cycle_Operations.pdf

363   Phil Goyeau. "Don't just manage payer denials, prevent them. 3M Health Care Academy." December 13, 2018. Accessed October 23, 2019. http://cthima.org/wp-content/uploads/2018/12/CTHIMA-Payer-Denial-Trends-Rocky-Hill-Dist-12.13.2018.pdf

364   Eric Benson. "Mismatched: How Patient Identification Errors are Costing Patients and Health Systems. Health IT Outcomes." November 29, 2017. Accessed October 3, 2019. https://www.healthitoutcomes.com/doc/mismatched-how-patient-identification-errors-are-costing-patients-and-health-systems-0001; and "Patient Identification Lessons Learned from ECRI Institute's 2016 Deep Dive." ECRI Institute. September 28, 2019. Accessed October 3, 2019. https://www.ecri.org/components/HRCAlerts/Pages/HRCAlerts092816_PatientID.aspx

365   Richard Hillestad, James H. Bigelow, and Basit Chaudhry, et al. "Identity Crisis: An Examination of the Costs and Benefits of a Unique Patient Identifier for the U.S. Health Care System. "Rand Corporation. 2008. Accessed October 4, 2019. https://www.rand.org/content/dam/rand/pubs/monographs/2008/RAND_MG753.pdf

366   Eric Benson. "Mismatched: How Patient Identification Errors are Costing Patients and Health Systems." Health IT Outcomes. November 29, 2017. Accessed October 4, 2019. https://www.healthitoutcomes.com/doc/mismatched-how-patient-identification-errors-are-costing-patients-and-health-systems-0001

367   Beth Jones Sanborn. "Change Healthcare analysis shows $262 billion in medical claims initially denied, meaning billions in administrative costs." June 27, 2017. Healthcare Finance News. June 27, 2017. Accessed October 5. 2019. https://www.healthcarefinancenews.com/news/change-healthcare-analysis-shows-262-million-medical-claims-initially-denied-meaning-billions

368   B.J. Sanborn. "Change Healthcare analysis." June 27, 2017.

369   B.J. Sanborn. "Change Healthcare analysis." June 27, 2017.

370   Pat Maccariella-Hafey. "CPT Coding: A Look at What's Coming in 2019. Health Information Associates." November 19, 2019. Accessed October 5, 2019. https://www.hiacode.com/education/a-look-at-whats-coming-in-2019-for-cpt/

371   Beth Jones Sanborn. "HIMSS Analytics survey shows patient want convenient payment options." Healthcare Finance News. June 8, 2018. Accessed October 5, 2019. https://www.healthcarefinancenews.com/news/himss-analytics-survey-shows-patients-want-convenient-payment-options

372   The Impact of Consumerism on Healthcare: Consumer Feedback Shows Progress on Hospital Business Office Interactions. Connance. October 2018. Accessed October 6, 2019. https://cdn2.hubspot.net/hubfs/634119/White%20Paper%20-%20The%20Impact%20of%20Consumerism%20on%20Healthcare%20-%20October%202018.pdf?__hssc=223962692.1.1556549010703&__hstc=223962692.ed91 7847dcc2518965f19e6172d4d0a9.1556549010701.1556549010701.1556549010701.1&__

373   TransUnion Healthcare. "News Reports about a Weakening Economy Impacting How Some Patients Seek Medical Treatment." September 17, 2019. Accessed September 30, 2019. https://newsroom.transunion.com/news-reports-about-a-weakening-economy--impacting-how-some-patients-seek-medical-treatment/

374   Beth Jones Sanborn. "HIMSS Analytics survey shows patient want convenient payment options." Healthcare Finance News. June 8, 2018. Accessed October 6, 2019. https://www.healthcarefinancenews.com/news/himss-analytics-survey-shows-patients-want-convenient-payment-options

375   TransUnion Healthcare. "News Reports about a Weakening Economy Impacting How Some Patients Seek Medical Treatment." September 17, 2019. Accessed September 30, 2019. https://newsroom.transunion.com/news-reports-about-a-weakening-economy--impacting-how-some-patients-seek-medical-treatment/

376   "Paying Doctors Upfront: Point-of-Service Collections." Comprehensive Primary Care. January 13, 2017. Accessed December 6, 2019. https://comprehensiveprimarycare.com/paying-doctors-upfront-point-of-service-collections/

377   Kelly Gooch. "Survey: Nearly 70% of patients more likely to pay bill if they receive cost estimate on day of service." Becker's Hospital CFO Report. December 5, 2017. Accessed October 23, 2019. https://www.beckershospitalreview.com/finance/survey-finds-nearly-70-of-patients-more-likely-to-pay-bill-if-they-receive-cost-estimate-on-day-of-service.html

378   "Healthcare Banking: Key Trends in Healthcare Patient Payments." J.P. Morgan. 2013. Accessed October 7, 2019. https://www.jpmorganchina.com.cn/jpmpdf/1320610345938.pdf

379   Jessica Kim Cohen. "Some hospitals are already offering price estimates." Modern Healthcare. July 30, 2019. Accessed October 7, 2019. https://www.modernhealthcare.com/payment/some-hospitals-are-already-offering-price-estimates

380   J.K. Cohen. "Some hospitals are already offering price estimates." July 30, 2019.

381   Jacqueline LaPointe. "36% of Providers Never Address Patient Financial Responsibility." Rev Cycle Intelligence. August 29, 2017. Accessed October 23, 2019. https://revcycleintelligence.com/news/36-of-providers-never-address-patient-financial-responsibility

382   "More Hospitals Are Promoting Loans and Credit Cards. Is That Good for Patients?" February 26, 2018. Accessed December 6, 2018. https://www.advisory.com/daily-briefing/2018/02/26/bank-loans

383   Lee Masterson. "Intermountain, Geisinger shift focus to patients in revenue cycle." February 7, 2018. Accessed October 23, 2019. https://www.healthcaredive.com/news/intermountain-geisinger-shift-focus-to-patients-in-revenue-cycle/515484/

384   Insurance Discovery Solutions. TransUnion. (n.d.) Accessed October 7, 2019. https://www.transunion.com/product/healthcare-insurance-discovery

385   Medicare Program; Reporting and Returning of Overpayments. 42 CFR 401, 42 CFR 405. February 12, 2016. https://www.federalregister.gov/documents/2016/02/12/2016-02789/medicare-program-reporting-and-returning-of-overpayments

386   Data from CHS Cost Reports (HCRIS Data). Accessed October 23, 2019. https://www.cms.gov/Research-Statistics-Data-and-Systems/Downloadable-Public-Use-Files/Cost-Reports/

387   Emily Gee. "The High Price of Hospital Care." Center for American Progress. June 26, 2019. Accessed October 8, 2019. https://www.americanprogress.org/issues/healthcare/reports/2019/06/26/471464/high-price-hospital-care/

388   "Maximizing Medicare Reimbursement: Understanding the Three Types of Medicare Bad Debt." TransUnion Healthcare blog post. March 21, 2019. Accessed October 8, 2019. https://www.transunion.com/blog/maximizing-medicare-reimbursement-understanding-the-three-types-of-medicare-bad-debt

389   "Maximizing Medicare Reimbursement: Understanding the Three Types of Medicare Bad Debt." TransUnion Healthcare blog post. March 21, 2019. Accessed October 8, 2019. https://www.transunion.com/blog/maximizing-medicare-reimbursement-understanding-the-three-types-of-medicare-bad-debt

390   "Medicare Bad Debt. Medicare Cost Reporting." TransUnion Healthcare. (n.d.) Accessed October 8, 2019. https://www.transunion.com/product/medicare-cost-reporting

391   "Medicare Disproportionate Share (DSH). Medicare Cost Reporting." TransUnion Healthcare. (n.d.) Accessed October 9, 2019. https://www.transunion.com/product/medicare-cost-reporting

392   "Uncompensated Hospital Care Cost Fact Sheet." American Hospital Association. January 2019. Accessed July October 9, 2019. https://www.aha.org/system/files/2019-01/uncompensated-care-fact-sheet-jan-2019.pdf

393   "Hospital Loses its Section 501(c)(3) Status Due to Noncompliance with Section 501(r)." The National Law Review. November 3, 2018. Accessed October 23, 2019. https://www.natlawreview.com/article/hospital-loses-its-section-501c3-status-due-to-noncompliance-section-501r

394   *Caddyshack.* Warner Bros. Entertainment. 1980.

395   Andrea Downing Peck. "Because of expended numbers of patients with high-deductible health plans, patients are now responsible for 30% of hospital revenues." Dark Daily. September 22, 2017. Accessed October 9, 2019. https://www.darkdaily.com/because-of-expanded-numbers-of-patients-with-high-deductible-health-plans-patients-are-now-responsible-for-30-of-hospital-revenues-920/

396   Matthew Bayley, Sarah Calkins, Ed Levine and Monisha Machado-Pereira. "Hospital revenue cycle operations: Opportunities created by the ACA" [PDF document]. May 2013. Accessed October 9, 2019. http://healthcare.mckinsey.com/sites/default/files/793544_Hospital_Revenue_Cycle_Operations.pdf

397   Christine Buttorff, Teague Ruder and Melissa Bauman. "Multiple Chronic Conditions in the United States." Rand Corporation. 2017. Accessed July 19, 2019. https://www.rand.org/content/dam/rand/pubs/tools/TL200/TL221/RAND_TL221.pdf

398   Americans' Views of Healthcare Costs, Coverage and Policy. Issue Brief. West Health Institute/NORC Survey on Healthcare Costs, Coverage and Policy. NORC at the University of Chicago. March 2018. Accessed October 26, 2019. http://www.norc.org/PDFs/WHI%20Healthcare%20Costs%20Coverage%20and%20Policy/WHI%20Healthcare%20Costs%20Coverage%20and%20Policy%20Issue%20Brief.pdf

399   Timothy M. Dall, Wenya Yang, Karin Gillespie, Michelle Mocarski, Erin Byrne, Inna Cintina, Kaleigh Beronja, April P. Semilla, William Iacobucci and Paul F. Hogan. "The Economic Burden of Elevated Blood Glucose Levels in 2017: Diagnosed and Undiagnosed Diabetes, Gestational Diabetes, and Prediabetes." Diabetes Care. April 2019. Accessed November 4, 2019. https://doi.org/10.2337/dc18-1226

400   Timothy M. Dall, Wenya Yang, Karin Gillespie, Michelle Mocarski, Erin Byrne, Inna Cintina, Kaleigh Beronja, April P. Semilla, William Iacobucci and Paul F. Hogan. "The Economic Burden of Elevated Blood Glucose Levels in 2017: Diagnosed and Undiagnosed Diabetes, Gestational Diabetes, and Prediabetes." Diabetes Care. April 2019. Accessed November 4, 2019. https://doi.org/10.2337/dc18-1226

401   "4 basic health insurance terms 96% of Americans don't understand." PolicyGenius. January 24, 2018. Accessed October 27, 2019. https://www.policygenius.com/health-insurance/health-insurance-literacy-survey/

402   "4 basic health insurance terms." PolicyGenius. January 24, 2018.

403   Thomas Bodenheimer and Christine Sinsky. "From Triple to Quadruple Aims: Care for the Patient Requires Care of the Provider." Annals of Family Medicine. November/December 2014, Vol. 12, No. 6, 573–576. Accessed October 26, 2019. http://www.annfammed.org/content/12/6/573.full

404   Anna D. Sinaiko, Ateev Mehrotra, and Neeraj Sood. "Cost-Sharing Obligations, High-Deductible Health Plan Growth, and Shopping for Health Care: Enrollees With Skin in the Game." *JAMA Intern Med.* 2016;176(3):395–397. Accessed April 24, 2019. doi:10.1001/jamainternmed.2015.7554

405   TransUnion Healthcare. "News Reports about a Weakening Economy Impacting How Some Patients Seek Medical Treatment." September 17, 2019. Accessed September 30, 2019. https://newsroom.transunion.com/news-reports-about-a-weakening-economy--impacting-how-some-patients-seek-medical-treatment/

406   Carol K. Kane. "Updated Data on Physician Practice Arrangements: Inching Toward Hospital Ownership." Policy Research Perspectives. American Medical Association. 2015. Accessed October 20, 2019. https://www.m3globalresearch.com/img/resources/AMA_PRP_Physician_Practice_Arrangements.pdf; and Carol K. Kane. "Updated Data on Physician Practice Arrangements: For the First Time, Fewer Physicians are Owners Than Employees." Policy Research Perspectives. American Medical Association. July 2019. Accessed October 20, 2019. https://www.ama-assn.org/system/files/2019-07/prp-fewer-owners-benchmark-survey-2018.pdf

407   Peter Ubel. "Doctors must discuss the cost of care with their patients." MedPageToday's KevinMD.com. July 10, 2014. Accessed October 26, 2019. https://www.kevinmd.com/blog/2014/07/doctors-must-discuss-cost-care-patients.html

408   Jacqueline LaPointe. "Medical Billing Complexity Highest for Medicaid Fee-for-Service." RevCycleIntelligence. April 4, 2018. Accessed October 18, 2019. https://revcycleintelligence.com/news/medical-billing-complexity-highest-for-medicaid-fee-for-service ; and Joshua D. Gottlieb, Adam Hale Shapiro and Abe Dunn. "The Complexity of Billing and Paying for Physician Care." Health Affairs. April 2018. Accessed October 18, 2019. https://doi.org/10.1377/hlthaff.2017.1325

409   Castell. Intermountain's New Comprehensive Health Platform Company. 2019. Accessed November 4, 2019. https://intermountainhealthcare.org/about/transforming-healthcare/innovation/castell/

410   Castell. Intermountain's New Comprehensive Health Platform Company. 2019

411   Health Maintenance Organization (HMO). Glossary. Healthcare.gov. (n.d.) Accessed October 26, 2019. https://www.healthcare.gov/glossary/health-maintenance-organization-hmo/#targetText=Health%20Maintenance%20Organization%20(HMO),to%20be%20eligible%20for%20coverage.

412   Exhibit 5.1, Distribution of health plan enrollment for covered workers, by plan type, 1988-2015 [PNG file]. The Henry J. Kaiser Family Foundation. 2015 Employer health benefits survey, 2015.Accessed October 26, 2019. http://kff.org/report-section/ehbs-2015-section-five-market-shares-of-health-plans/

413   Jonathan Wiik. *Healthcare Revolution: The Patient Is the New Payer.* 2017.

414   Kaiser Family Foundation. KFF Employer Health Benefits Survey, 2018. Figure 5.2 Distribution of Health Plan Enrollment for Covered Workers, by Plan Type and Firm Size, 2018. Accessed October 26, 2019. https://www.kff.org/report-section/2018-employer-health-benefits-survey-section-5-market-shares-of-health-plans/attachment/figure-5-2-2/

415   Drew Altman, Kaiser Family Foundation. "Narrow health care networks aren't actually that common." Axios. October 12, 2018. Accessed October 29, 2019. https://www.axios.com/narrow-health-care-networks-arent-actually-that-common-daeb99fb-45dc-43d2-895b-f99c72a2426a.html

416   Summary of Findings. Employer Health Benefits 2019. Kaiser Family Foundation. Accessed October 29, 2019. http://files.kff.org/attachment/Summary-of-Findings-Employer-Health-Benefits-2019

417   Summary of Findings. Employer Health Benefits 2019. Kaiser Family Foundation.

418   Summary of Findings. Employer Health Benefits 2019. Kaiser Family Foundation.

419   Drew Altman, Kaiser Family Foundation. "Narrow health care networks aren't actually that common." Axios. October 12, 2018. Accessed October 29, 2019.

https://www.axios.com/narrow-health-care-networks-arent-actually-that-common-daeb99fb-45dc-43d2-895b-f99c72a2426a.html ; and Liz Hamel, Jamie Firth and Mollyann Brodie. Kaiser Health Tracking Poll: February 2014. Kaiser Family Foundation. February 26, 2014. Accessed October 29, 2019. https://www.kff.org/health-reform/poll-finding/kaiser-health-tracking-poll-february-2014/

420   Angie Stewart. "3 ways payers are aggressively driving patients to ASCs." Becker's ASC Review. April 5, 2019. Accessed October 28, 2019. https://www.beckersasc.com/asc-coding-billing-and-collections/3-ways-payers-are-aggressively-driving-patients-to-ascs.html

421   Table 3.1: Trends in Inpatient Utilization in Community Hospitals, 1995 – 2016. Supplementary Data Tables, Utilization and Volume. Trendwatch Chartbook 2018. American Hospital Association. Accessed October 21, 2019. https://www.aha.org/system/files/2018-06/2018-AHA-Trendwatch-Chartbook-Appendices.pdf

422   Laura Dyrda. "12 things to know about site-neutral payments." Becker's Hospital CFO Report. February 9, 2017. Accessed October 10, 2019. https://www.beckershospitalreview.com/finance/12-things-to-know-about-site-neutral-payments.html

423   L. Dyrda. "12 things to know about site-neutral payments." February 9, 2017.

424   Site-Neutral Payment. American Hospital Association. (n.d.) Accessed October 10, 2019. https://www.aha.org/site-neutral/outpatient-pps

425   L. Dyrda. "12 things to know about site-neutral payments." February 9, 2017; and Jacqueline LaPointe. "Site-neutral payments for hospital clinic visits starting in 2019." RevCycleIntelligence. November 2, 2018. Accessed October 10, 2019. https://revcycleintelligence.com/news/site-neutral-payments-for-hospital-clinic-visits-starting-in-2019

426   Rich Daly. "Court tosses $380 million site-neutral payment cut." HFMA. September 24, 2019. https://www.hfma.org/topics/news/2019/09/court-tosses--380-million-site-neutral-payment-cut.html

427   R. Daly. "Court tosses $380 million site-neutral payment cut." 2019.

428   Fact Sheet. CY 2020 CY 2020 Medicare Hospital Outpatient Prospective Payment System and Ambulatory Surgical Center Payment System Final Rule (CMS-1717-FC). November 1, 2019. Accessed November 6, 2019. https://www.cms.gov/newsroom/fact-sheets/cy-2020-medicare-hospital-outpatient-prospective-payment-system-and-ambulatory-surgical-center-0

429   Kenneth Simon. The 2018 in-patient only list. Bulletin of the American College of Surgeons. May 1, 2018. Accessed October 29, 2019. http://bulletin.facs.org/2018/05/the-2018-inpatient-only-list/

430   Debbie Sconce. "Total knee arthroplasty – no longer inpatient only." Becker's Hospital Review. April 17, 2018. Accessed November 6, 2019. https://www.beckershospitalreview.com/hospital-physician-relationships/total-knee-arthroplasty-no-longer-inpatient-only.html

431   David Blumenthal, Lovisa Gustafsson and Shawn Bishop. "To Control Health Care Costs, U.S. Employers Should Form Purchasing Alliances." Harvard Business Review. November 2, 2018. Accessed November 4, 2019. https://hbr.org/2018/11/to-control-health-care-costs-u-s-employers-should-form-purchasing-alliances

432   Bruce Japsen. "Walmart's First Healthcare Services 'Super Center' Opens." Forbes. September 13, 2019. Accessed November 4, 2019. https://www.forbes.com/sites/brucejapsen/2019/09/13/walmarts-first-healthcare-services-super-center-opens/#2f5fcf7e79d2

433   B. Japsen. "Walmart's First Healthcare Services 'Super Center' Opens." September 13, 2019.

434   Consumer-centric health community. The future of health: How innovation will blur traditional health care boundaries. Deloitte. (n.d.) Accessed November 4, 2019.

https://www2.deloitte.com/us/en/pages/life-sciences-and-health-care/articles/future-of-health.html?id=us:2ps:3gl:fohc2:awa:lshc:101819:ad4:aud-551708264859:kwd-326136523131:%2Bhealth%20%2Bcare%20%2Binnovation&gclid=Cj0KCQjwr-tBRCMARIsAN413WTS3XcPp2iA4e0DqW0fEYCaOO-Jlghs8H4PhYQwjPZAUsTEg05_QBcaAr7fEALw_wcB

435   Executive Order 13765 of January 20, 2017. Minimizing the Economic Burden of the Patient Protection and Affordable Care Act Pending Repeal. Federal Register, Vol 82, No. 14. January 24, 2017. Accessed October 29, 2019. https://www.govinfo.gov/content/pkg/FR-2017-01-24/pdf/2017-01799.pdf

436   Chris Donovan and Adam Kelsey. "Fact-checking Trump's 'repeal and replace' Obamacare timeline." March 24, 2017. ABC News. Accessed October 29, 2019. https://abcnews.go.com/Politics/fact-checking-trumps-repeal-replace-obamacare-timeline/story?id=46360908

437   "The Affordable Care Act in 2019: Still alive." PwC (U.S.) 2019. Accessed October 29, 2019. https://www.pwc.com/us/en/industries/health-industries/top-health-industry-issues/aca-in-2019.html

438   Selena Simmons-Duffin. "Trump is Trying Hard to Thwart Obamacare. How's That Going?" All Things Considered. NPR. October 14, 2019. Accessed October 29, 2019. https://www.npr.org/sections/health-shots/2019/10/14/768731628/trump-is-trying-hard-to-thwart-obamacare-hows-that-going

439   Texas, et. al., v. U.S. (ACA Constitutionality Challenge). Groom Benefits Brief. September 26, 2019. Accessed October 29, 2019. https://www.groom.com/resources/texas-et-al-v-u-s-aca-constitutionality-challenge/

440   Selena Simmons-Duffin. "Heads Up: A Ruling On The Latest Challenge to the Affordable Care Act is Coming." NPR. October 12, 2019. Accessed October 29, 2019. https://www.npr.org/sections/health-shots/2019/10/12/769038397/heads-up-a-ruling-on-the-latest-challenge-to-the-affordable-care-act-is-coming

441   "Potential Impact of Texas v. U.S. Decision on Key Provisions of the Affordable Care Act." Kaiser Family Foundation. March 26, 2019. Accessed October 29, 2019. https://www.kff.org/health-reform/fact-sheet/potential-impact-of-texas-v-u-s-decision-on-key-provisions-of-the-affordable-care-act/

442   "Medicaid enrollment changes following the ACA. Medicaid and CHIP Payment Access Commission (MACPAC)." April 2019. Accessed October 29, 2019. https://www.macpac.gov/subtopic/medicaid-enrollment-changes-following-the-aca/

443   Kathleen Gifford, Eileen Ellis, Aimee Lashbrook, Mike Nardone, Elizabeth Hinton, Robin Rudowitz, Maria Diaz and Marina Tian. "A View from the States: Key Medicaid Policy Changes: Results from a 50-State Medicaid Budget Survey for State Fiscal Years 2019 and 2020." Kaiser Family Foundation. October 18, 2019. Accessed October 29, 2019. https://www.kff.org/medicaid/report/a-view-from-the-states-key-medicaid-policy-changes-results-from-a-50-state-medicaid-budget-survey-for-state-fiscal-years-2019-and-2020/

444   Larisa Antonisse, Rachel Garfield, Robin Rudowitz and Madeline Guth. The Effects of Medicaid Expansion under the ACA: Updated Findings from a Literature Review. Issue Brief. Kaiser Family Foundation. August 15, 2019. Accessed October 29, 2019. https://www.kff.org/medicaid/issue-brief/the-effects-of-medicaid-expansion-under-the-aca-updated-findings-from-a-literature-review-august-2019/

445   Susan L. Hayes, Akeiisa Coleman, Sara R. Collins, and Rachel Nuzum. "The Fiscal Case for Medicaid Expansion. To The Point: Quick Takes on Health Care Policy and Practice." The Commonwealth Fund. February 15, 2019. Accessed October 29, 2019. https://www.commonwealthfund.org/blog/2019/fiscal-case-medicaid-expansion

446   Robert Pear. "Trump Administration Says States May Impose Work Requirements for Medicaid." The New York Times. January 11, 2018. Accessed October 30, 2019. https://www.nytimes.com/2018/01/11/us/politics/medicaid-work-requirements.html

447   Landscape of Approved vs. Pending Section 115 Medicaid Demonstration Waivers, October 9, 2019. Kaiser Family Foundation. Accessed October 30, 2019.

https://www.kff.org/medicaid/issue-brief/medicaid-waiver-tracker-approved-and-pending-section-1115-waivers-by-state/#Table2

448   Work Requirement Waivers: Approved and Pending as of October 9, 2019. Medicaid Waiver Tracker: Approved and Pending Section 115 Waivers by State. Kaiser Family Foundation. October 9, 2019. Accessed October 30, 2019. https://www.kff.org/medicaid/issue-brief/medicaid-waiver-tracker-approved-and-pending-section-1115-waivers-by-state/#Table2; and *Charles Gresham, et. al., v. Alex M. Azar II, et. al.,* Civil Action No. 18-1900 (JEB), US District Court for the District of Columbia. March 27, 2019. Accessed October 30, 2019. https://ecf.dcd.uscourts.gov/cgi-bin/show_public_doc?2018cv1900-58

449   Jacqueline Froelich. "In Arkansas, Thousands of People have lost Medicaid Coverage over New Work Rule." All Things Considered. NPR. February 18, 2019. Accessed October 30, 2019. https://www.npr.org/sections/health-shots/2019/02/18/694504586/in-arkansas-thousands-of-people-have-lost-medicaid-coverage-over-new-work-rule

450   Amy Goldstein. "Indiana backs away from Medicaid work requirements." The Washington Post. October 31, 2019. Accessed November 7, 2019. https://www.washingtonpost.com/health/indiana-backs-away-from-medicaid-work-requirements/2019/10/31/b2504256-fc04-11e9-8190-6be4deb56e01_story.html

451   Vanessa C. Forsberg. "Overview of Health Insurance Exchanges. Congressional Research Service. June 20, 2018. Accessed October 30, 2019. https://fas.org/sgp/crs/misc/R44065.pdf

452   Insurance Marketplace Types, 2019. Kaiser Family Foundation. Accessed October 30, 2019. https://www.kff.org/health-reform/state-indicator/state-health-insurance-marketplace-types/?currentTimeframe=0&sortModel=%7B%22colId%22:%22Location%22,%22sort%22:%22asc%22%7D

453   Potential Impact of Texas v. U.S. Decision on Key Provisions of the Affordable Care Act. Kaiser Family Foundation. March 26, 2019. Accessed October 30, 2019. https://www.kff.org/health-reform/fact-sheet/potential-impact-of-texas-v-u-s-decision-on-key-provisions-of-the-affordable-care-act/

454   S. Simmons-Duffin. "Trump is Trying Hard to Thwart Obamacare." 2019.

455   S. Simmons-Duffin. "Trump is Trying Hard to Thwart Obamacare." 2019.

456   Rachel Fehr, Cynthia Cox and Larry Levitt. "Insurer Participation on ACA Marketplaces, 2014-2019." Kaiser Family Foundation. November 14, 2018. Accessed October 31, 2019. https://www.kff.org/health-reform/issue-brief/insurer-participation-on-aca-marketplaces-2014-2019/

457   R. Fehr et al. "Insurer Participation on ACA Marketplaces, 2014-2019." November 14, 2018.

458   R. Fehr et al. "Insurer Participation on ACA Marketplaces, 2014-2019." November 14, 2018.

459   R. Fehr et al. "Insurer Participation on ACA Marketplaces, 2014-2019." November 14, 2018.

460   Kelsey Waddill. "More Payers Will Join ACA Health Insurance Marketplace In 2020." Health Payer Intelligence. September 19, 2019. Accessed November 6, 2019. https://healthpayerintelligence.com/news/more-payers-will-join-aca-health-insurance-marketplace-in-2020

461   Health Care Payment Learning & Action Network. "Measuring Progress: Adoption of Alternative Payment Models in Commercial, Medicaid, Medicare Advantage, and Medicare Fee-for-Service Programs." October 31, 2018. Accessed October 29, 2019. https://hcp-lan.org/2018-apm-measurement/

462   Centers for Medicare & Medicaid Services. "CMS' Value-Based Programs." Last modified May 17, 2019. Accessed October 31, 2019. https://www.cms.gov/medicare/quality-initiatives-patient-assessment-instruments/value-based-programs/value-based-programs.html

463   "HHS to Deliver Value-Based Transformation in Primary Care." Innovation models. HHS News. April 22, 2019. Accessed October 31, 2019. https://www.cms.gov/newsroom/press-releases/hhs-news-hhs-deliver-value-based-transformation-primary-care

464   Fiscal Year (FY) 2019 Medicare Hospital Inpatient Prospective Payment System (IPPS) and Long-Term Acute Care Hospital (LTCH) Prospective Payment System Final Rule (CMS-1694-F), 83 Fed. Reg. 41144 (Aug. 17, 2018). *Federal Register: The Daily Journal of the United States*. Accessed October 31, 2019. https://www.federalregister.gov/d/2018-16766 see also: 42 C.F.R. Parts 412, 413, 424 and 495.

465   Executive Order on Improving Price and Quality Transparency in American Healthcare to Put Patients First. Section 3, (c). President Donald J. Trump. June 24, 2019. Accessed October 31, 2019. https://www.whitehouse.gov/presidential-actions/executive-order-improving-price-quality-transparency-american-healthcare-put-patients-first/

466   AHIP: https://www.ahip.org/wp-content/uploads/AHIP-OPPS-Plan-Comment-Letter-9-27-2019-1.pdf; AAMC: https://www.aamc.org/system/files/2019-09/ocomm-org-FINALAAMCCY2020OPPSProposedRuleCommentLetter%209_26%20%282%29.pdf; AHA: https://www.aha.org/system/files/media/file/2019/09/aha-comments-cms-outpatient-pps-asc-proposed-rule-cy-2020-9-27-19.pdf; FAH: https://www.fah.org/fah-ee2-uploads/website/documents/FAH_CY2020_OPPS_Comment_Letter_FINAL.pdf; HFMA: https://www.hfma.org/content/dam/hfma/document/comment_letter/PDF/62016.pdf. AHP, AAMC, AHA and FAH letters. September 27, 2019. Accessed October 31, 2019.

467   "Industry Skeptical About New Price Transparency Rules." Managed Healthcare Executive. October 7, 2019. Accessed October 31, 2019. https://www.managedhealthcareexecutive.com/news/industry-skeptical-about-new-price-transparency-rules ; and Advis Healthcare Survey: Price Transparency. 2019. Accessed October 31, 2019. https://advis.com/advis-in-the-news/advis-healthcare-survey2-fall2019/

468   Susan Morse. "CMS releases final and proposed rules on price transparency bound to get provider and payer pushback." Healthcare Finance News. November 15, 2019. Accessed November 18, 2019. https://www.healthcarefinancenews.com/node/139433

469   S. Morse. "CMS releases final and proposed rules." November 15, 2019.

470   S. Morse. "CMS releases final and proposed rules." November 15, 2019; and Transparency in Coverage Proposed Rule (CMS- 9915 –P). Fact Sheet. CMS.gov. November 15, 2019. Accessed November 18, 2019. https://www.cms.gov/newsroom/fact-sheets/transparency-coverage-proposed-rule-cms-9915-p

471   Susan Morse. "American Hospital Association, provider groups to sue over final rule." Healthcare Finance News. November 18, 2019. Accessed November 18, 2019. https://www.healthcarefinancenews.com/node/139439

472   *American Hospital Association et al* v. *Azar*. Case No. 1:19-CV-03619. December 4, 2019. Accessed December 22, 2019. https://www.aha.org/system/files/media/file/2019/12/hospital-groups-lawsuit-over-illegal-rule-mandating-public-disclosure-individually-negotiated-rates-12-4-19.pdf%20.pdf

473   Karen Pollitz. "Surprise Medical Bills." Kaiser Family Foundation. March 17, 2016. Accessed November 1, 2019. https://www.kff.org/private-insurance/issue-brief/surprise-medical-bills/

474   Issue brief: Balance Billing. American Medical Association. 2016. Accessed November 1, 2019. https://www.ama-assn.org/media/14691/download

475   Karen Pollitz, Matthew Rae, Gary Claxton, Cynthia Cox and Larry Levitt. "An examination of surprise medical bills and proposals to protect consumers from them." Peterson-Kaiser Health System Tracker. October 16, 2019. Accessed November 1, 2019. https://www.healthsystemtracker.org/brief/an-examination-of-surprise-medical-bills-and-proposals-to-protect-consumers-from-them/

476   K. Pollitz et al. "An examination of surprise medical bills." October 16, 2019. Accessed November 1, 2019.

477   Remarks by President Trump on Ending Surprise Medical Billing. White House Briefing Statement. May 9, 2019. Accessed November 1, 2019.

https://www.whitehouse.gov/briefings-statements/remarks-president-trump-ending-surprise-medical-billing/

478   Karen Pollitz, Matthew Rae, Gary Claxton, Cynthia Cox and Larry Levitt. "An examination of surprise medical bills and proposals to protect consumers from them." Peterson-Kaiser Health System Tracker. October 16, 2019. Accessed November 1, 2019. https://www.healthsystemtracker.org/brief/an-examination-of-surprise-medical-bills-and-proposals-to-protect-consumers-from-them/

479   Rachel Roubein. "Health groups backed dark money campaign to sink 'surprise' billing fix." Politico. September 13, 2019. Accessed November 1, 2019. https://www.politico.com/story/2019/09/13/health-groups-dark-money-hospital-bills-legislation-1495697

480   R. Roubein. "Health groups backed dark money campaign." September 13, 2019.

481   R. Roubein. "Health groups backed dark money campaign." September 13, 2019.

482   Avik Roy. "How Arbitration for Surprise Medical Bills Leads to Runaway Costs and Higher Premiums." Forbes. September 26, 2019. Accessed November 1, 2019. https://www.forbes.com/sites/theapothecary/2019/09/26/how-arbitration-for-surprise-medical-bills-leads-to-runaway-costs-higher-premiums/#295337204442

483   Samantha McGrail. "Surprise Billing Law in NY Leading to Higher Healthcare Costs." RevCycleIntelligence. October 31, 2019. Accessed November 6, 2019. https://revcycleintelligence.com/news/surprise-billing-law-in-ny-leading-to-higher-healthcare-costs

484   "Medicare Advantage (Part C) private health plans." Medicareresources.org. (n.d.) Accessed November 1, 2019. https://www.medicareresources.org/medicare-benefits/medicare-advantage/

485   "Understanding Medicare Advantage Plans." Centers for Medicare & Medicaid Services. (n.d.) Accessed November 2, 2019. https://www.medicare.gov/Pubs/pdf/12026-Understanding-Medicare-Advantage-Plans.pdf

486   "Understanding Medicare Advantage Plans." Centers for Medicare & Medicaid Services. (n.d.)

487   "Understanding Medicare Advantage Plans." Centers for Medicare & Medicaid Services. (n.d.)

488   Phil Galewitz. "Medicare Advantage growing as new insurers compete to sell to seniors." USA Today. October 15, 2018. Accessed November 2, 2019. https://www.usatoday.com/story/news/2018/10/15/medicare-advantage-enrollment-growing-affordable-care-act-obamacare-insurance-plans/1618652002/

489   P. Galewitz. "Medicare Advantage growing." October 15, 2018.

490   Fact Sheet: 2020 Part C and D Star Ratings. CMS.gov. (n.d.) Accessed November 2, 2019. https://www.cms.gov/Medicare/Prescription-Drug-Coverage/PrescriptionDrugCovGenIn/Downloads/2020-Star-Ratings-Fact-Sheet-.pdf

491   "Medicare Advantage Plans: The good, the bad and the ugly." RWC, LLC. April 27, 2018. Accessed November 2, 2019. https://reedwilsoncase.com/medicare-advantage-plans-the-good-the-bad-and-the-ugly/

492   Michael Adelberg and Kristin Rodriguez. "Medicare Advantage is nudging aside 'old Medicare' with a free ride, a warm meal, and a handyman." STAT. April 3, 2019. Accessed November 2, 2019. https://www.statnews.com/2019/04/03/medicare-advantage-nudging-aside-old-medicare/

493   Alex M. Azar II. "The Root of the Problem: America's Social Determinants of Health." From remarks made at the Hatch Foundation for Civility and Solutions. November 14, 2018, Washington D.C. Accessed November 2, 2019. https://www.hhs.gov/about/leadership/secretary/speeches/2018-speeches/the-root-of-the-problem-americas-social-determinants-of-health.html

494   Michael Adelberg and Kristin Rodriguez. "Medicare Advantage is nudging aside 'old Medicare' with a free ride, a warm meal, and a handyman." STAT. April 3, 2019. Accessed November 2, 2019. https://www.statnews.com/2019/04/03/medicare-advantage-nudging-aside-old-medicare/

495   Medicare Advantage. Kaiser Family Foundation. June 6, 2019. Accessed November 3, 2019. https://www.kff.org/medicare/fact-sheet/medicare-advantage/

496   The Office of the National Coordinator for Health Information Technology. "Percent of Hospitals, By Type, that Possess Certified Health IT." Health IT Dashboard. (2015). Accessed November 3, 2019 from https://dashboard.healthit.gov/quickstats/pages/certified-electronic-health-record-technology-in-hospitals.php

497   "Medicare and Medicaid Promoting Interoperability Program." CMS.gov. August 14, 2019. Accessed November 3, 2019. https://www.cms.gov/Regulations-and-Guidance/Legislation/EHRIncentivePrograms/Basics.html

498   "Certified EHR Technology." CMS.gov. May 8, 2019. Accessed November 3, 2019. https://www.cms.gov/Regulations-and-Guidance/Legislation/EHRIncentivePrograms/Certification.html

499   "Certified EHR Technology." May 8, 2019. https://www.cms.gov/Regulations-and-Guidance/Legislation/EHRIncentivePrograms/Certification.html

500   Mandy Roth. "In EMR Market Share Wars, Epic and Cerner Triumph Yet Again." HealthLeaders. April 30, 2019. Accessed November 3, 2019. https://www.healthleadersmedia.com/innovation/emr-market-share-wars-epic-and-cerner-triumph-yet-again

501   "HHS Proposes New Rules to Improve the Interoperability of Electronic Health Information." HHS.gov. February 11, 2019. Accessed November 3, 2019. https://www.hhs.gov/about/news/2019/02/11/hhs-proposes-new-rules-improve-interoperability-electronic-health-information.html

502   Rebecca Pifer. "Industry cheers spirit but not fine print in HHS interoperability rules." June 5, 2019. HealthcareDive. Accessed November 3, 2019. https://www.healthcaredive.com/news/industry-cheers-spirit-but-not-fine-print-in-hhs-interoperability-rules/556099/

503   Interoperability and Patient Access for MA Organization and Medicaid Managed Care Plans, State Medicaid Agencies, CHIP Agencies and CHIP Managed Care Entities, Issuers of QHPs in the Federally-facilitated Exchanges and Health Care Providers (CMS-9115-P). Accessed November 3, 2019. https://www.regulations.gov/docket?D=CMS-2019-0039 ; and 21st Century Cures Act: Interoperability, Information Blocking, and the ONC Health IT Certification Program. Accessed November 3, 2019. https://www.regulations.gov/docket?D=HHS-ONC-2019-0002

504   AHA Comment Letter on RIN 0955-AA01. AHA. June 3, 2019. Accessed November 3, 2019. https://www.documentcloud.org/documents/6128300-AHACommentLetteronONCProposedRule060319.html

505   "US NFP & public hospitals' annual medians show expense growth topping revenues for second year." Moody's. August 28, 2018. Accessed November 3, 2019. https://www.moodys.com/research/Moodys-US-NFP-public-hospitals-annual-medians-showexpense-growth--PBM_1139331

506   Jack O'Brien. "Nonprofit hospital operating margins improve for first time since 2016." HealthLeaders. September 3, 2019. Accessed November 3, 2019. https://www.healthleadersmedia.com/finance/nonprofit-hospital-operating-margins-improve-first-time-2016

507   J. O'Brien. "Nonprofit hospital operating margins." September 3, 2019.

508   Jonathan Lapook. "How well did 'Star Trek' do in predicting the future of medicine?" CBS News. September 21, 2017. Accessed November 1, 2019. https://www.cbsnews.com/news/star-trek-predicted-future-of-medicine/

509   Jeff Heenan-Jalil. "'Star Trek' tricorder becomes reality (and other healthcare innovations)." Medical Economics. November 27, 2018. Accessed November 1, 2019. https://www.medicaleconomics.com/med-ec-blog/star-trek-tricorder-becomes-reality-and-other-healthcare-innovations

510   "Empowering personal healthcare." Qualcomm Tricorder XPRIZE. (n.d.) Accessed November 1, 2019. https://tricorder.xprize.org/prizes/tricorder

511 "Family-led team takes top prize in qualcomm tricorder xprize competition for consumer medical device inspired by Star Trek®." April 13, 2017. Accessed November 1, 2019. https://tricorder.xprize.org/prizes/tricorder/articles/family-led-team-takes-top-prize-in-qualcomm-tricor

512 DXTERTM: A New Kind of Consumer Medical Device. Basil Leaf Technologies. (n.d.) Accessed November 1, 2019. http://www.basilleaftech.com/dxter

513 DXTERTM: A New Kind of Consumer Medical Device. Basil Leaf Technologies.

514 Dr. Basil Harris. Basil Leaf Technologies website. (n.d.) Accessed November 1, 2019. http://www.basilleaftech.com/

515 "Number of U.S. Retail Health Clinics Will Surpass 2,800 by 2017." Accenture Forecasts. Accenture. November 12, 2015. Accessed November 1, 2019. https://newsroom.accenture.com/news/number-of-us-retail-health-clinics-will-surpass-2800-by-2017-accenture-forecasts.htm

516 Table 76. Visits to physician offices, hospital outpatient departments, and hospital emergency departments, by age, sex, and race: United States, selected years 2000–2015. Health, United States, 2017. National Center for Health Statistics. Centers for Disease Control and Prevention. 2017. Accessed November 1, 2019. https://www.cdc.gov/nchs/data/hus/2017/076.pdf

517 "Facts & FAQs." Walgreens. (n.d.). Accessed November 1, 2019. https://news.walgreens.com/fact-sheets/frequently-asked-questions.htm

518 "CVS Health at a Glance." CVS Health. (n.d.). Accessed November 15, 2019. https://cvshealth.com/about/facts-and-company-information

519 "Understanding Retail Clinic Patients." Civis Analytics. 2018. Accessed November 2, 2019. https://www.civisanalytics.com/wp-content/uploads/2018/11/RetailClinics_Whitepaper2018_v9.pdf

520 "Understanding Retail Clinic Patients." Civis Analytics. 2018.

521 "Retail clinics market will surpass $8 billion by 2028." Future Market Insights. March 27, 2019. Accessed November 2, 2019. https://www.globenewswire.com/news-release/2019/03/27/1774088/0/en/Retail-Clinics-Market-will-Surpass-US-8-billion-by-2028-Future-Market-Insights.html

522 "Understanding Retail Clinic Patients." Civis Analytics. 2018. Accessed November 2, 2019. https://www.civisanalytics.com/wp-content/uploads/2018/11/RetailClinics_Whitepaper2018_v9.pdf

523 "Understanding Retail Clinic Patients." Civis Analytics. 2018.

524 Alyssa Rege. "Patient wait times in America: 9 things to know." Becker's Hospital Review. June 9, 2017. Accessed November 2, 2019. https://www.beckershospitalreview.com/hospital-physician-relationships/patient-wait-times-in-america-9-things-to-know.html

525 Ken Terry. "How to compete with retail clinics." Medical Economics, Vol. 96, Issue 16. August 12, 2019. Accessed November 15, 2019. https://www.medicaleconomics.com/news/how-compete-retail-clinics

526 K. Terry. "How to compete with retail clinics." August 12, 2019.

527 2019 Fair Health Healthcare Indicators® and the FH Medical Price Index®. Fair Health. 2019. Accessed November 15, 2019. https://s3.amazonaws.com/media2.fairhealth.org/whitepaper/asset/FH%20Healthcare%20Indicators%20and%20FH%20Medical%20Price%20Index%202019%20-%20A%20FAIR%20Health%20White%20Paper.pdf

528 Ken Terry. "How to compete with retail clinics." Medical Economics, Vol. 96, Issue 16. August 12, 2019. Accessed November 15, 2019. https://www.medicaleconomics.com/news/how-compete-retail-clinics ; and 2019 Fair Health Healthcare Indicators® and the FH Medical Price Index®. Fair Health. 2019. Accessed November 15, 2019. https://s3.amazonaws.com/media2.fairhealth.org/whitepaper/asset/FH%20Healthcare%20Indicators%20and%20FH%20Medical%20Price%20Index%202019%20-%20A%20FAIR%20Health%20White%20Paper.pdf

529   "Retail clinics market will surpass $8 billion by 2028." Future Market Insights. March 27, 2019. Accessed November 2, 2019. https://www.globenewswire.com/news-release/2019/03/27/1774088/0/en/Retail-Clinics-Market-will-Surpass-US-8-billion-by-2028-Future-Market-Insights.html

530   Price list. MinuteClinic. CVS. April 1, 2019. Accessed November 2, 2019. https://www.cvs.com/minuteclinic/services/price-lists; and Price menu. Walgreens. (n.d.) Accessed November 1, 2019. https://www.walgreens.com/topic/healthcare-clinic/price-menu.jsp

531   Price list. MinuteClinic. CVS. April 1, 2019.

532   Price list. MinuteClinic. CVS. April 1, 2019.

533   "Understanding Retail Clinic Patients." Civis Analytics. 2018. Accessed November 2, 2019. https://www.civisanalytics.com/wp-content/uploads/2018/11/RetailClinics_Whitepaper2018_v9.pdf

534   "Understanding Retail Clinic Patients." Civis Analytics. 2018.

535   "The Evolving Role of Retail Clinics." RAND Corporation, RB-9491-2. 2016. Accessed November 4, 2019. https://www.rand.org/pubs/research_briefs/RB9491-2.html

536   Thomas S. Nesbitt. "The Evolution of Telehealth: Where Have We Been and Where Are We Going? The Role of Telehealth in an Evolving Health Care Environment: Workshop Summary." National Academies Press (US). November 20, 2012. Accessed November 3, 2019. https://www.ncbi.nlm.nih.gov/books/NBK207141/

537   T.S. Nesbitt. "The Evolution of Telehealth." November 20, 2012.

538   T.S. Nesbitt. "The Evolution of Telehealth." November 20, 2012. Accessed November 3, 2019; and History of Telepsychiatry. American Psychiatric Association. (n.d.) https://www.psychiatry.org/psychiatrists/practice/telepsychiatry/toolkit/history-of-telepsychiatry

539   Telehealth Index: 2019 Consumer Survey. American Well. 2019. Accessed November 4, 2019. https://static.americanwell.com/app/uploads/2019/07/American-Well-Telehealth-Index-2019-Consumer-Survey-eBook2.pdf

540   Telehealth Index: 2019 Consumer Survey. American Well. 2019.

541   Telehealth Index: 2019 Consumer Survey. American Well. 2019.

542   "Providers Push for Telehealth While Patient Uptake Lags." Avizia. December 18, 2017. Accessed November 4, 2019. https://www.businesswire.com/news/home/20171218005231/en/Providers-Push-Telehealth-Patient-Uptake-Lags

543   "Telehealth Services." Medicare Learning Network Booklet. CMS. January 2019. Accessed November 4, 2019. https://www.cms.gov/Outreach-and-Education/Medicare-Learning-Network-MLN/MLNProducts/downloads/TelehealthSrvcsfctsht.pdf?utm_campaign=2a178f351b-EMAIL_CAMPAIGN_2019_04_19_08_59&utm_term=0_ae00b0e89a-2a178f351b-353229765&utm_content=90024810&utm_medium=social&utm_source=facebook&hss_channel=fbp-372451882894317

544   John D. Fanburg and Jonathan J. Walzman. "Telehealth and the law: the challenge of reimbursement." September 12, 2018. Medical Economics, V. 95, Issue 20. Accessed November 4, 2019. https://www.medicaleconomics.com/article/telehealth-and-law-challenge-reimbursement

545   "Telehealth Services." Medicare Learning Network Booklet. CMS. January 2019. Accessed November 4, 2019. https://www.cms.gov/Outreach-and-Education/Medicare-Learning-Network-MLN/MLNProducts/downloads/TelehealthSrvcsfctsht.pdf?utm_campaign=2a178f351b-EMAIL_CAMPAIGN_2019_04_19_08_59&utm_term=0_ae00b0e89a-2a178f351b-353229765&utm_content=90024810&utm_medium=social&utm_source=facebook&hss_channel=fbp-372451882894317

546   "Telehealth Services." Medicare Learning Network Booklet. CMS. January 2019

547   "2019 State of the States: Coverage and Reimbursement." American Telemedicine Association. July 18, 2019. Accessed November 4, 2109.

https://www.americantelemed.org/initiatives/2019-state-of-the-states-report-coverage-and-reimbursement/

548 "State Telehealth Laws & Reimbursement Policies." Center for Connected Health Policy: The National Telehealth Policy Resource Center. Fall 2019. Accessed November 4, 2019. https://www.cchpca.org/sites/default/files/2019-10/50%20State%20Telehealth%20Laws%20and%20Reibmursement%20Policies%20Report%20Fall%202019%20FINAL.pdf

549 "State Telehealth Laws & Reimbursement Policies Report." 2019.

550 Rob Waugh. "There are now more mobile phones on the planet than there are people." Yahoo News UK. April 30, 2019. Accessed November 15, 2019. https://news.yahoo.com/now-mobile-phones-planet-people-191456148.html

551 Mobile Fact Sheet. Internet & Technology. Pew Research Center. June 12, 2019. Accessed November 4, 2019. https://www.pewresearch.org/internet/fact-sheet/mobile/

552 Monica Anderson. "Mobile Technology and Home Broadband 2019." Pew Research Center, Internet & Technology. June 13, 2019. Accessed November 4, 2019. https://www.pewresearch.org/internet/2019/06/13/mobile-technology-and-home-broadband-2019/

553 Samantha McDonald. "The Average American Spends More Than Three Hours a Day on Their Phone—Here's What That Means for Retailers." Footwear News. June 5, 2019. Accessed November 5, 2019. https://footwearnews.com/2019/business/retail/americans-smartphone-usage-retail-1202788408/

554 S. McDonald. "The Average American Spends More Than Three Hours a Day on Their Phone.". June 5, 2019.

555 S, McDonald. "The Average American Spends More Than Three Hours a Day on Their Phone." June 5, 2019.

556 Telehealth Index: 2019 Consumer Survey. American Well. 2019. Accessed November 5, 2019. https://static.americanwell.com/app/uploads/2019/07/American-Well-Telehealth-Index-2019-Consumer-Survey-eBook2.pdf

557 Telehealth IndexAmerican Well. 2019.

558 Sheena Butler-Young. "The No. 1 Reason People Use Mobile Shopping Apps is Actually Very Old-Fashioned." Footwear News. May 29, 2019. Accessed November 5, 2019. https://footwearnews.com/2019/business/retail/mobile-shopping-app-ecommerce-business-tips-1202786356/

559 S. Butler-Young. "The No. 1 Reason People Use Mobile Shopping Apps." 2019.

560 S. Butler-Young. "The No. 1 Reason People Use Mobile Shopping Apps." 2019.

561 Jacqueline LaPointe. "Healthcare Orgs Still Rely on Paper-Based Medical Billing." RevCycle Intelligence. May 10, 2018. Accessed November 5, 2019. https://revcycleintelligence.com/news/healthcare-orgs-still-rely-on-paper-based-medical-billing

562 J. LaPointe. "Healthcare Orgs Still Rely on Paper-Based Medical Billing." May 10, 2018.

563 Wayne Wood. "Think it's flu? Now you can ask Alexa." My Southern Health. Vanderbilt University Medical Center. February 21, 2018. Accessed November 6, 2019. https://www.mysouthernhealth.com/alexa-flu-tool/

564 W. Wood. "Think it's flu? Now you can ask Alexa." February 21, 2018.

565 Mayo Clinic First Aid. Mayo Clinic. (n.d.). Accessed November 6, 2019. https://www.mayoclinic.org/voice/apps

566 Mayo Clinic First Aid. Mayo Clinic. (n.d.).

567 Mayo Clinic First Aid. Mayo Clinic. (n.d.).

568 Bret Kinsella. "U.S. Smart Speaker Ownership Rises 40% in 2018 to 66.4 Million and Amazon Echo Maintains Market Share Lead Says New Report from Voicebot." Voicebot.ai. March 7, 2019. Accessed November 6, 2019/ https://voicebot.ai/2019/03/07/u-s-smart-speaker-ownership-rises-40-in-2018-to-66-4-million-and-amazon-echo-maintains-market-share-lead-says-new-report-from-voicebot/

569 B. Kinsella. "U.S. Smart Speaker Ownership." March 7, 2019.

570 B. Kinsella. "U.S. Smart Speaker Ownership." March 7, 2019.

571   Bret Kinsella. "Smart Speaker Installed Base to Surpass 200 Million in 2019, Grow to 500 Million in 2023 – Canalys." Voicebot.ai. April 15, 2019. Accessed November 6, 2019. https://voicebot.ai/2019/04/15/smart-speaker-installed-base-to-surpass-200-million-in-2019-grow-to-500-million-in-2023-canalys/

572   Bryan Montany. "More than 900,000 smart speakers to be used in healthcare facilities by 2021." IHS Markit. April 26, 2018. Accessed November 6, 2019. https://technology.ihs.com/602327/more-than-900000-smart-speakers-to-be-used-in-healthcare-facilities-by-2021

573   Ava Mutchler. "A Timeline of Voice Assistant and Smart Speaker Technology From 1961 to Today." Voicebot.ai. March 28, 2018. Accessed November 15, 2019. https://voicebot.ai/2018/03/28/timeline-voice-assistant-smart-speaker-technology-1961-today/

574   Beth Snyder Bulik. "Otsuka's dose-tracking digital pill charts its first course to market with Magellan." FiercePharma. September 5, 2018. Accessed November 6, 2019. https://www.fiercepharma.com/marketing/otsuka-digital-pill-tracker-takes-another-step-toward-reality-magellan-health-deal

575   B.S. Bulik. "Otsuka's dose-tracking digital pill." September 5, 2018.

576   "Otsuka Announces First Collaboration Agreement to Bring the ABILIFY MYCITE® System to the US Market." Otsuka. August 30, 2018. Accessed November 6, 2019. https://www.otsuka-us.com/discover/articles-1208

577   Dan Reilly. "How this U.S. startup plans to save lives, lower medical bills." Fortune. September 28, 2015. Accessed November 1, 2019. https://fortune.com/2015/09/28/medical-startup-plans/

578   "What is MDsave? FAQ." Mdsave.com (n.d.) Accessed November 6, 2019. https://www.mdsave.com/faq?id=heading-1

579   "About MDsave." MDsave. (n.d.). Accessed Novembver 7, 2019. https://www.mdsave.com/patients

580   "Tonsillectomy under age 12." MDsave. Accessed November 7, 2019. https://www.mdsave.com/procedures/tonsillectomy-under-age-12/d785f4c4#new-search

581   "Find Procedures in the United States." MDsave. (n.d.) Accessed November 7, 2019. https://www.mdsave.com/united-states

582   Donna Rosato. "How Paying Your Doctor in Cash Could Save You Money: Even if you have health insurance, sometimes you are better off not using it." Consumer Reports. May 4, 2018. Accessed November 7, 2019. https://www.consumerreports.org/healthcare-costs/how-paying-your-doctor-in-cash-could-save-you-money/; and Holly Fletcher. "Want to save on a medical procedure? There's an app for that." Tennessean. September 7, 2016. Accessed November 7, 2019. https://www.tennessean.com/story/money/industries/health-care/2016/09/07/mdsave-marketplace-lets-people-shop-for-medical-service-online/89714258/

583   "Can I apply my MDsave purchase to my deductible? FAQ." Mdsave.com (n.d.) Accessed November 7, 2019. https://www.mdsave.com/faq?id=heading-20

584   "Dan Reilly. "How this U.S. startup plans to save lives, lower medical bills." Fortune. September 28, 2015. Accessed November 7, 2019. https://fortune.com/2015/09/28/medical-startup-plans/

585   "For employers. How MDsave works." MDsave. (n.d.). Accessed November 7, 2019. https://www.mdsave.com/employers

586   "How GoodRx Works." GoodRx. (n.d.) Accessed November 7, 2019. https://www.goodrx.com/how-goodrx-works

587   "How GoodRx Works." GoodRx. (n.d.)

588   Kristen V. Brown. "GoodRx buys HeyDoctor in Expansion into Telemedicine." Bloomberg. September 26, 2019. Accessed November 7, 2019. https://www.bloomberg.com/news/articles/2019-09-26/goodrx-acquires-heydoctor-in-expansion-into-virtual-medicine?utm_source=google&utm_medium=bd&cmpId=google

589   K.V. Brown. "GoodRx buys HeyDoctor in Expansion into Telemedicine." September 26, 2019.

590   "How does GoodRx make money?" GoodRx. (n.d.). Accessed November 7, 2019.
       https://www.goodrx.com/how-goodrx-works
591   "Our Team: Scott Marlette." GoodRx. (n.d.) Accessed November 8, 2019.
       https://www.goodrx.com/about
592   "Not-so-GoodRx, Part II." Crazyrxman blog. May 2, 1017. Accessed November 1, 2019.
       http://crazyrxman.blogspot.com/2017/05/not-so-goodrx-part-ii.html
593   Kristen V. Brown. "GoodRx buys HeyDoctor in Expansion into Telemedicine."
       Bloomberg. September 26, 2019. Accessed November 8, 2019.
       https://www.bloomberg.com/news/articles/2019-09-26/goodrx-acquires-heydoctor-in-
       expansion-into-virtual-medicine?utm_source=google&utm_medium=bd&cmpId=google
594   The CMS Innovation Center. Centers for Medicare & Medicaid Services (CMS). (n.d.)
       Accessed November 8, 2019. https://innovation.cms.gov/
595   "'What is CMMI?' and 11 other FAQs about the CMS Innovation Center." February 27,
       2018. Accessed November 8, 2019. https://www.kff.org/medicare/fact-sheet/what-is-cmmi-
       and-11-other-faqs-about-the-cms-innovation-center/
596   "'What is CMMI?' and 11 other FAQs about the CMS Innovation Center." February 27,
       2018.
597   "Explaining Health Care Reform: Medical Loss Ratio (MLR)." Kaiser Family Foundation.
       February 29, 2012. Accessed November 8, 2019. https://www.kff.org/health-reform/fact-
       sheet/explaining-health-care-reform-medical-loss-ratio-mlr/
598   Jonathan Wiik. *Healthcare Revolution: The Patient Is the New Payer.* 2017.
599   Asher, T., Love, M. and Wilson, B. "Wouldn't It Be Nice." [Recorded by The Beach Boys].
       On *Pet Sounds* [CD]. Los Angeles: Capital Records. 1966.
600   TransUnion Healthcare. "News Reports about a Weakening Economy Impacting How
       Some Patients Seek Medical Treatment." September 17, 2019. Accessed October 27, 2019.
       https://newsroom.transunion.com/news-reports-about-a-weakening-economy--impacting-
       how-some-patients-seek-medical-treatment/
601   TransUnion Healthcare. "News Reports about a Weakening Economy." 2019.
602   Patient Friendly Billing ®. Healthcare Financial Management Association (HFMA). 2019.
       Accessed October 27, 2019. https://www.hfma.org/patientfriendlybilling/
603   Regulatory Overload Report. American Hospital Association. November 3, 2017. Accessed
       October 16, 2019. https://www.aha.org/guidesreports/2017-11-03-regulatory-overload-
       report#
604   Regulatory Overload Report. American Hospital Association. November 3, 2017.
605   Regulatory Overload Report. American Hospital Association. November 3, 2017.
606   Regulatory Overload Report. American Hospital Association. November 3, 2017.
607   CMS Data Navigator Glossary of Terms. (n.d.) Accessed October 17, 2019.
       https://www.cms.gov/Research-Statistics-Data-and-
       Systems/Research/ResearchGenInfo/Downloads/DataNav_Glossary_Alpha.pdf
608   Charlie Hoban, Minoo Javanmardian, Lucy X. Liu, Tom Robinson and Chris Schrader.
       "The Sparks Are Flying: Lighting a fire under healthcare." Oliver Wyman Health
       Innovation Journal, Volume 2. December 2018. Accessed October 17, 2019.
       https://www.oliverwyman.com/our-expertise/insights/2018/dec/health-innovation-
       journal/lighting-a-fire-under-healthcare/the-sparks-are-flying--lighting-a-fire-under-
       healthcare.html
609   Pat Currie. "The changing role of hospitals as healthcare evolves." Hands-on Health Care
       Discussions by Baylor Scott & White Health. September 11, 2018. Accessed October 18,
       2019. https://scrubbing.in/the-changing-role-of-hospitals-as-healthcare-evolves/
610   John Elflein. "Hospital Occupancy rate in the U.S. from 1975 to 2017." *Statistica.* Last
       edited March 18, 2019. Accessed June 25, 2019.
       https://www.statista.com/statistics/185904/hospital-occupancy-rate-in-the-us-since-2001/
611   Ana Lechintan. "April's smart KPI: % Hospital Bed Occupancy Rate." The KPI Institute.
       April 18, 2019. Accessed October 17, 2019.
       https://www.performancemagazine.org/smartkpi-hospital-bed-occupancy-

rate/#targetText=Market%20data%20from%20our%20database,needed%2C%20possibly%20crucial%2C%20healthcare.; and James Allen. "What is the Ideal Hospital Occupancy Rate?" The Hospital Medical Director. June 3, 2017. Accessed October 17, 2019. https://hospitalmedicaldirector.com/what-is-the-ideal-hospital-occupancy-rate/

612   CON – Certificate of Need State Laws. National Conference of State Legislatures. February 28, 2019. Accessed October 18, 2019. http://www.ncsl.org/research/health/con-certificate-of-need-state-laws.aspx

613   CON – Certificate of Need State Laws. National Conference of State Legislatures. February 28, 2019.

614   Jonathan Wiik. *Healthcare Revolution: The Patient Is the New Payer*. 2017.

615   Clean Claim Rate (CL-1). Map Keys for Hospitals and Health Systems. HFMA. (n.d.) Accessed October 18, 2019. https://www.hfma.org/MAP/mapkeys

616   Laine Dowling. "5 Secrets Hiding in Your Hospital's Revenue Cycle Metrics." Change Healthcare blog. February 10, 2017. Accessed October 18, 2019. https://www.changehealthcare.com/blog/secrets-hiding-hospitals-revenue-cycle-metrics; and Mary Guarino. "How to Improve Your Clean Claims Rate." HIMSS. October 19, 2010. Accessed October 17, 2019. https://www.himss.org/resource-news/how-improve-your-clean-claims-rates#

617   Jacqueline LaPointe. "Tracking Key Hospital Revenue Cycle Metrics to Up Profitability." RevCycleIntelligence. March 17, 2017. Accessed October 18, 2019. https://revcycleintelligence.com/news/tracking-key-hospital-revenue-cycle-metrics-to-up-profitability

618   Lori Zindl. "12 Things Keeping Hospital CFOs Awake at Night." OutSource, Inc. April 2, 2018. Accessed October 18, 2019. https://www.os-healthcare.com/blog/12-things-keeping-hospital-cfos-awake-at-night

619   President George W. Bush. Text of President Bush's 2004 State of the Union Address. *The Washington Post*. January 20, 2004. Accessed October 18, 2019. http://www.washingtonpost.com/wp-srv/politics/transcripts/bushtext_012004.html

620   Jacqueline LaPointe. "NY Hospital Settles with Cerner Over $38M Medical Billing Problem." RevCycleIntelligence. March 20, 2019. Accessed October 19, 2019. https://revcycleintelligence.com/news/ny-hospital-settles-with-cerner-over-38m-medical-billing-problem

621   J. LaPointe. "NY Hospital Settles with Cerner Over $38M Medical Billing Problem." March 20, 2019.

622   Katheleen Morre. "Audit: Bad billing system costs Glens Falls Hospital $38 million in revenue." The Post-Star. March 7, 2019. Accessed October 19, 2019. https://poststar.com/news/local/audit-bad-billing-system-costs-glens-falls-hospital-million-in/article_4b430f4f-859f-59ba-bac0-5e886c8b9d85.html

623   K. Moore. "Glens Falls Hospital settled with company over billing problems." 2019.

624   Jacqueline LaPointe. "NY Hospital Settles with Cerner Over $38M Medical Billing Problem." RevCycleIntelligence. March 20, 2019. Accessed October 19, 2019. https://revcycleintelligence.com/news/ny-hospital-settles-with-cerner-over-38m-medical-billing-problem

625   Jeff Kiger. "Mayo Clinic reports 'a very good' 2018, despite Epic costs." Post Bulletin. February 18, 2019. Accessed October 27, 2019. https://www.postbulletin.com/news/local/mayo-clinic-reports-a-very-good-despite-epic-costs/article_9b7d4f3c-33b0-11e9-829f-f7dca8cdcf01.html

626   J. Kiger. "Mayo Clinic reports 'a very good' 2018, despite Epic costs." 2019.

627   Shelby Livingston. "Will blockchain save the healthcare system?" Modern Healthcare. February 9, 2019. Accessed October 20, 2019. https://www.modernhealthcare.com/article/20190209/TRANSFORMATION02/190209953/will-blockchain-save-the-healthcare-system

628   S. Livingston. "Will blockchain save the healthcare system?" February 9, 2019.

629   "About us." Synaptic Health Alliance. (n.d.) Accessed October 20, 2019. https://www.synaptichealthalliance.com/about-us

630 Richard Mark Kirkner. "How blockchain has strange bedfellows singing kumbaya." July 5, 2019. Accessed October 20, 2019. https://www.managedcaremag.com/archives/2019/7/how-blockchain-has-strange-bedfellows-singing-kumbaya

631 "About us." Synaptic Health Alliance. (n.d.) Accessed October 20, 2019. https://www.synaptichealthalliance.com/about-us

632 Shubham Singhal and Stephanie Carlton. "The era of exponential improvement in healthcare?" McKinsey & Company Healthcare Systems & Services. May 2019. Accessed October 27, 2019. https://www.mckinsey.com/industries/healthcare-systems-and-services/our-insights/the-era-of-exponential-improvement-in-healthcare

633 The W. Edwards Deming Institute. W. Edwards Deming Quotes. (n.d.) Accessed October 20, 2019. https://quotes.deming.org/authors/W._Edwards_Deming/quote/3734

GLOSSARY ENDNOTES

i "What is considered fraud, waste, or abuse?" Officer of Inspector General, U.S. Agency for International Development. April 16, 2018. Accessed November 10, 2019. https://oig.usaid.gov/node/221

ii Accountable Care Organizations (ACO). Centers for Medicare & Medicaid Services (CMS). October 2, 2019. Accessed November 10, 2019. https://www.cms.gov/Medicare/Medicare-Fee-for-Service-Payment/ACO/index.html?redirect=/Aco/

iii "About the AHA." American Hospital Association (AHA). (n.d.) Accessed November 10, 2019. http://www.aha.org/about/index.shtml

iv Jatinder Bali, Rohit Garg and Renu T. Bali. "Artificial intelligence (AI) in healthcare and biomedical research: Why a strong computational/AI bioethics framework is required." Indian Journal of Ophthalmology. January 2019; 67(1):3-6. Accessed November 10, 2019. https://www.ncbi.nlm.nih.gov/pmc/articles/PMC6324122/

v Blockchain. Glossary. Bankrate. (n.d.) Accessed November 10, 2019. https://www.bankrate.com/glossary/b/blockchain/

vi James K. Elrod and John L. Fortenberry, Jr. "Centers of excellence in healthcare institutions: what they are and how to assemble them." BMC Health Services Research. July 11, 2017. (Suppl 1): 425. Accessed November 10, 2019. DOI: 10.1186/s12913-017-2340-y

vii Children's Health Insurance Program Overview. National Conference of State Legislatures. January 10, 2019. Accessed November 10, 2019. http://www.ncsl.org/research/health/childrens-health-insurance-program-overview.aspx

viii Clean Claim Rate (CL-1). Map Keys for Hospitals and Health Systems. HFMA. (n.d.) Accessed October 18, 2019. https://www.hfma.org/MAP/mapkeys

ix Laine Dowling. "5 Secrets Hiding in Your Hospital's Revenue Cycle Metrics." Change Healthcare blog. February 10, 2017. Accessed October 18, 2019. https://www.changehealthcare.com/blog/secrets-hiding-hospitals-revenue-cycle-metrics; and Mary Guarino. "How to Improve Your Clean Claims Rate." HIMSS. October 19, 2010. Accessed October 17, 2019. https://www.himss.org/news/how-improve-your-clean-claims-rates#targetText=The%20average%20U.S.%20hospital%20has,from%20about%2075%2D85%25.&targetText=Healthcare%20providers%20should%20focus%20on,rules%20research%20and%20discovery%20plan

x   Cost Sharing Reduction (CSR). Healthcare.gov. Accessed August 16, 2019.
         https://www.healthcare.gov/glossary/cost-sharing-reduction/
xi   Kristen Lee. "Current Procedural Terminology (CPT) code definition." HealthIT/Tech
         Target. 2017. Accessed November 10, 2019.
         https://searchhealthit.techtarget.com/definition/Current-Procedural-Terminology-CPT
xii   Diagnosis Related Group (DRG). HMSA Provider Resource Center. July 13, 2018.
         Accessed November 10, 2019. https://hmsa.com/portal/provider/zav_pel.fh.DIA.650.htm
xiii   "Disproportionate share hospital payments." Medicaid and CHIP Payment and Access
         Commission (MACPAC). (n.d.) Accessed November 10, 2019.
         https://www.macpac.gov/subtopic/disproportionate-share-hospital-payments/
xiv   "What is an electronic health record (EHR)?" HealthIT.gov. September 10, 2019. Accessed
         November 10, 2019. https://www.healthit.gov/faq/what-electronic-health-record-ehr
xv   Emergency Medical Treatment & Labor Act (EMTALA). Centers for Medicare &
         Medicaid Services (CMS). (n.d.) Accessed November 10, 2019.
         https://www.cms.gov/regulations-and-guidance/legislation/emtala/
xvi   Health plans & benefits: ERISA. U. S. Department of Labor. (n.d.) Accessed November 10,
         2019. https://www.dol.gov/general/topic/health-plans/erisa
xvii   Federal Poverty Level (FPL). Glossary. Healthcare.gov. (n.d.) Accessed November 10,
         2019. https://www.healthcare.gov/glossary/federal-poverty-level-fpl/
xviii   "What is considered fraud, waste, or abuse?" Officer of Inspector General, U.S. Agency for
         International Development. April 16, 2018. Accessed November 10, 2019.
         https://oig.usaid.gov/node/221
xix   "What is considered fraud, waste, or abuse?" Officer of Inspector General, U.S. Agency for
         International Development. April 16, 2018.
xx   "Amazon, Berkshire Hathaway, and JPMorgan Chase & Co. to partner on U.S. employee
         health care." Haven. January 30, 2018. Accessed November 10, 2019.
         https://havenhealthcare.com/media/abj-partner-health-care
xxi   "About HHS." U.S. Department of Health and Human Services. (n.d.) Accessed November
         11, 2019. https://www.hhs.gov/about/index.html#
xxii   U.S. Department of the Treasury. Internal Revenue Service (IRS). (2016). IRS Publication
         969, Health Savings Accounts (HSAs). March 6, 2019. Accessed November 10, 2019.
         https://www.irs.gov/publications/p969/ar02.html#en_US_2016_publink1000204020
xxiii   High Deductible Health Plan (HDHP). Glossary. HealthCare.gov. (n.d.) Accessed
         November 19, 2019. https://www.healthcare.gov/glossary/high-deductible-health-plan/
xxiv   Readmissions Reduction Program (HRRP). Centers for Medicare & Medicaid Services
         (CMS). (n.d.) Accessed November 10, 2019. https://www.cms.gov/medicare/medicare-fee-
         for-service-payment/acuteinpatientpps/readmissions-reduction-program.html
xxv   Insurance Discovery. TransUnion. 2019. Accessed November 10, 2019.
         https://www.transunion.com/product/escan-insurance-discovery.page
xxvi   ICD-10-CM. National Center for Health Statistics. Centers for Disease Control and
         Prevention. October 17, 2019. Accessed November 19, 2019.
         https://www.cdc.gov/nchs/icd/icd10cm.htm
xxvii   Drew E. Altman. "Explaining KFF." KFF.org. August 2019. Accessed November 2019.
         https://www.kff.org/presidents-message/
xxviii   Long-term care hospitals (LTCHs). American Hospital Association (AHA). (n.d.) Accessed
         November 10, 2019. https://www.aha.org/advocacy/long-term-care-pps
xxix   Medicare and Medicaid Promoting Interoperability Program. CMS.gov. August 14, 2019.
         Accessed November 3, 2019. https://www.cms.gov/Regulations-and-
         Guidance/Legislation/EHRIncentivePrograms/Basics.html
xxx   "What is MACRA and MIPS?" Practice Fusion blog. June 3, 2016. Accessed November
         19, 2019. https://www.practicefusion.com/blog/what-is-macra-and-mips/
xxxi   Medical Necessity Law and Legal Definition. USLegal.com. (n.d.) Accessed November 10,
         2019. https://definitions.uslegal.com/m/medical-necessity/

xxxii   How do Medicare Advantage Plans work? Medicare.gov. (n.d.) Accessed November 19,
         2019. https://www.medicare.gov/sign-up-change-plans/types-of-medicare-health-
         plans/medicare-advantage-plans/how-do-medicare-advantage-plans-work
xxxiii   "Understanding Medicare Advantage Plans." Centers for Medicare & Medicaid Services.
         (n.d.) Accessed November 2, 2019. https://www.medicare.gov/Pubs/pdf/12026-
         Understanding-Medicare-Advantage-Plans.pdf
xxxiv   Bad Debt. Noridian Medicare. August 16, 2018. Accessed November 19, 2019.
         https://med.noridianmedicare".com/web/jea/audit-reimbursement/audit/bad-debt
xxxv   "What Marketplace health insurance plans cover. Healthcare.gov. (n.d.). Accessed
         November 11, 2019. https://www.healthcare.gov/coverage/what-marketplace-plans-cover/
xxxvi   Outpatient Prospective Payment System (OPPS). Glossary. MedicareInteractive.org. (n.d.).
         Accessed November 11, 2019. https://www.medicareinteractive.org/glossary/outpatient-
         prospective-payment-system-opps
xxxvii   Programs to Evaluate Payment Patterns Electronic Report (PEPPER). Compliance Projects.
         CMS.gov. June 20, 2018. Accessed August 27, 2019. https://www.cms.gov/Research-
         Statistics-Data-and-Systems/Monitoring-Programs/Medicare-FFS-Compliance-
         Programs/Data-Analysis/index.html
xxxviii "What is population health?" Population Health Training. Centers for Disease Control and
         Prevention. July 23, 2019. Accessed November 19, 2019.
         https://www.cdc.gov/pophealthtraining/whatis.html
xxxix   U.S. Department of Health and Human Services. Office of the Secretary. 45 CFR Subtitle
         A, § 160.103, https://www.gpo.gov/fdsys/pkg/CFR-2010-title45-vol1/pdf/CFR-2010-
         title45-vol1-sec160-103.pdf
xl   Revenue Cycle Management. Healthcare Business Management Association (HBMA).
         (n.d.) Accessed November 11, 2019. https://www.hbma.org/content/about/medical-billing-
         revenue-cycle-management
xli   Robotic Process Automation (RPA). Intelligent Information Management Glossary. The
         Association for Intelligent Information Management (AIIM). (n.d.) Accessed November 11,
         2019. https://www.aiim.org/What-is-Robotic-Process-Automation#
xlii   Samantha Artiga and Elizabeth Hinton. "Beyond Health Care: The Role of Social
         Determinants in Promoting Health and Health Equity." Kaiser Family Foundation. May 10,
         2018. Accessed June 25, 2019. https://www.kff.org/disparities-policy/issue-brief/beyond-
         health-care-the-role-of-social-determinants-in-promoting-health-and-health-equity/
xliii   "What is Value-Based Healthcare?" NEJM Catalyst. January 1, 2017. Accessed November
         19, 2019. https://catalyst.nejm.org/what-is-value-based-healthcare/
xliv   "What is considered fraud, waste, or abuse?" Officer of Inspector General, U.S. Agency for
         International Development. April 16, 2018. Accessed November 10, 2019.
         https://oig.usaid.gov/node/221

INDEX

ABOUT THE AUTHOR

Jonathan G. Wiik, MHA, MBA has 25 years of healthcare experience in acute care, health IT and insurance settings. He started his career as a hospital transporter and held various roles (clinical operations, patient access, billing, case management and more) at a large, not-for-profit, acute care hospital, before serving as the hospital's chief revenue officer. He also served in various roles at a prominent commercial payer. His cumulative expertise gives him vast knowledge of—and keen insight into—the inner workings of the revenue cycle across the continuum of care.

In his current role as principal of healthcare strategy at TransUnion Healthcare, Wiik is responsible for support and consultation on business development opportunities, and works closely with the market and hospitals on industry best practices for revenue cycle management. He's considered an industry expert on healthcare finance, legislation, revenue cycle management and strategic transformation.

Wiik is an active advocate of legislative changes that evolve the healthcare industry. He's the author of *Healthcare Revolution: The Patient Is the New Payer* and frequently speaks as a thought leader at state and national events and conferences.

He's an officer on the Colorado HFMA Board and previously served as a board member for the American College of Healthcare Executives (ACHE) and Colorado Association of Healthcare Executives (CAHE). He holds a bachelor's degree in sports medicine and master's degrees in healthcare administration and business.

Jonathan enjoys spending time in the Colorado outdoors with his wife and two very energetic, red-headed boys. He's also a certified white water rafting instructor and an avid traveler.